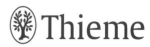

# Pre-Medicine

## The Complete Guide for Aspiring Doctors

**Joel Thomas, MD**
Diagnostic Radiology Resident
Washington University School of Medicine
St. Louis, Missouri, USA

**Phillip Wagner, MD**
Internal Medicine Faculty
The Johns Hopkins Hospital
Baltimore, Maryland, USA

**Ray Funahashi, MD**
CEO and Co-Founder of The Labkind Project
Peter H. Diamandis A360 Fellow
Head of Clinical Affairs at Gesund.ai
Boston, Massachusetts, USA

**Nitin Agarwal, MD**
Assistant Professor of Neurological Surgery and Orthopedic Surgery
Director of Neurotrauma
Department of Neurological Surgery
Washington University School of Medicine
St. Louis, Missouri, USA

42 Illustrations

Thieme
New York • Stuttgart • Delhi • Rio de Janeiro

**Library of Congress Cataloging-in-Publication Data** is available with the publisher.

**Important note**: Medicine is an ever-changing science undergoing continual development. Research and clinical experience are continually expanding our knowledge, in particular our knowledge of proper treatment and drug therapy. Insofar as this book mentions any dosage or application, readers may rest assured that the authors, editors, and publishers have made every effort to ensure that such references are in accordance with **the state of knowledge at the time of production of the book**.

Nevertheless, this does not involve, imply, or express any guarantee or responsibility on the part of the publishers in respect to any dosage instructions and forms of applications stated in the book. **Every user is requested to examine carefully** the manufacturers' leaflets accompanying each drug and to check, if necessary in consultation with a physician or specialist, whether the dosage schedules mentioned therein or the contraindications stated by the manufacturers differ from the statements made in the present book. Such examination is particularly important with drugs that are either rarely used or have been newly released on the market. Every dosage schedule or every form of application used is entirely at the user's own risk and responsibility. The authors and publishers request every user to report to the publishers any discrepancies or inaccuracies noticed. If errors in this work are found after publication, errata will be posted at www.thieme.com on the product description page.

Some of the product names, patents, and registered designs referred to in this book are in fact registered trademarks or proprietary names even though specific reference to this fact is not always made in the text. Therefore, the appearance of a name without designation as proprietary is not to be construed as a representation by the publisher that it is in the public domain.

Thieme addresses people of all gender identities equally. We encourage our authors to use gender neutral or gender- equal expressions wherever the context allows.

Thieme Medical Publishers, Inc.
333 Seventh Avenue, 18th Floor
New York, NY 10001, USA
www.thieme.com
+1 800 782 3488, customerservice@thieme.com

Cover design: © Thieme
Cover image source: © Thieme
Typesetting by TNQ Technologies, India

Printed in Germany by Beltz Grafische Betriebe      5 4 3 2 1

ISBN: 978-1-68420-507-3

Also available as an e-book:
eISBN (PDF): 978-1-68420-508-0
eISBN (epub): 978-1-68420-509-7

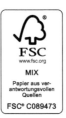

FSC
www.fsc.org
MIX
Papier aus ver-
antwortungsvollen
Quellen
FSC® C089473

# Contents

## Section I: The Pre-Med Primer

**1. The 30,000-Foot View**
*Ray Funahashi and Joel Thomas*

**2. What Medical Schools Look For**
*Joel Thomas*

# Contents

## Section II: Succeeding as a Pre-Medical Student

# Contents

# Contents

# Contents

## Section III: Applying to Medical School

# Contents

# Contents

## Section IV: Medical School and Career Insights

## 43.    Real Talk on Succeeding in Medical School ................................. 320

*Joel Thomas*

## 44.    A Peek at the Residency Application Process ................................. 331

*Joel Thomas and Neal K. Ramchandani*

## 45.    A Day in the Life in Medicine. ........................................... 338

*Joel Thomas, Phillip Wagner, Ray Funahashi, Nitin Agarwal, and Vamsi Reddy*

## 46.    Nonclinical Careers. ................................................... 344

*Ray Funahashi*

## Contents

# Preface

So you want to get into medical school?

Great! Welcome to the years leading up to it: the **pre-med** (pre-medical) years of your life.

We know there can be much uncertainty during this time about how to prepare, when to take the MCAT, how to do well in your science classes—it can all be overwhelming. The journey will be challenging, but we did our best to pass down the pearls of wisdom we learned from our own journeys, as well as from pre-meds who came before you and succeeded—even after having failed at first.[1]

Within this book, we lay out strategies which we believe to be most advantageous for pre-medical success. We're fully aware that not every recommendation will apply in the same way for every pre-med. Therefore, we encourage you to weigh our recommendations against your personal circumstances, the most up-to-date scientific evidence, and the judgment of your mentors. Additionally, there is no single best way for each pre-med to get into medical school. As such, we encourage you to track your progress, to remain open-minded about opportunities for improvement, and to experiment with our suggestions when you can safely do so.[2] Making informed decisions is crucial because—unfortunately—there are no guarantees to the process of getting into medical school, and it is dangerously easy to inadvertently destroy your chances.

So why choose this book out of the sea of available pre-med resources?

- *We address the hard, uncomfortable questions*: Should you major in something easier to get a higher GPA? Does going to a more prestigious college matter for medical school admissions? Why do doctors have the highest rate of suicide among any profession even though matriculating medical students have similar—if not better—mental health than the general population? Why do so many medical students ignore their schools' lectures (for which they're paying around $60,000 yearly) to study at home from outside resources? Is it even financially worth it to become a physician nowadays?
  - These topics cannot be answered with a quick Google search. They require engagement with multiple opposing viewpoints and careful data analysis. We do much of this legwork for you, but we also provide you with resources for further research on your own.
  - Many other books about medical school simply gloss over these issues, even though they're some of the most important considerations for anyone seriously considering a life in medicine.
  - We bring together multiple authors with different life experiences and perspectives. As such, we feel that our conclusions on these issues are broadly applicable to students from different backgrounds.
- We have a proven track record of success using our own methods. We all went to a US News Top 20 medical school and/or trained at a Doximity Top 20 residency program.
- We are deeply committed to evidence-based recommendations. You will find a source for virtually every claim in this book. We are also careful to avoid several discouraging trends in nonfiction: cherry-picking data to fit claims as well as citing sources that vaguely support the claim made (if at all). Rest assured, we have scrupulously read every primary source cited in this book, and we also took the time to perform multiple reviews of early drafts to remove claims and sources that were not sufficiently supported by the authors' consensus. We also qualify the strength of our "surviving" recommendations, as well as the level of confidence we have in the sources themselves. Additionally, for every claim that we make, we made a good-faith effort to explore alternative recommendations to avoid cherry-picking information that naively supports our intuitions. We also took care to use open-ended search strategies (e.g., "What are the pros and cons of spaced repetition?" vs. "spaced repetition benefits") when researching to assess the broad body of evidence surrounding the topics—rather than just the data supporting our intuitions and preferences. Nonetheless, we **still** invite you to be skeptical and

---

[1] One of the co-authors poignantly attests to this. Ray Funahashi's major motivation for writing this book was to minimize the mistakes made by future applicants, as he personally did not get into a single medical school during his first application cycle. In retrospect, he realized that he simply lacked clear, cohesive guidance on the overall application process and spent a painstaking amount of time integrating material from various blogs and forums to ultimately gain admission in the next cycle. He hopes that no one else will fail to get into medical school for the same reasons he originally faced.

[2] For example, trying a new study strategy several weeks before a low-stakes quiz, NOT the weekend before the final exam.

scientifically rigorous when reading through our recommendations. *If you find any claim in this book that seems off-base or unsupported by science, we encourage you to contact us to discuss.*

- We don't care about making money. We encourage anyone who cannot afford to pay for this book to reach out to the authors for help in finding an affordable option from the Publisher. Our first and foremost goal is getting this information out to whoever my need it.
- We are committed to updating this book as a living, breathing document that evolves with the medical landscape. We know that many of the recommendations in this book will become outdated shortly because medicine constantly changes. The authors have resolved to regularly update the book's recommendations throughout their careers, and this book will update in real-time with its companion website: premedicine.info

Congratulate yourself on taking a serious step toward a career in medicine. Whether you read this book cover-to-cover or jump ahead to the sections that interest you, we sincerely wish you the best of luck in your future endeavors. Hopefully we'll see you in the doctors' lounge someday.

## Disclaimer

The opinions expressed in this text do not reflect those of the institutions at which we trained or worked, and are ours alone.

Each of the authors' viewpoints were subject to editorial feedback and criticism, but they are ultimately their own. We know that despite how much we tried to be respectful, considerate, and accurate, that some of these opinions will not necessarily address the uniqueness of every reader's experience or situation. We know that this book would not have been created—or be anywhere as helpful as we think it can be—without input from a variety of voices and perspectives. We also see no reason why that input should stop. If you are concerned that one of the opinions or recommendations put forth in this text is inaccurate, malicious, incomplete, or hurtful, please reach out and discuss it with us.

Thank you for reading.

*Joel Thomas, MD*
*Phillip Wagner, MD*
*Ray Funahashi, MD*
*Nitin Agarwal, MD*

# How to Read This Book

This book contains a *lot* of information. It is meant to be a comprehensive tome that covers every major aspect of the path to becoming a physician, from exploring your initial interest in medicine, succeeding as a pre-medical student, maximizing time between college and medical school (if relevant), applying to medical school, picking a medical school, succeeding in medical school, applying for residency, picking a medical specialty, and finding professional satisfaction in medicine as the field constantly evolves. As such, there are a number of different ways you[3] can read this book:

If you're already committed to becoming a physician, then we recommend reading the book cover-to-cover. You will likely not retain everything, but you will catch important glimpses of concepts and perspectives you may not have been aware of. You can always return to those sections for additional detail when you're ready.

If you're already committed to becoming a physician *and* in a high school, then start with Chapter 7, Guaranteed Admission Programs and Early Assurance Programs to read about ways to get admitted to a medical school as a high school student. Many readers might be unaware that these programs even exist.

If you're already committed to becoming a physician *and* early in undergrad, then you should also start with Chapter 7, Guaranteed Admission Programs and Early Assurance Programs to read about early assurance programs (i.e., conditional acceptance to medical school early in college). Many readers might be unaware that these programs even exist. You will also benefit from the other chapters in Section II: Succeeding as a Pre-Medical Student that meticulously discuss each major aspect of building a competitive application (e.g., volunteering, research, MCAT, personal wellness, mentorship).

If you're already committed to becoming a physician *and* approaching graduation, then you should read Section III: Applying to Medical School in detail to get a perspective on every major aspect of the application process, as well as potential plans (B, C, D, etc.) if you don't get accepted. Alternatively, if you don't plan to apply to medical school at the end of college, then you should read Chapter 16, Gap Years, Employment, Graduate Degrees, and Post-Baccalaureate Fellowships to explore the best options for the time between graduation and medical school.

If you're struggling with personal wellness, self-doubt, anxiety, or depression, then we recommend *starting* with Chapter 5, Building Your Narrative; Chapter 6, Common Pre-Med Diseases and How to Treat Them; and Chapter 18, Self-Care and Wellness for avenues to explore on your own. That said, this book is no substitute for professional medical and psychological counsel.

If you're still simply exploring medicine as a potential career, then we recommend reading Section I: The Pre-Med Primer to get a birds-eye view of the process of becoming a physician. We also recommend skimming through Section II: Succeeding as a Pre-Medical Student to get a better perspective of the various commitments you will have to juggle for several years. We also recommend reading Chapter 41, Real Talk on a Medical Career; Chapter 42, Real Talk on the Medical School Experience; Chapter 43, Real Talk on Succeeding in Medical School; Chapter 45, A Day in the Life in Medicine; and Chapter 47, Stories of Inspiration for rich, detailed accounts of the day-to-day life in medicine, ranging from the mundane to the extraordinary. We also recommend Chapter 46, Nonclinical Careers and Appendix B: Medical Specialties and Subspecialties for a comprehensive (but by no means exhaustive) list of the tremendous variety of options available for practicing medicine.

If you're already in medical training (e.g., medical student, resident, or even attending physician), then we recommend reading Section IV: Medical School and Career Insights and even Appendix B: Medical Specialties and Subspecialties for perspective and discussion on evolving issues in medicine and professional fulfillment.

# Acknowledgments

We are deeply grateful to the following reviewers who provided insightful comments and critiques on earlier drafts of this work.

- Carolyn Ayers, MD: Internal Medicine/Pediatrics resident, Indiana University
- Reetwan Bandyopadhyay: Pre-med Undergraduate, University of Pittsburgh
- Elizabeth Cook, MD: Transitional Year Resident, Indiana University; Dermatology Resident, Medical College of Wisconsin
- Abigail Gerig: Software Engineer
- Anna Grobengieser: High school student interested in medical school
- Brandon J. Kiley, MD: Psychiatry Resident, Washington University School of Medicine
- Philip King, PharmD: Clinical Pharmacist, Indiana University; Assistant Professor, Pharmacy Practice College of Pharmacy and Health Sciences, Butler University
- Amaan Rahman: BS/MD Student, University of Pittsburgh
- Neal K. Ramchandani, MD: General Surgery Resident, Vascular Surgery Fellow, Indiana University
- Kenneth Shiao, MD: Transitional Year Resident, Indiana University; Diagnostic Radiology Resident, Emory University

# Contributors

**Nitin Agarwal, MD**
Assistant Professor of Neurological Surgery and
    Orthopedic Surgery
Director of Neurotrauma
Department of Neurological Surgery
Washington University School of Medicine
St. Louis, Missouri, USA

**Landon Cluts, MD**
Research Coordinator
Department of Orthopaedic Surgery
University of Pittsburgh School of Medicine
Pittsburgh, Pennsylvania, USA

**Ray Funahashi, MD**
CEO and Co-Founder of The Labkind Project
Peter H. Diamandis A360 Fellow
Head of Clinical Affairs at Gesund.ai
Boston, Massachusetts, USA

**Samyuktha Melachuri, MD**
Resident
Department of Ophthalmology
University of Pittsburgh School of Medicine
Pittsburgh, Pennsylvania, USA

**Christian Morrill, MD**
Research Fellow
Department of Pediatric Urology
Brady Urological Institute at Johns
    Hopkins University
Baltimore, Maryland, USA

**Chinweoke Osigwe, BA**
Medical Student
University of Pittsburgh School of Medicine
Pittsburgh, Pennsylvania, USA

**Neal K. Ramchandani, MD**
Vascular Surgery Fellow
Department of Vascular and General Surgery
Indiana University
Indianapolis, Indiana, USA

**Vamsi Reddy, MD**
Consultant
McKinsey & Company
New York, New York, USA

**Eva Roy, MD**
Resident
Division of Plastic and Reconstructive Surgery
Brigham & Woman's Hospital
Harvard University
Boston, Massachusetts, USA

**Jorna Sojati, BS, MS**
Medical Student
Department of Medicine
University of Pittsburgh School of Medicine
Pittsburgh, Pennsylvania, USA

**Joel Thomas, MD**
Diagnostic Radiology Resident
Washington University School of Medicine
St. Louis, Missouri, USA

**Phillip Wagner, MD**
Internal Medicine Faculty
The Johns Hopkins Hospital
Baltimore, Maryland, USA

# Section I

## The Pre-Med Primer

# 1 The 30,000-Foot View

*Ray Funahashi and Joel Thomas*

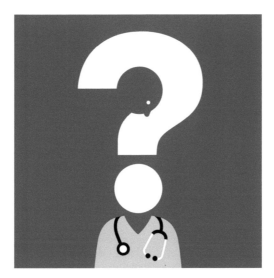

Whether you're already committed to or still contemplating a career in medicine, understanding the birds-eye view to becoming a physician is paramount.

You might be surprised to learn that applying to medical school requires years of preparatory work from required courses and grades to volunteering, shadowing, and extracurricular activities. There are also many unwritten rules, like working with the "pre-medical committee/advisors/office" at your college and carefully timing your application.

Feeling overwhelmed? Don't worry! We'll explain all of these things step-by-step so that you will feel well-prepared and poised for success. Below, we outline the basic pathways to medical school and becoming a physician. We will describe each step in more detail in the subsequent chapters, so focus on understanding the big picture for now. *You've got this.*

How do you become a physician in the United States? Let's get started!

## 1.1 Step 1. Get a Bachelor's Degree

All medical schools in the United States require you to have a bachelor's degree (B.S. or B.A.) from an accredited college or university (they require you complete 90 credits before you apply, and that you will complete your bachelor's before enrollment). The degree can be in any major. Yes, whether you are a biology major or a philosophy major, it doesn't directly affect your chances of getting into medical school.

Additionally, some applicants take additional time to pursue another degree, work, or do research after finishing their bachelor's to become more competitive applicants. More on this later.

On the other hand, if you're in high school and committed to becoming a physician (and have thoroughly explored that commitment), then you can apply to Guaranteed Admissions Programs to secure a spot in medical school at the time you enter college. More on this in Chapter 7, Guaranteed Admission Programs and Early Assurance Programs.

### 1.1.1 Complete Required Classes

In addition to receiving a bachelor's degree, completing certain classes in the sciences, humanities, and mathematics is a prerequisite to applying to medical school. These classes can be—and often are—done while working toward a bachelor's degree. The usual length of time for this step is 1.5 to 2 years if doing this in the context of an ongoing bachelor's degree, and 1 year if completing a post-baccalaureate pre-medical program. In general, it takes most people 4 years if they need to complete a bachelor's degree, although students in some Guaranteed Admission Programs can save up to 2 years off the process and complete their undergraduate studies in 2 years instead of the usual 4.

### Common Prerequisite Classes for Applying to Medical School

- One year of **Biology** with laboratory.
- One year of **General Chemistry** with laboratory.
- One semester to one year of **Organic Chemistry** with laboratory.
- One year of **Physics** with laboratory.
- One year of **English.**
- One semester of **Biochemistry.**

One year = 2 semesters, or 6–8 credits, depending on the course and your school's academic credit system.
    Some schools require additional classes such as **Statistics, Calculus, Genetics, Sociology,** and **Psychology.**
    Some schools will accept Advanced Placement (AP) credit and some won't. Some schools require one year of organic chemistry, whereas others will accept one semester of organic chemistry + one semester of biochemistry.
    *Since these requirements are a moving target (i.e., liable to change over time), we recommend discussing with your pre-med advisor and/or checking the admission requirements on individual schools' websites before creating your academic schedule.*

You might be surprised to note that you're not required to complete any "medical" courses as an undergraduate, (e.g., anatomy, physiology, microbiology, and immunology). This is because all medical students will cover these subjects in the first 2 years of medical school, but in extreme detail and focus on clinical applications. The undergraduate years are instead designed to develop your general scientific thinking to develop a scaffold for clinical decision-making and application of science in medicine.

If you didn't complete these required classes, you have options to complete them by taking them through a pre-medical post-baccalaureate (post-bac) program (see Chapter 16, *Gap Years, Employment, Graduate Degrees, and Post-Baccalaureate Fellowships*).

You should have a good — ideally great (close to 4.0) — GPA, especially in your science classes (*more in Chapter 10, Obtaining a Solid GPA*).

## 1.1.2 Engage in "Recommended" (Essentially Required) Activities

Most medical schools want to see that applicants have the following:

### Clinical Exposure

How do you know if you want to become a physician if you have never been exposed to medicine from a career perspective? Medical schools expect applicants to have either (ideally both) **shadowed a physician in person or worked/volunteered in a setting where they worked with patients and/or physicians**. In case you were wondering, being a patient yourself doesn't fulfill this expectation.

### Volunteering and Service

Medicine is a field where you are caring for others. Accordingly, medical schools expect applicants to demonstrate this through **volunteering over a significant period of time**. Volunteering should be longitudinal and personally meaningful.

For example, an applicant who volunteers for several years at his/her local food shelter and communicates personal meaning from the experience demonstrates a more compelling commitment to service than an applicant who volunteers to clean the local park for a week and can't articulate any transformative insight after doing so. Medicine is a 24/7 vocation, and showing you can commit to something matters.

## Research Experience

The practice of clinical medicine actively evolves through scientific discovery, and many medical schools are also academic research institutions. Most—if not all—value students who have demonstrated critical thinking using the scientific method. In addition, as a doctor you will be a lifelong learner. This means that you will have to be able to consistently appraise and critique the latest research when making day-to-day clinical decisions. The research you get involved in doesn't have to be medical—it can be in any academic field from philosophy to theoretical mathematics.

Schools don't necessarily expect you to become a researcher or conduct research once you are in medical school, but they still value those who at least have had the experience.[1]

# 1.2 Step 2. Take the Medical College Admissions Test (MCAT)

MCAT stands for Medical College Admissions Test, and it is a standardized computer-based exam that tests critical thinking and comprehension across physical sciences (physics and chemistry), biological sciences (biology and organic chemistry), psychology and sociology, and verbal reasoning. This is the "big test" that you may have heard other pre-meds talk about. Taking this test is a prerequisite to applying to medical school, and doing well is essentially a requirement for acceptance into medical schools.

Your MCAT score is one of the most important factors in your application's competitiveness besides your GPA because medical schools will have a soft (and sometimes hard) cutoff on reviewing applications based on the MCAT score. That means some schools will have automatic cutoff scores that will preclude certain applicants from having their applications even be *seen* by reviewers.

Generally, this test requires you to have a strong grasp on the scientific concepts central to the required coursework we have discussed. Your college classes should cover the majority of what you need to know, but you will most likely need to buy a MCAT review book or review materials to make sure you can focus efficiently on the right content. Some people choose to enroll in preparation classes, which are generally very expensive.

Basically, the MCAT questions give you information or evidence in a written passage or graph/table form. Sometimes this information will be baffling on purpose. You will need to understand how to identify the relationship between the new information given and scientific concepts you already know.

When you take this exam is up to you, but most people finish their science classes first and then dedicate weeks to months of study time to prepare to take the exam prior to June of the year before starting medical school. For traditional applicants, this would be around the end of their junior year of their undergraduate degree.

The timing of when to take this exam will vary based on your situation, especially if you are not applying to medical school straight out of college. Those applicants that have already graduated—or plan on taking time off but have not taken the test—will have to find a time that makes sense for them and when they want to apply.

The exam is graded with a numerical score that will *permanently* remain on your record. Generally, most medical schools will accept MCAT scores from the last 2 to 3 years. However, some schools may accept older scores. Schools also vary on how they determine the time cutoffs. Some schools count the time backward from the date of expected matriculation, while others count the time backward from time of application.

If you score poorly on this exam, you *can* retake the exam, but taking this exam more than twice is not encouraged. In addition, each MCAT score will likely appear on the exam transcript sent to schools; thus, schools will likely see a poor initial attempt followed by an improved score. It's ultimately up to individual schools' discretion what they do with multiple scores; the Association of American Medical Colleges (AAMC, i.e., the collective organization of US MD schools) has no hard requirements for Admissions Committees (ADCOMs).

How do you study for and score high on this exam? Don't worry, we'll tell you all about how to study for and score well on this exam in Chapter 17, Crushing the MCAT.

---

[1] Especially for students interested in the most competitive specialties, (i.e., dermatology, orthopaedic surgery, plastic surgery, otolaryngology, and neurosurgery). Incidentally, undergraduate research activity in these fields may also be helpful for gaining acceptance to residency programs in these fields down the line.

## 1.3 Step 3. Complete Online Applications to Medical Schools, Attend Interviews, and Get Accepted

Because **the process from application to acceptance takes an entire year** (see Chapter 20, The Big Picture), proper planning and timing is essential.

Ideally, you send your application to medical schools in June (one year prior to the fall of the year you want to matriculate), interview at schools in the subsequent fall or winter, and decide where to attend in April/May.

There are two parts to the application: Primary Application and Secondary Application.

### 1.3.1 The Primary Application

Also see Chapter 28, Primary Application: AMCAS, AACOMAS, and TMDSAS). This is what you prepare first and it includes the following:
- School transcript(s).
- MCAT test score.
- Manually categorizing the classes you have taken.
- Recommendation letters.
- Personal statement essay.
- Listing out your activities, short essays describing them, and listing hours involved in each.
- A list of medical schools you are applying to.

**Quick Note about Letters of Recommendation**

You will need to have Letters of Recommendation sent on your behalf as part of your application. The majority of these letters are typically from professors you've worked with at your school.

One recommendation letter, however, should come from your school's **"pre-medical committee,"** if there is one. This is a group of advisors at your school, typically formed by several professors. They are like gatekeepers that prescreen pre-med students at your school. Read more in Chapter 23, Letters of Recommendation.

**Quick Note about MD and DO**

Did you know medical schools come in two flavors? Allopathic (MD: Doctor of Medicine) and Osteopathic (DO: Doctor of Osteopathy). All you need to know right now is that you can be a physician with either degree.

Both curriculums overlap, and most patients don't know the difference between an MD doctor and DO doctor. You can apply to either or both MD and DO schools. Read more in Chapter 24, DO, MD, and International Schools.

### 1.3.2 The Secondary Application (Secondaries)

This is explained further in Chapter 33, Secondary Application. It is an online application that becomes available to you once your Primary Application is received, and it is specific to the schools to which you applied. Most of your schools will send you a link to complete a secondary application unless you were screened out (e.g., your stats weren't good enough).

The secondary application generally includes the following:
- More questions about you and your background.
- Additional essays for you to write about, for example: *why do you want to come to XYZ medical school?*

Because you will be receiving these essays to complete from most of your schools around the same time *and* you have to complete them quickly, it can get a little overwhelming. And yes, most secondaries will have a fee.

But there's good news! The essay prompts do not change much from year to year, and you can usually find the prompts on the Internet. This means you can prepare your essays ahead of time before you receive the actual secondary. In addition, many schools tend to have similar questions/prompts, so you can have somewhat of a workable template for yourself.

### 1.3.3 Admissions Interviews

Yes! The schools have reviewed both your primary and secondary application, and they liked you on paper. Now they want to interview you to see if you are the real deal. You will receive these invitations via email or through an online portal where you submitted your secondary.

Interview season runs from about late September through early February. Schools may differ slightly.

This chapter was originally written prior to the COVID-19 pandemic, when interviews were exclusively in-person and associated with extensive costs from travel and lodging. Since the COVID-19 pandemic, the logistics of medical school interviews have been evolving, with multiple admissions cycles switching to 100% online interviews. The future for medical school interviews is still uncertain, but many of the basic facts of the interview experience still persist. It's a nerve-wracking time of constant email and forum-checking, and every ping from your phone kicks up your blood pressure. Luckily we have tips on maintaining your sanity through the application cycle. Read more about logistical tips for the application and interview trail in Chapter 22, Before You Begin: Application Cycle Prophylaxis and Chapter 35, Interview Trail Travel and Attire.

Interviews can be with faculty and/or medical students. They come in a few different flavors like **Traditional** (e.g., "What brought you to this point?" "Why do you want to become a doctor?" "Come to our school," etc.) or **Multiple Mini-Interviews** (**MMI**), which offer a large number of mini-interviews at multiple stations in succession. These shorter interviews may include problem solving and eliciting your take on ethical dilemmas. Read more about acing your interviews in Chapter 34, Interviews.

### 1.3.4 Acceptance

Finally, the application process is coming to a close! Schools have notified you of acceptance offers and you have chosen THE ONE (as per Chapter 38, Acceptance and Decisions: What Really Matters When Choosing the One School). Maybe you had waited diligently on several waiting lists and employed the strategies in Chapter 36, Wait-List and Update Letters in the meantime. Nonetheless, you're going to be a medical student! In the coming months, you will make arrangements to relocate and apply for financial aid (Chapter 37, Financial Aid and Chapter 39, Before and After Matriculation).

Many students will take on loans to finance the large cost of tuition and living expenses. You will fill out a FAFSA form for financial aid and work with your medical school's financial aid office to arrange your loans and potential grants/scholarships.

## 1.4 Step 4. Attend Medical School

### 1.4.1 First and Second Years

After a brief orientation period getting to know your new school and classmates, you will hit the ground running with the books… or online videos and flashcard apps. Strap yourself in for long study hours!

Curricula slightly vary among schools, but generally, **in your first and second year** you will study **basic biomedical sciences with classroom lectures, anatomy cadaver lab,** and online learning. You also will learn the basic physical examination and some patient interviewing skills. Of note, medical education is rapidly advancing, and many schools are experimenting with progressive, more interactive learning methods. Read more in Chapter 42, Real Talk on the Medical School Experience and Chapter 43, Real Talk on Succeeding in Medical School.

#### What Are Basic Sciences?

As a pre-med, we refer to basic science as chemistry, biology, physics, and the subsubjects that are included under those subjects (e.g., microbiology).

As a medical student, we refer to basic science as the subjects covered (to the extent) on the Step 1 USMLE exam. These include anatomy, microbiology, cell and molecular biology, pathology, physiology, behavioral sciences, pharmacology, biochemistry, genetics, immunology, nutrition, epidemiology, and biostatistics.

### MS = Medical Student

You might hear med students referred to as **MS1 or M1.** The M or MS stand for Medical Student, and the number refers to what year of medical school they are currently in. So an MS1 or M1 is a first-year student, MS2 or M2 a second-year student, and so on.

MS1 → First-year medical student.
MS2 → Second-year medical student.
MS3 → Third-year medical student.
MS4 → Fourth-year medical student.

Likewise, residents are referred to as **PGY1, PGY2, etc.,** for "postgraduate year 1," "postgraduate year 2," etc.

## 1.4.2 Take the USMLE Step 1 (or COMLEX-USA Level 1) Exam

To progress through medical school and residency, you have to pass the medical licensing exams. Of note, there are two major pathways by which this is done: the U.S. Medical Licensing Exams (USMLE) for MD students, and the COMLEX-USA exams for DO students. There are four USMLE exams in total: Step 1, Step 2 Clinical Knowledge (CK), Step 2 Clinical Skills (CS), and Step 3. The COMLEX-USA exams are analogous but also cover osteopathic medicine; however, many DO students choose to also take the USMLE to make themselves more competitive for ACGME (i.e., MD) residency programs (more in Chapter 44, A Peek at the Residency Application Process).

In medical school, you take Step 1, Step 2 CK, and Step 2 CS. In residency, you take Step 3. These exams not only give you a numerical score but also have a pass/fail threshold. They also have a "score once" policy, meaning that if you fail the exam you can retake them, but if you pass, even if you pass with the slimmest of margins, you may never retake it.

Traditionally, between the end of your second and into your third year of medical school, you will take the Step 1 exam. However, some schools have their students take it after the first year, and other schools have pushed it to the end of third year. Step 1 is a basic science-focused exam. This 8-hour exam had been considered the "biggest exam" of medical school, as it had traditionally been one of the most—if not *the most*—important variable for placement into competitive residency programs (analogous to the MCAT for medical school admissions). However, the National Board of Medical Examiners (NBME) decided to transition Step 1 to a pass/fail scoring system. The implications of this for residency program placement (as well as its impact on the relative weights of other aspects of evaluating applicants, e.g., clerkship scores, medical school rank, research productivity) are speculative at the time of writing, unfortunately.[2,3,4]

## 1.4.3 Pass/Fail USMLE Step 1: A Deeper Dive

Step 1 was essentially the MCAT of medical school: the single most important standardized marker of your academic aptitude that could make or break your application to competitive residency programs. Students spent countless hours studying for this exam—often at the expense of their in-house exam material—to make themselves maximally competitive. The NBME, however, concluded that this disproportionate emphasis on a single exam—that may not even reliably predict one's aptitude as a physician—majorly contributed to stress and poor mental health among medical students. As a result, the exam was made pass/fail.

---

[2] Aziz F, Bechara CF. USMLE Step 1 Scoring System Change to Pass/Fail –Implications for International Medical Graduates. JAMA Surg 2020;155(12):1098–1099. Available at: https://jamanetwork.com/journals/jamasurgery/article-abstract/2769849. Accessed July 8, 2022.

[3] Neville AL, Smith BR, de Virgilio C. USMLE Step 1 Scoring System Change to Pass/Fail –An Opportunity for Change. JAMA Surg 2020;155(12):1093–1094. Available at: https://jamanetwork.com/journals/jamasurgery/article-abstract/2769846. Accessed July 8, 2022.

[4] Humphrey HJ, Woodruff JN. The Pass/Fail Decision for USMLE Step 1 –Next Steps. JAMA 2020;323(20):2022–2023. Available at: https://jamanetwork.com/journals/jama/article-abstract/2766393. Accessed July 8, 2022.

So what are the implications? Again, it's not completely clear yet, but many speculate that Step 2 CK—taken at the end of third year or the beginning of fourth year—will take the place of Step 1 as the standardized measure of academic aptitude. This could prove disastrous for someone who spent 3 years preparing for a highly competitive specialty (e.g., orthopaedic surgery) only to receive a score that would essentially remove them from the running, arguably invalidating 3 years of grueling work. Medical school prestige could also be weighed much more, making the MCAT significantly more important for eventual residency placement (as more prestigious schools tend to have higher average MCAT scores). Number of publications, abstracts, and presentations may also become more important for competitive residency, incentivizing applicants in these fields to pursue research years to build their CVs even further. Ultimately, *we urge readers to stay up-to-date on the developing downfield effects of this change*, as it may impact your decisions on which medical schools to ultimately attend, especially if you're thinking about a competitive specialty.

Indeed, the preliminary available data appears consistent with our predictions, as a survey of residency program directors in 2020[5] revealed that medical school prestige and Step 2 CK scores will become more important, given the lack of objective Step 1 scores to distinguish among applicants.

## 1.4.4 Complete Core Clerkships, aka Get a Taste of the Different Specialties

For your third and fourth years, you will complete clerkships in the major various hospital medical specialties (internal medicine/general adult medicine, pediatrics, obstetrics and gynecology, surgery, psychiatry, family medicine). A clerkship, also referred to as a "rotation," is a period of a few weeks (typically 4–8 wk), where you spend time being a team member in a particular specialty. You will be supervised while seeing patients, examining them, and coming up with diagnoses and treatments with the team. During your clerkship years, your schedule will entirely consist of rotations. This means every few weeks, you will be moving on to a new rotation.

Clerkships are considered one of the most stressful aspects of medical school; at the same time, what one *does* on a clerkship is incredibly nebulous and hard to truly understand until one is actively participating in one.[6] Please carefully read the clerkship section in Chapter 42, Real Talk on the Medical School Experience and Chapter 43, Real Talk on Succeeding in Medical School to gain a deeper understanding of what this essential component of medical education is like.

### Clerkships aka Rotations

Core clerkships are mandatory. Elective clerkships are not.

Every medical school will have a **core set of clerkships** you complete. These may or may not include:

| | | |
|---|---|---|
| Internal Medicine | Surgery | Obstetrics and Gynecology (OB/GYN) |
| Neurology | Pediatrics | Psychiatry |
| Family Medicine | Anesthesiology | Emergency Medicine |
| Ophthalmology | Ear Nose Throat (ENT) aka Otolaryngology | |

---

[5] Makhoul AT, Pontell ME, Kumar NG, Drolet BC. Objective Measures Needed—Program Directors' Perspectives on a Pass/Fail USMLE Step 1. N Engl J Med 2020; 382:2389–2392. Available at: https://www.nejm.org/doi/full/10.1056/NEJMp2006148. Accessed July 8, 2022.

[6] You may read extensively about the clerkship experience prior to starting them, but will likely not start to fully understand the scope of what you are getting yourself into until maybe a week into the clerkship!

At the end of each clerkship, you take a **Shelf Exam**, which are 2-hour exams with USMLE-style questions. They're like mini-Step 2 exams. You will take these exams at your medical school.

### 1.4.5 Electives

In your MS3 year and especially in your MS4 year, you can take various elective rotations. The specialties and topics will vary from school to school. You may also have the opportunity to go abroad/international rotations as well!

### 1.4.6 Take the USMLE Step 2 Exam (CK and CS)

During or after your third year (MS3), you will take the **USMLE Step 2 board exam** (or COMLEX Step 2). There are two separate exams that make up Step 2:

There is **Step 2 Clinical Knowledge (CK)** (or the similar COMLEX Step 2 CE for DO students), a 9-hour exam which focuses on clinical diagnostics and treatment knowledge.

For MD students, there also used to be **Step 2 Clinical Skills (CS)** (or the similar COMLEX Step 2 PE for DO students), which was an 8-hour patient encounter exam. This exam was discontinued in January 2021 during the COVID-19 pandemic. As of May 2021, COMLEX Step 2 PE is still suspended; keep an eye out for major developments by the NBOME!

### 1.4.7 Complete an Acting Internship (AI), aka Pretending to Be a First-Year Resident

Another requirement for graduating from medical school is completing an acting internship (AI/sub-I) in your MS4 year. You can think of this as sort of an audition to become a resident/intern in the specialty you are interested in. You are given more independence and responsibility for caring for patients.

You choose your AI from a few options offered at your school. For example, if you are interested in applying to an Internal Medicine residency, you will do an Internal Medicine AI rotation.

### 1.4.8 Complete Away Rotations (Optional)

Some specialties, (e.g., Emergency Medicine [EM]), basically require you to have done a rotation in the specialty at an institution other than your own. This means if you want to apply to EM, you need to do a "home" EM rotation at your own school, and then an "Away" EM rotation at a different school.

You arrange these opportunities with an online application database.

## 1.5 Step 5. Apply to Residency

You apply to residency in the specialty of your choice in the last year of medical school. Keep in mind that there are numerous subspecialties—sometimes more than twenty—within each of the specialties listed below. These are not listed here.

## Medical Specialties

Every medical student up until third year will have essentially the same education. In the fourth year of medical school you start customizing your education with elective rotations geared toward your specialty of interest.

Here are some common specialties you might apply to for residency:

| | | |
|---|---|---|
| Internal Medicine (IM) | General Surgery | Obstetrics & Gynecology (OB/GYN) |
| Neurology | Neurological Surgery | Pediatrics (Peds) |
| Family Medicine | Orthopedic Surgery | Psychiatry |
| Urology | Pathology (i.e., anatomic pathology, clinical pathology, or both) | Ophthalmology |
| Anesthesiology | Emergency Medicine (EM) | Otolaryngology (ENT) |
| Plastic Surgery | Cardiothoracic Surgery | Dermatology |
| Diagnostic and/or Interventional Radiology | Radiation Oncology | Vascular Surgery |
| IM-Peds Combined | Physical Medicine & Rehabilitation (PM&R) | Transitional/Preliminary (program) |
| Medical Genetics | Preventative Medicine | Nuclear Medicine |

The **residency application** process is also quite involved, similar in ways to applying to medical schools. You will have to complete an online application, obtain recommendation letters, and travel to attend interviews. Unlike the medical school application, however, you get to rank your preference of programs at which you interviewed, and the residency programs will rank you among other interviewees. Read more in Chapter 44, A Peek at the Residency Application Process (although we recommend additional reading material for a comprehensive understanding of this process).

## 1.5.1 Match Day

After the interview season ends, there is a computer-based matching result that is revealed nationally in March called Match Day, when you will find out what program you and your classmates have matched at. There will be a ceremony (and hopefully parties!).

Once you match with a residency, you have to attend that designated program with few exceptions. Once you graduate medical school you are now technically a "doctor" with an MD or DO degree, but without license to treat patients on your own. That privilege comes after completing residency.[7]

---

[7] Strictly speaking, after completing intern year and passing USMLE/COMLEX-USA Step 3. One year of residency (i.e., intern year) with licensing is enough to practice independently as a "general practitioner," but you will face significant obstacles in getting reimbursed by insurance companies and covered by malpractice insurance without board certification/eligibility in a specialty such as internal medicine. Nonetheless, entrepreneurial-minded physicians *have* carved out unique niches with a single year of residency (e.g., cosmetics, rural medicine, serving prison populations, etc.).

## 1.6 Step 6. Complete Residency

You will attend the residency program at a hospital where you matched for clinical training. You will be paid modestly while you work as a **resident physician**—a doctor who is in basic training. Residency programs are between 3 and 7 years depending on the medical specialty. Residency training is grueling and may include very long work hours (+/− 80 h/wk) and include scheduled overnight shifts.

Of note, not all medical specialties force you to work extreme hours. Residency programs in psychiatry, dermatology, diagnostic radiology, physical medicine and rehabilitation, and radiation oncology—among others—often allow trainees to work closer to 40 to 60 hours per week during training. Consider these specialties if you discover in medical school that you likely will not be able to tolerate 3 to 7 years of 80-hour workweeks.

After graduating from residency, passing your board exams, and obtaining your state medical license, you are considered a "full-fledged" doctor capable of practicing independently with full privileges (e.g., reimbursement by insurance companies, malpractice coverage), either privately or at a hospital. Completing residency programs are required for becoming a physician who can treat patients with qualified independent authority.

### 1.6.1 But Wait. Why Do I Have to Attend Residency? Isn't Medical School Where You Learn Medicine and Become a Doctor?

Yes and no. Medical schools give you a broad and basic foundation of knowledge and clinical skills that is common across most clinical specialties. For example, you spend the first two years (1 or 1.5 years at some schools) learning the basic science underpinning modern medical care. In third and fourth year of medical school you actually participate in patient care in hospitals while doing your clinical rotations, but the bottom line is that there is too much medical information and skills to cover. Residency programs provide the in-depth and specialized clinical training you need to gain expertise in a specific field to become a competent physician.

## 1.7 Step 7. Complete Fellowships (Optional)

Some people choose to subsequently attend fellowship programs (which are like "advanced residencies") for further specialized training. Some people also choose not to apply to a residency program and instead pursue alternative careers in academic research or other fields.

Sometimes a fellowship is necessary to ultimately practice in your chosen specialty. For example, to become a hand surgeon, you may need to complete an Orthopedic residency program (5 years) and a Hand Surgery fellowship (1–2 years). Likewise, some specialties are becoming so specialized that fellowship training is *de facto* necessary for securing employment. For example, virtually all diagnostic radiologists and pathologists complete fellowship training, bumping up the average length of training to 6 and 5 to 6 years, respectively.

In the case of hand surgery, there could also be alternative paths such as completing a General Surgery residency (5–7 years) or Plastic Surgery residency (5–9 years depending on your training pathway, the longest being a 5+2 years of academic general surgery with research years, followed by a 2-year plastic and reconstructive surgery fellowship), and then go on to complete the Hand Surgery fellowship.

Many of the most well-known medical specialties (e.g., ICU doctor, cardiologist) require fellowship training. A great advantage of becoming a physician is that your doctoral training and years of intensive on-the-job training give you the flexibility to carve your own niche and create your own areas of practice. Refer to Appendix C, Medical Specialties and Subspecialties for an in-depth exploration of the 200+ available medical subspecialties.

## 1.8 Step 8. Become an Attending Physician

Congratulations! You finally finished all that training! You are now an attending physician, a full-fledged independent physician.

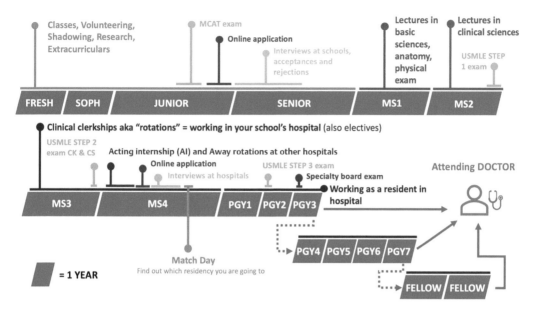

Fig. 1.1

Here's a general map that summarizes your journey (▶ Fig. 1.1). Note that depending on your life circumstances and career goals, this map may look very different. For example, you may become a fellow in an internal medicine sub-specialty as a PGY-4, versus a fellow in diagnostic radiology as a PGY-6.

## 1.9 Summary

Altogether, the path to becoming an independently practicing physician involves:
- Bachelor's degree in any major, as long as ~2 years of pre-reqs are completed. You will also do *de facto* required extracurriculars (clinical experience, volunteering, +/– personal hobbies and research).
  - Cultivate strong mentorships to get good letters of recommendation.
  - Maintain a strong GPA and do *not* get in trouble with the law or your university.
- MCAT—prepare for weeks—months and get a decent score.
- Apply to medical schools online, attend interviews, and matriculate at a medical school.
  - Alternatively, take time before medical school, e.g., 1 or more gap years or even another career entirely (as many non-traditional applicants do) OR post-bac programs/graduate degrees.
- Attend medical school for 4 to 8 years (depending on whether you pursue dual-degrees).
  - Pass USMLE Steps 1 and 2.
  - Figure out what specialty you want to go into and excel in rotations.
- Apply to residency programs online, attend interviews, match at a residency program.
- Attend residency for 3 to 7 years.
- +/– Attend fellowship for further training (typically 1–3 y).
- Now you are an Attending Physician!

# 2 What Medical Schools Look For

*Joel Thomas*

## 2.1 What Are the Goals of Medical Schools?

Medical schools want to admit students whom they can reliably craft into caring, competent physicians. Here are some mission statements from schools themselves.

"To nurture a diverse, inclusive community dedicated to alleviating suffering and improving health and well-being for all through excellence in teaching and learning, discovery and scholarship, and service and leadership." (Harvard Medical School)

"To educating physicians who will form and lead the integrated healthcare delivery and research teams of tomorrow; discovering new knowledge that will define the future of clinical care through investigation from the laboratory to the bedside, and into the community; and setting the standard for quality, compassionate and efficient patient care for our community and for the nation." (Jefferson Medical College)

Before we dive deep into what medical schools look for in applicants, let's explore two very different approaches to the pre-medical years.

## 2.2 How Many Students Approach the Pre-Medical Years

Bill has always wanted to become a doctor. The idea of driving a Lamborghini greatly appeals to him, and he dreams of the respect he would garner as the chief of pediatric neurosurgery. He's not particularly passionate about science, but he majors in biology because it's what "all the pre-med kids are doing." He crams for his tests the night before and manages to pull a 3.6 GPA through an admirable force of will. He is incredibly frustrated with his MCAT prep, however, because he failed to develop a conceptual understanding or long-term retention of his course material. He volunteers at the local hospital because it was the first clinical volunteering opportunity he found online. However, he hates it because "they don't even let you do anything." Because he put the bare minimum into his courses, he remained a nameless face among the sea of the pre-med students. Suffice to say, his letters of recommendation were suboptimal. His personal statement accurately reflected his commitment to medicine, as he was unable to articulate any unique, personal reasons for pursuing a career in medicine beyond vague interests in "science" and "helping people." Don't be like Bill.

## 2.3 How YOU Will Approach the Pre-Medical Years

Shea started college without any clear direction. She liked reading, so she took many English and comparative literature courses in her first few semesters. However, she also took introductory biology to fulfill her school's general education requirement. To her surprise, she loved the material and eventually pursued enough courses to double major in English and biology. She enjoyed the idea of bridging the humanistic themes in literature with biology, and therefore she reached out to the pre-med advising department. After careful consideration of all her options to explore a medical career, she began volunteering at a free clinic, where she forged strong relationships with the physicians on site. She excelled in her courses—largely due to her personal interest coupled with consistent studying—and received an excellent score on the MCAT. Her medical school interviewers could clearly see her passion for medicine as she earnestly spoke about her favorite physician-writers and her desire to join their ranks. She continued to develop her interests in medical school and beyond, writing humanities pieces for the *Journal of the American Medical Association* and other publications.

While Shea's unique interests and life experiences made her a successful applicant to medical school, they are just that: unique. Don't force yourself to pursue the same path that she did, as there are many different but equally valid roads to acceptance. Build up the 6 pillars and pursue what makes you happy. Along the way, you may even discover that happiness lies in a nonmedical career. If so, do some serious self-reflection, as the pre-medical years should be a time for identity formation. Not everyone will be happy as a physician, and that is perfectly fine. Moreover, as you may have inferred, the road to becoming a physician requires juggling multiple commitments and deadlines. In the next few chapters, we will discuss key tips for consolidating this seemingly overwhelming amount of information.

Keeping these two contrasting approaches in mind, we now explore a key question: *what are medical schools looking for in applicants and why?*

## 2.4  The 6 Pillars

While some schools may emphasize specific attributes, there are certain *core competencies*[1] desired by *all* medical schools. We have organized these attributes into groupings, which we call the 6 Pillars of a Great Applicant.

Just a heads up: there is a *lot* of detail in this chapter, as it lays the foundation for your pre-medical career. Don't worry if you don't get it all in the first pass. We will continue to refer to these "6 pillars" throughout the book.

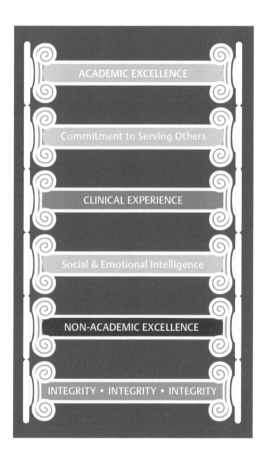

### 2.4.1  Pillar 1: Academic Excellence (aka Good Grades and Test Scores)

Medical school is a *lot* of studying. No—really—it's a *lot* of studying, and at most schools, your role will be a full-time test-taker for the first 2 years. The material isn't any more conceptually difficult than upper-level undergraduate biology courses, but the sheer volume and pace is unprecedented. In 3 weeks, a medical school biochemistry course may cover more material than *2 semesters* of undergraduate

---

[1] Core Competencies for Entering Medical Students. Available at: https://www.aamc.org/admissions/dataandresearch/ 477182/corecompetencies.html. Accessed July 8, 2022.

**Table 2.1** Acceptance rates to US MD Programs by GPA

| Total GPA | Acceptance rate (%) |
| --- | --- |
| >3.79 | 61.9 |
| 3.60–3.79 | 43.4 |
| 3.40–3.59 | 30.4 |
| 3.20–3.39 | 22.1 |
| 3.00–3.19 | 16.8 |
| 2.80–2.99 | 11.4 |

2019–2022 (Aggregated) Acceptance Rates to US MD Programs by GPA, All Applicants

| | |
| --- | --- |
| **Average GPA** | 3.74 ± 0.25 |
| **Average science GPA (GPA using science courses only)** | 3.67 ± 0.31 |

2021–2022 Average GPA and science GPA for US MD Program Matriculants

biochemistry. The only way to stay on top of this is by studying 4 to 8 hours virtually every day. Thus, medical schools want applicants who can excel in their undergraduate courses—particularly the sciences, particularly with a high GPA that demonstrates sustained excellence over years (▶ Table 2.1). The mean GPA ± standard deviation (SD) for matriculants in 2021 to 2022 for US MD programs was 3.74 ± 0.25, and mean GPA ± SD using only science courses (i.e., "science GPA") was 3.67 ± 0.31.[2] While there is no "pre-med" major, all matriculants must complete specific prerequisite courses in general, organic, ± biochemistry; physics, biology, and mathematics.[3] Scientific acumen can also be demonstrated through helping with research projects, as we'll talk about in later chapters.

The importance of attending a "prestigious" undergraduate institution is harder to assess. While medical schools[4] "selectivity of undergraduate institution" as "lowest importance" (similar to applicants' gender and age) when directly surveyed, attending a prestigious undergraduate institution typically makes it significantly easier to find productive research groups, engaging clinical opportunities at an affiliated academic medical center, and well-funded extracurricular opportunities among other things. Attending an elite university also gives you the benefits of tapping into a powerful alumni network, which may prove more helpful if you decide against attending medical school down the line. Additionally, while extremely impressive students attend every institution, "elite" colleges attract a disproportionate number of unusually driven and accomplished individuals (e.g., future Nobel prize winners) who would truly push you beyond your perceived limits. That said, the pressures of being surrounded by such a driven and accomplished cohort may not be appropriate for everyone. All things held equal, however, we recommend attending the most prestigious undergraduate institution that accepts you for these more intangible benefits. See Chapter 4, The Types of Pre-Medical Students and Paths to Medical School for additional discussion on attending a prestigious undergraduate school.

## How Does a GPA Below 3.0 Affect My Chances of Acceptance?

You should understand the context for these statistics, particularly outlier statistics such as GPA's below 3.0 gaining acceptance. For example, some students with GPAs lower than 3.0 will enroll in post-baccalaureate

---

[2] Table A-17: MCAT and GPAs for Applicants and Matriculants to U.S. MD-Granting Medical Schools by Primary Undergraduate Major, 2021–2022. Available at: https://www.aamc.org/media/6061/download. Accessed July 8, 2022.
[3] https://students-residents.aamc.org/choosing-medical-career/article/admission-requirements-medical-school/
[4] Table 1: Using MCAT® Data in 2023 Medical Student Selection. Available at: https://www.aamc.org/system/files/2022-06/2023%20MCAT%20Data%20Selection%20Guide%20Online.pdf. Accessed July 8, 2022.

programs and subsequently obtain near-perfect GPAs to gain admission into medical school. However, their GPAs will be averaged for aggregate, official statistics such as "Acceptance Rates to US MD Programs by GPA." As such, a 9.3% acceptance rate for GPAs between 2.80 and 2.99 should be interpreted with a grain of salt.

You'll also need to be good at taking standardized tests (i.e., the MCAT), hopefully on your first attempt. There are two reasons for this. First, the difficulty of courses can vary widely from school to school, as well as within schools. Standardized tests (as the name suggests) are the best available tool to quickly distinguish the capabilities of applicants of different academic backgrounds. Let's say Bob only took the easiest courses for his major beyond the pre-medical requirements, while Janice over-loaded on quantum electrodynamics and poststructural critical theory whenever possible. If they both have the same GPA, then a standardized test provides additional information for admissions committees to differentiate between them. The second reason is that you will take a *lot* of standardized tests throughout your medical career. Importantly, one of the most (if not *the* most) important factors for residency placement[5] is your score on the standardized United States Medical Licensing Exam (USMLE) Step 2 CK (up until several years ago, it was USMLE Step 1, now a pass/fail exam). This test is taken after clinical rotations and evaluates your clinical knowledge. As described in Chapter 1, The 30,000-Foot View, this exam will likely serve as the graded standardized test that residency program directors will use to evaluate applicants.

Of course, it doesn't end there, as you'll also take standardized shelf exams at the end of each rotation in your third year, Steps 1 and 3 for the USMLE, and specialty-specific exams during residency and beyond to maintain board certification in your field. Be aware that the average MCAT ± SD in 2021 to 2022 for matriculants to MD programs was a 511.9 ± 6.6, or the 84th percentile.

Unfortunately, medical schools have found that nothing predicts success on standardized testing like your performance on previous standardized tests. Specifically, there is good evidence to suggest that those with high MCAT scores have high Step scores. Medical schools want you to score well on your shelf and Step exams so that you get into a good residency (and make their school look more competitive by comparison). So, whether fair or not, you should get used to the importance this career path places on standardized testing.

## 2.4.2 Pillar 2: Commitment to Serving Others

As a physician, you will guide people through the most harrowing moments of their lives while connecting with them on a deeply personal level. You will do this despite being hungry, sleep-deprived, uncertain in your ability to help, or some combination thereof. Despite increasing bureaucratic demands that pull clinicians away from the bedside, the fundamental role of the physician remains unchanged: to sometimes cure, to often relieve, and to always comfort.[6]

You might be the most empathetic, caring person on the planet, but it will be difficult for schools to assess this unless you have concrete evidence of sustained commitments to serving others. While volunteering in a clinical setting would also provide clinical experience (see #3), you have a tremendous amount of freedom to pursue whatever opportunity to help your community that appeals to you. Because volunteering opportunities can vary greatly in terms of what you're allowed to do (e.g., walking dogs in the morning at the animal shelter, helping build houses through Habitat for Humanity), we recommend dipping your toes in many different settings until you find something that deeply resonates with you i.e., something memorable you can continue to come back to and discuss years later, despite having that organic chemistry test or research project looming over your head.

Ideally, you'll identify a true calling to serve your community: something that you *enjoy doing* as opposed to just ticking off a checkbox on your application. You will have been involved with this cause for at least a year or two, even if it's just a few hours every weekend. Maybe you had the opportunity to step outside the college bubble to engage with people unlike yourself, such as homeless communities or new immigrants. Along the way, you also forged a strong working relationship with a supervisor who writes you a letter of recommendation highlighting your outstanding interpersonal skills.

---

5 Results of the 2018 NRMP Program Director Survey. Available at: https://www.nrmp.org/wp-content/uploads/2018/07/NRMP-2018-Program-Director-Survey-for-WWW.pdf. Accessed July 8, 2022.

6 Kumar A, Allaudeen N. To Cure Sometimes, to Relieve Often, to Comfort Always. JAMA Intern Med 2016;176(6):731–732. Available at: https://jamanetwork.com/journals/jamainternalmedicine/article-abstract/2516767. Accessed July 8, 2022.

Over time, you've also periodically engaged in self-reflection (actual life lessons *as well as* personal statement fodder) to assess what service means to you and how you were able to go above and beyond for others despite the pull of your personal responsibilities. Most importantly, you'll gain access to different experiences and perspectives, all while being able to make someone else's life a little easier.

## 2.4.3  Pillar 3: Clinical Experience

If you don't have any experience with the day-to-day practice of medicine, medical schools will not take your motivations seriously. Medicine is still a highly romanticized profession, and it's easy to be captivated by the superattractive TV neurosurgeon who swoops in to save the day without breaking a sweat. However, it's vital to get a realistic understanding of what it's like to be a physician and to work in a healthcare setting in general. *The reality is that a significant percentage of practicing physicians (up to 60–70% in some surveys!)*[7,8] *would not recommend a career in medicine.* This is a profoundly important fact to internalize, and we encourage you to gain both breadth and depth in your clinical experiences to honestly assess whether you could thrive in such settings for the rest of your life. Could you realistically see yourself tolerating working 80 hours (possibly more when accounting for workplace hour falsification[9]) every week for years in residency in such an environment? Could you tolerate years of waking up in the middle of the night as a 50-year-old to see a patient in the emergency department?

Much like volunteering, **clinical experience**[10] can be gained in a variety of settings. In fact, you can even knock out two birds with one stone by volunteering in a clinical setting: many hospitals and nursing facilities have volunteering opportunities available. Be aware that the opportunities for active engagement may vary widely. Without any actual medical training or certification, you're more of a liability than an asset to any healthcare organization, and your involvement with patient care will likely be very limited (if not outright boring). Don't let this discourage you! You will be surprised by how much of a difference you can make for patients through friendly banter, corny jokes, and taking the extra time to find the best-looking turkey sandwich. Again, medical schools value longitudinal experience, so years of hospital volunteering for 4 hours per week will go farther than 100 hours crammed in a single summer before applying. If you want even further involvement with patient care, you can apply for a part-time healthcare job in college (e.g., EMT, nursing assistant). We do not recommend doing this just for the sake of strengthening your application, however, as you can gain enough clinical experience through longitudinal volunteering experiences.

Physician **shadowing**[11] has also become a *de facto*—if not actual—requirement for admission. True to the name, you will be following a physician and observing what they do on a typical day. This is a valuable opportunity because you might be surprised to discover how physicians actually spend most of their time. For example, on an inpatient medicine service, you might observe that the nurses and nurse assistants have the most direct face-time with patients at the bedside, while the physicians spend most of their time in workrooms poring over lab values and imaging, writing orders, calling consultant physicians to coordinate care, and reviewing prior health records. Your undergraduate institution may have formal relationships with physicians in the area for shadowing opportunities, but we also recommend personally reaching out to physicians via phone or email to arrange shadowing opportunities. Simply introduce yourself as a student interested in applying to medical school who's eager to shadow and learn about the career.

Unfortunately, many schools do not have clear guidelines for how much shadowing is sufficient. Some schools will have explicit requirements, e.g., the University of Utah states that, "Competitive applicants

---

[7] Beresford L. Among Physicians, 59% Would Not Recommend a Medical Career. Available at: https://www.the-hospitalist.org/hospitalist/article/125660/among-physicians-59-would-not-recommend-medical-career. Accessed July 8, 2022.

[8] The Future of Healthcare: A National Survey of Physicians. Available at: https://www.thedoctors.com/future. Accessed July 8, 2022.

[9] Byrne JM, Loo LK, Giang DW. Duty Hour Reporting: Conflicting Values in Professionalism. Available at: http://www.jgme.org/doi/pdf/10.4300/JGME-D-14-00763.1. Accessed July 8, 2022.

[10] Glossary.

[11] Glossary.

will have shadowed a variety of physicians for at least 24 hours."[12] Our recommendation, again, is to gain breadth and depth by shadowing a variety of specialties over the many years of your pre-medical education, as the introspections you glean from the experiences will likely mature as your personal motivations evolve over time. Some applicants choose to shadow a single physician over an extended period to develop a strong working relationship reflected in a letter of recommendation. While not necessary (except for some osteopathic schools requiring a letter from an osteopathic physician), this may enhance your application if it's something you're eager to pursue.

### 2.4.4 Pillar 4: Social and Emotional Intelligence

You will hear this theme repeatedly throughout your medical education, so the sooner you internalize it, the better: modern medicine is a team sport. While leadership ability is vital to succeeding as a physician (e.g., guiding the new interns as the resident), you also need to be able to defer expertise and authority to others (e.g., trusting the judgment of the cardiologist you consulted).

So how do you demonstrate to admissions committees that you're a team player? The most straightforward approach is taking on a leadership position in a student organization and *actually doing things*. That is, being one of four copresidents for the Pre-medical Association won't cut it if you just sat back and let everyone else do the work. As a leader, you should ideally motivate your teammates to be the best versions of themselves and provide regular guidance without micromanaging them. You should challenge yourself and take on new responsibilities and opportunities. A healthy amount of adversity should be freely welcomed, mostly for the sake of personal growth and experience, but also being able to knock behavioral interview questions ("Tell me about a time you overcame a challenge") out of the park.

At the same time, you should also develop a sense of comfort in deferring leadership to others and learning from their expertise. Throughout much of medical school, you will receive direct feedback from supervising physicians. As such, you should be able to take criticism well, even if it's not delivered tactfully. Moreover, many schools are emphasizing team-based learning (TBL), and some schools even evaluate applicants' performance in **TBL**[13] settings on interview day. While medical school tends to attract "Type A" individuals who are eager to take the lead, no one wants to be in a TBL environment in which everyone's fighting to be heard. On a personal level, you should cultivate the ability to pick up on social cues such as *reciprocity*: identifying that split-second when it's safe to chime in with your opinion without cutting anyone off. On a more tangible, demonstrable level, you should have extracurricular experiences in which you worked in a nonleadership capacity, as well.

While long-term involvement in student organizations suggests some baseline level of social competence, the best evidence will come from your letters of recommendation. A letter of recommendation is a seal of approval from a respected community member who has worked with many other students (and can assess where you stand and provide relative perspective on who you are). An ideal letter demonstrates that others can closely work with you for long periods of time over many years. This is extremely reassuring to admissions committees because many applicants can muster up enough social charm to appear socially adjusted for several hours on interview day, and existing literature reports that medical school applicants are liable to distort their own image to gain acceptance.[14] In contrast, it would take an impressive amount of manipulation to deceive a professor or supervisor into thinking that you're a decent person after closely working with them for years. Thus, we recommend identifying mentors early and forging strong relationships with them. See professors at office hours and stick around if they seem open to it (again, develop that social intuition!). Work closely with a research supervisor. Don't be afraid to get to know your mentors as people, but be mindful of professional boundaries. If you consistently demonstrate a genuine desire to learn from your mentors, work hard, and communicate your professional aspirations (i.e., becoming a physician), you will almost certainly have a strong letter of support for medical school.

---

[12] The Office of Admissions. Available at: https://medicine.utah.edu/students/programs/md/admissions/. Accessed July 8, 2022.

[13] Glossary.

[14] Griffin B, Wilson IG. Faking good: self-enhancement in medical school applicants. Medical Education 2012;46(5):485–490. Available at: https://onlinelibrary.wiley.com/doi/full/10.1111/j.1365-2923.2011.04208.x. Accessed July 8, 2022.

## 2.4.5 Pillar 5: Non-Academic Excellence–Passion and Deep Achievement

Medical schools want to produce physicians who will excel in their areas of interest, whether it be clinical medicine, healthcare administration, research, public outreach, etc. Because the best predictor of future success is past success, we encourage you to continue your personal hobbies and excel in them in some demonstrable way. For example, if you like to play the guitar, try to write original music or play shows! Developing your personal interests will make you a more interesting person, which provides conversation fodder for interviews and talking to patients. Despite how impersonal and numbers-focused the application process may appear at times, schools really are interested in you as a person. It's refreshing to see, for example, that the biography pages of medical residents at many programs will highlight their personal interests and hobbies.

We also recommend being a "pointy" applicant. You've probably heard that you need to be "well-rounded" to get into medical school. This is true to an extent: you need to demonstrate academic excellence, clinical exposure, a commitment to serving others, and social intelligence at minimum, but it greatly helps to have an edge that distinguishes you from the thousands of other applicants who also have those same characteristics. The average admission rate for US MD programs is 7%,[15] and a common question on the interview trail—spoken or unspoken—is "Why should we admit you over the thousands of other applicants to this program?" Exploring your personal interest in working with underserved populations, for example, would be one way to distinguish yourself from the pack, especially if you can demonstrate that passion through fluency in Spanish and volunteering experiences at Hispanic clinics, for example.

Of course, it's much easier to excel at things that you actually like. Whenever possible, choose extracurriculars that appeal to you; don't just join clubs because they would look nice on your resume. You're more likely to put effort into things that you enjoy, and you might discover or create opportunities that you hadn't originally considered. Moreover, cultivating hobbies that you enjoy will allow you to decompress amid the many stressors of a medical career.

## 2.4.6 Pillar 6: Integrity

The last five qualities were things that you *should* do. For most applicants, this section will focus on things that you *shouldn't* do. To state the obvious, you should be a decent person. However, having certain "**red flags**" on your application will make it incredibly difficult—if not outright impossible—to gain admission to medical school. The reality is that every school receives thousands of applications to fill a class of approximately 100 students. Selecting among qualified applicants is hard enough, so autorejecting applicants with red flags makes the process significantly easier for admissions.

So what are these "red flags"? Broadly speaking, they're any documented history of breaking the rules. These include criminal history, institutional action (i.e., breaking university rules), and dishonorable discharge from the military. Most students aren't intimately familiar with the sheer number of ways to break their university or state's rules, however. Ignorance of the law excuses no one, and medical school admissions is no exception.

Imagine the following scenario. You just received an interview invite to a school in Virginia. You're driving in from Maryland, and you're cruising along 70 and 80 mph on the interstate highways because the trip is punishingly long and everyone else is doing it. The next thing you know, you're pulled over by the police and hit with a misdemeanor charge for going over 20 mph in Virginia.[16] We highlight this example because Virginia is an oddity, in that going 20 mph over the speed limit can grant you a criminal record. Most applicants wouldn't know this, and many may accidentally incriminate themselves while crossing state lines!

Now, will a medical school necessarily toss your application for a speeding misdemeanor? Who knows. It will depend on who's reading your application, but simply being forced to check the "criminal activity" box on your application brands you with a scarlet letter that colors how admissions will evaluate your

---

[15] 10 Med Schools With the Lowest Acceptance Rates. Available at: https://www.usnews.com/education/best-graduate-schools/the-short-list-grad-school/articles/2018-04-03/10-medical-schools-with-the-lowest-acceptance-rates. Accessed July 8, 2022.

[16] https://www.dmv.virginia.gov/drivers/#points_6.asp

application. Even if your crime is minor, schools have thousands of other qualified applicants to choose from. Why should they choose you over the sea of applicants who managed to keep a clean slate? In addition, simply having to check the "criminal record" box adds needless anxiety to an already anxiety-provoking application process.

Thus, we encourage you to be very familiar with the laws in your state and university. Take the time to review your school's code of conduct and be mindful of common ways that college students get in trouble. Err on the side of caution in unfamiliar situations; if a classmate asks you for information about old test questions and you're unsure if this would violate academic dishonesty, play it safe and politely decline. Use a plagiarism check before you submit any assignment via Turnitin or similar software. You'd be surprised how easy it is to accidentally plagiarize material that you had read at one point, and once you're suspected of academic dishonesty, it can be agonizingly difficult to clear your name. Moreover, while criminal charges presume innocence until proven guilty, your university's code of conduct may not be as lenient for suspected infractions. Lastly, if you do find yourself on the wrong side of the law, *keep your mouth shut* until you have a lawyer available (including asking for advice on the Internet with identifying information). Once you're in the hot seat with law enforcement, it is incredibly easy to accidentally incriminate yourself—*even if you're innocent*. Stay calm and let the legal experts do their job.

We also cannot understate the importance of using social media responsibly. As you've probably seen with recent celebrity and politician scandals: *the Internet is forever*. It's not unheard of for admissions committees to do a quick Google or Facebook search on you to easily identify applicants to reject for unprofessional behavior. Many patients Google physicians, so the ability to maintain a professional online identity is a reasonable expectation for admissions committees. Avoid having inappropriate photos of yourself in plain sight. If the damage has already been done, there are fortunately resources available for damage control.[17] We recommend doing an extensive search of your name (add your school to the search if you have a common name) on search engines and social media to identify any possible red flags.

We also advise caution when speaking publicly about sociopolitical issues. It's normal to care deeply about these topics, and many people communicate that passion via social media. That said, there can be a significant potential downside for your career with controversial postings, and the standards for acceptability are always evolving. Things that are considered relatively mild now may not be looked upon so favorably in 5 or 10 years. Again, *the Internet is forever*. Always assess the benefit of public discussion online with the risk of your comment aging poorly and potentially affecting your professional reputation down the line.

While you obviously want to avoid any red flags on your application, a scarlet letter is not necessarily the end of the world. For one thing, not all red flags are weighted equally. Nonetheless, you will be fighting an uphill battle. Your medical school application will have a section to explain the circumstances of what happened. It is vital that you review your response with advisors and demonstrate that this was a one-off event that does not represent your general character. Convince the reader that you've learned humility from an isolated lapse in judgment. Be very mindful of your tone (i.e., avoid even accidentally suggesting that it "wasn't your fault"). In severe cases, you may need to take some time off between the event and applying to medical school to convince admissions that you're a different person now. However, with perseverance, medical school will still be in your sights.

These 6 pillars will be your foundation. You can pursue other interests if you want, but your application will fail if you miss any of these. For example, the fencing club might be a wonderful fit for you, but you need to ask yourself if it would be the best use of your limited time if you've never set foot in a clinical setting or if you're barely passing your chemistry course.

## 2.5 For Lovers of Hard Data

In a 2021 report, the American Association of Medical Colleges (AAMC) revealed data from ADCOMs at 130 medical schools, summarizing which factors were most important for receiving acceptance at medical school (▶ Table 2.2).[18]

---

[17] 10 Med Schools With the Lowest Acceptance Rates. Available at: https://www.usnews.com/education/best-graduate-schools/the-short-list-grad-school/articles/2018-04-03/10-medical-schools-with-the-lowest-acceptance-rates. Accessed July 8, 2022.

[18] https://www.aamc.org/media/18901/download

**Table 2.2** Mean importance ratings of academic, experiential, demographic, and interview. Data used by admissions committees to make decisions about which applicants receive interview invitations and acceptance offers[1]

| Mean importance ratings[2] | Academic mtrics | Experiences | Demographics | Other data |
|---|---|---|---|---|
| Highest Importance Ratings (≥3.0) | 1. GPA: cumulative biology, chemistry, physics, and math<br>2. MCAT total score<br>3. GPA: grade trend<br>4. GPA: cumulative total<br>5. GPA: cumulative total from postbaccalaureate pre-medical program<br>6. MCAT total score trend<br>7. Completion of pre-medical course requirements | • Community service/volunteer: medical/clinical<br>• Community service/volunteer: not medical/clinical<br>• Physician shadowing/clinical observation<br>• Leadership | • U.S. citizenship/permanent residency (public)[3]<br>• State residency (public)[3]<br>• Rural/urban, underserved background | • Interview results[4] |
| Medium Importance Ratings (≥2.5 and <3.0) | • Completion of challenging upper-level science courses<br>• GPA: cumulative "all other" (not biology, chemistry, physics, and math) | • Paid employment: medical/clinical<br>• Research/lab<br>• Other extracurricular activities<br>• Military service | • Race/ethnicity<br>• U.S. citizenship/permanent residency (private)[3]<br>• Parental education/occupation/socioeconomic status (SES) | |
| Lowest Importance Ratings (<2.5) | • Degree from graduate or professional program<br>• Completion of challenging non-science courses<br>• Selectivity of undergraduate institution(s)<br>• Undergraduate major | • Teaching/tutoring/teaching assistant<br>• Paid employment: not medical/clinical<br>• Intercollegiate athletics<br>• Honors, awards, recognitions<br>• Conferences attended, presentations, posters, publications | • First-generation immigrant status<br>• Fluency in multiple languages<br>• Gender<br>• English language learners<br>• State residency (private)[3]<br>• Legacy status<br>• Selectivity of undergraduate institution(s)<br>• Community college attendance<br>• Age | |

[1] Admissions officers at 130 medical schools completed a 2015 AAMC survey on the use and importance of data in admissions decision-making. The survey asked, "How important were the following data about academic preparation, experiences, attributes/personal competencies, biographic/demographic characteristics, and interview results in identifying the applicants to [interview, offer an acceptance]?"

[2] Importance was rated on a scale ranging from 1 to 4 ("Not Important," "Somewhat Important," "Important," and "Very Important," respectively). For each variable, we computed an overall mean importance rating based on admissions officers' ratings of importance for making decisions about whom to interview and whom to accept (the mean importance rating for the interview variable is the exception to this rule because interview data were not available until applicants were invited to interview). We chose to classify variables using overall mean importance ratings because their mean importance ratings were similar for the interview and the acceptance phases. Variables are ordered by overall mean importance rating.

[3] Overall mean importance ratings for public and private institutions were significantly different from one another.

[4] Only available at the admissions stage where admissions committees make a decision to offer an acceptance.

Note that this is not an exhaustive list; lack of disciplinary action on your record is *extremely* important to gaining acceptance, but it was not explicitly mentioned in this survey. Nonetheless, it's consistent with pillars 1 to 6, and we will continue to refer to the pillars throughout this book.

## 2.6 Summary

The path to becoming a physician is highly individualized and varies greatly with personal life circumstances. However, all pre-medical students should consider the following "pillars" as they go along the journey:

1. **Academic excellence**: Get the highest GPA and MCAT possible, ideally at a prestigious undergraduate institution.
2. Demonstrate a **commitment to serving others**, ideally through some cause that genuinely moves you and allows a longitudinal commitment over years (e.g., volunteering at a shelter every weekend).
3. Get **clinical experience** (i.e., direct patient contact). Ideally this is through some cause that genuinely moves you and allows a longitudinal commitment over years. This should also include some physician shadowing.
4. Demonstrate **social and emotional intelligence**, (e.g., through leadership roles), excellent letters of recommendation.
5. **Nonacademic excellence**: Again, ideally this will be through some cause that genuinely moves you.
6. **Integrity:** Don't acquire a record of institutional or criminal violations. Keep in mind that ignorance doesn't necessarily protect you; there are many laws and regulations you might not be aware of that are surprisingly easy to violate. Be mindful of your local, state, federal, and institutional policies. When, in doubt, play it safe.

# 3 The Pre-Med Principles

*Ray Funahashi and Joel Thomas*

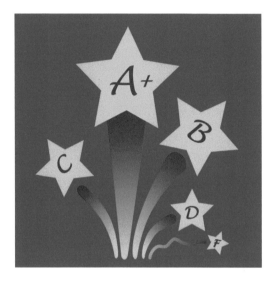

With the 6 Pre-Med Pillars in mind, we recommend the following *Pre-Med Principles*. These are 6 hard-and-fast rules you should always remember when making important decisions throughout your pre-medical career.[1]

## 3.1 Protect Your GPA and Integrity

Per Chapter 2.4.1, *Pillar 1: Academic Excellence (aka Good Grades and Test Scores)*, the path to becoming a physician entails consistently passing a seemingly endless barrage of high-stake exams. As such, medical schools want students with longstanding records of academic excellence. A strong cumulative GPA (ideally >3.8) is paramount, and a poor GPA will bar you from consideration at the vast majority of medical schools. In fact, we believe that—**aside from your physical and mental health—your GPA should be your *single biggest priority* as a pre-medical student**. Read that last sentence again: do *not* chase a high GPA at the cost of your physical and mental health. We understand that it's an easy trap to fall into: a few all-nighters here or there for "that big test" becomes several sessions a month, quickly leading you down the path of needing these strategies to simply maintain your performance.

We also want to emphasize—again—that **maintaining a spotless disciplinary record is critical**. You should always be mindful of university and legal policies, which should help guide your day-to-day decision-making as a pre-med (e.g., "Is it *really* the best move for me to go to this party this weekend to participate in undergrad drinking, knowing that police regularly raid parties and may arrest underage drinkers?").

### 3.1.1 Your Well-Being > GPA

If you find yourself potentially falling into a pattern of poor sleep hygiene, excessive weight gain or loss, depression or anxiety, the use of study drugs, etc., then take a serious moment to reflect on your priorities and trajectory. If caught early enough, you may simply be able to restructure your thoughts and behaviors (e.g., through CBT [cognitive behavioral therapy]). Make your health habits absolute priorities: regular sleep, diet, exercise, and social contact with people who make you feel good should not be neglected— *literally schedule them into your calendar if you need to.* Read more in Chapter 18, Self-Care and Wellness.

---

[1] Individual chapters in Section II: Succeeding as a Pre-Medical Student expand on the Pre-Med Principles.

If you continue to struggle on your own, reach out to trusted friends and family. Your school likely has counseling available at little to no cost. You may also need to take some time off from school to attend to your personal health. We absolutely encourage you to do so, as your application will be much stronger if you excelled in your courses after a medical leave of absence versus performing poorly while struggling with your well-being.

If you find that you're still struggling with mental or physical ailments, you will likely need to seek professional counsel; keep in mind that a minority of state medical licensing applications have stigmatizing questions against any history of mental illness. At the end of the day, your well-being is more important than theoretical distant risks to your future career, but we want you to be aware of cases and circumstances in which medical trainees experienced significant stigma and career consequences for rightfully seeking out treatment for their mental health.[2,3]

We offer the following tips for protecting your GPA:

- *Don't blow off your freshman year:* You can absolutely tank your entire medical school application in your first semester. While medical schools understand that the transition to college is difficult and appreciate upward GPA trends over time, it will be difficult to recover your cumulative GPA from the impact of even a single semester GPA of 2.0.
  - At the same time, keep in mind that a single bad test or course is probably not the end of the world. Learn from your mistakes and take the appropriate steps (e.g., meeting with the professor, tutoring, querying online forums such as Student Doctor Network or reddit.com/r/premed) to immediately change your study strategy to avoid the same errors in the future.
- *Your major (mostly) doesn't matter:* If you're debating between majors that interest you similarly, and you cannot decide, *consider picking the one that is known to be easier at your school* (only if you really can't decide). Your undergraduate major has little to no impact on medical school admissions (see Chapter 8, Schools, Majors, and More).[4] While some ADCOMs may grant some leniency to a 3.7 in chemical engineering (versus—say—a 3.9 in biology), your application will probably be screened out by most medical schools if you obtain a sub 3.0 GPA in any discipline.
  - That said, you should absolutely consider your personal interests. For one thing, you are more likely to be engaged and deeply study the material if you are personally interested and motivated in your classes. Moreover, becoming active in extracurriculars related to your personal academic interests can be an excellent way to distinguish yourself among the applicant pool, as well as to carve a cohesive narrative for the ADCOM.
- *Repeating a course does not replace the initial grade:* Medical schools will request *all* grades, including prior attempts at a course. Thus, it's generally better to withdraw from a course in which you think you may receive a D or F.
- *Take a full course load every semester:* If an upcoming semester looks particularly overwhelming, buffer the academic pain with easy credits (e.g., independent study, physical education courses, etc.). Read more about optimizing your schedule in Chapter 9, Timing, Class Structure, and Personal Schedules.
- *Learn the material in your prerequisite science courses as well as possible:* Seriously, you should aim for deep understanding and the ability to integrate material across your science courses into a unified web of knowledge. This will be enormously helpful for the MCAT and the first several years of medical school.
  - *Don't just aim to do well in pre-reqs by memorizing and regurgitating information.* Seriously, don't cram and pull all-nighters.[5] Study a little bit every day, and do as many practice problems as possible. Active learning is your best friend for mastering the sciences: engaging only in passively reading your textbook or class notes while highlighting will seriously limit what you get out of these courses.
    - In addition, getting into the habit of doing a manageable amount of work *every day* will make the transition to medical school much easier. The material in medical school is not conceptually any

---

[2] Physician-Friendly States for Mental Health: A Review of Medical Boards. Available at: https://www.idealmedicalcare.org/physician-friendly-states-for-mental-health-a-review-of-medical-boards/. Accessed July 8, 2022.

[3] Samuel L. Doctors fear mental health disclosure could jeopardize their licenses. Available at: https://www.statnews.com/2017/10/16/doctors-mental-health-licenses/. Accessed July 8, 2022.

[4] Caveat: an uncommon major (e.g., art history) could be a talking point in essays (e.g., "How are you diverse?") and interviews, especially if you actively pursue extracurriculars related to this interest. This does *not* mean that you should pursue an uncommon major just for the sake of being unique. You need to actually be interested in the material.

[5] The author was a notorious crammer in college and realizes—in retrospect—that this was extremely inefficient and needlessly painful.

more difficult than upper-level biology work. However, the sheer volume of information forces even the most seasoned crammers to become every-day studiers.

- Do not take your prerequisite science courses at a community college. While there are many fantastic community college courses, many are not taught to the same rigor as a university-level science course. Whether or not you believe that to be true, ADCOMs generally perceive prerequisites taken at community colleges as less rigorous than the equivalents at universities, which may hurt your application.
   - If you *do* want to take courses at a community college, we recommend the general education requirements for graduation that are *not* medical school prerequisites.

## 3.2  Do Not Take the MCAT Until You Are at least Averaging Your Target Score on Official Practice Tests

Per Chapter 2.4.1 Pillar 1: Academic Excellence (aka Good Grades and Test Scores), your MCAT score is a big deal, as it allows the ADCOM to compare academic performance across schools with different curricula and degrees of academic rigor. Chapter 17, Crushing the MCAT discusses specifics on how to prepare for this exam, but be aware that you will need to study several hours per day for *2 to 3 months* to prepare for this exam, *assuming that you already obtained a first-principles conceptual understanding of the material the first time you learned it in your undergraduate courses.* If you simply memorized everything blindly just to pass the exams in your prerequisite courses, then you will likely need more than 2 to 3 months of preparation for the MCAT.

*The MCAT should be a one-and-done event.* Medical schools will see every MCAT score you have received when you apply. If you do poorly on the MCAT once and retake it later, schools will take this into consideration. That is, they may average the scores and question your ability to reliably pass—on your first attempt—the endless onslaught of medical licensing exams. Applicants should defer taking the MCAT until they are reasonably confident that they've given their best effort toward preparation and aren't consistently making improvements on practice tests. Do not be afraid to postpone your exam if needed; it is better to take an additional year to apply if you are able to obtain a strong MCAT score with the additional time. Likewise, you have the option of *voiding* your exam (i.e., canceling the exam mid-test without receiving a score) if you feel that you are doing uncharacteristically poorly.[6] We recommend using this option if you *genuinely* feel that your performance is significantly worse than expected, given your experience with full-length practice exams in realistic settings.[7]

The average applicant should not take the MCAT until they are consistently averaging at least the 62nd percentile[8] (a 505 in 2018) because the average score for matriculants to MD schools that year was a 512 (84th percentile) with 1 standard deviation below at 505 (62nd percentile). That said, we recognize that (1) most applicants cannot score above the 50th percentile (obviously, half score below it, and half above) and (2) that some applicants will be unlikely to *ever* achieve such a score, no matter how well they prepare. If you genuinely feel that this is the case for you and have also explored multiple avenues for improving your score (e.g., MCAT tutors/courses, medical school consultants, pre-med advising, a variety of educational materials), then it may be worthwhile to reassess your application and specific goals. Do you have significant extenuating factors that would make up for a lower MCAT score (e.g., significant extracurricular activities, under-represented minority (URM) status, extremely prestigious undergraduate school, etc.)? Are you trying to get into *any* US MD or DO school vs. a top 20 MD school vs. MD schools only? Consider getting additional evaluation of your application as a whole and what MCAT score would be sufficient to achieve your specific goals (e.g., via pre-med advisors, medical school admissions consultants, etc.). In some cases, it may be necessary to take time off to strengthen your application to make up for a lower but workable MCAT score. Others may consider changing their goals (e.g., "top 20 MD schools

---

[6]  Don't confuse this with the normal anxiety of taking the MCAT. Most people feel like they're doing terribly when they're taking the actual exam. As such, you should take as many full-length MCATs in settings that mimic the actual MCAT administrator to prepare yourself for this feeling of dread. Consider taking a practice exam *at* the testing center to get accustomed to the logistics and atmosphere of test day.

[7]  The author actually almost voided his MCAT because he felt that he was doing exceedingly poorly on the test. He ended up doing just fine!

[8]  Lower MCAT scores are less likely to be screened out by ADCOM if you're an under-represented minority, however. See Chapter 21, Before You Begin: Application Strength Analysis for additional information.

only" to "any MD school," "MD schools only" to "any medical school, including DO schools and Caribbean schools").

In the worst case scenario, you're unable to obtain a competitive MCAT score despite your best efforts. In this scenario, you may need to give up applying to medical school altogether and explore different career paths because medical school and beyond is characterized by nonstop standardized tests. Before coming to this conclusion, we recommend exploring multiple different avenues for individualized counseling, especially if you're absolutely committed to becoming a physician otherwise. This isn't supposed to be harsh—medical school and a medical career is a lot harder than the MCAT.

## 3.3  Be an Interesting Person with a Cohesive Narrative Evidenced by Breadth and Depth of Experience

Pillars 2 (Commitment to serving others), 3 (Clinical experience), and 5 (Passion and deep achievement) largely refer to your values, as well as the tangible evidence of those values (i.e., extracurricular activities). Significant extracurricular achievement—*combined with a high GPA and MCAT*[9]—is necessary for admission to medical school.

In addition, ADCOMs appreciate applicants who are introspective and can articulate their narrative, (i.e., their professionally styled life story.)[10] That is, your extracurricular involvement should complement and be consistent with your interests and values. For example, an applicant who grew up in an impoverished area and pursued multiple leadership roles in clubs focusing on poverty would likely be able to tell a more cohesive story (e.g., on interviews and essays) than an applicant who randomly participates in clubs without any compelling reasons (e.g., "I thought this club would look good on my resume"). Of course, don't let this stop you from pursuing the occasional nonacademic interest. If you want to do Fencing Club or Civil War Reenactments, go for it—just don't let it take away from your grades and test scores.

We offer the following tips when considering extracurricular involvement.

- *Protect your GPA:* Don't take on too many commitments at once. One of the hardest skills to develop is saying "no," especially when people ask politely for favors. Remember that your grades take priority. You should dip your toes into new extracurricular activities and ease yourself in once you're confident that your GPA will not suffer.
  - You can always add additional extracurriculars later, (e.g., taking a gap year and not having to worry about classes at the same time). Once your GPA drops, it's *much* harder to make up for it down the line.
  - Pre-med is a marathon, not a sprint. If you feel burnt out and need to prioritize your mental or physical health, then *do so*. The process generally only gets more stressful over time. More and more applicants take gap years; the median age at matriculation in 2020 to US medical schools was 23 years.[11]
- *Consider your actual interests:* Whenever possible, do things that you actually like and *spin them* toward helping your medical school application (instead of doing "stereotypical" pre-med things just for the sake of strengthening your application). Virtually every interest can be related to medicine if you're creative enough. For example, if you're a musician, consider starting a music group that plays for patients in the hospital. If you're an artist, consider donating your work to a hospital or giving free painting lessons to nursing home patients. If you hate bench research, consider qualitative narrative-based research (e.g., interviewing individual patients about their life experiences as is done in domestic violence research).
- *Don't spread yourself too thin:* ADCOMs want to hear about what you *actually did*, not what you signed up for. We recommend identifying three to six specific things that interest you and pursuing them deeply. You don't have to start them all at once during your freshman year. At minimum, you should have volunteering (ideally both clinical and nonclinical), shadowing, clinical experience (if not already done through volunteering), and research (essential for research-oriented schools and highly valued by most—if not all—medical schools).

---

[9]  That is, while a low GPA and MCAT will likely keep you out of medical school, a high GPA and MCAT alone are not sufficient for admission.

[10]  See Chapter 5, Building Your Narrative for additional information.

[11]  Matriculating Student Questionnaire: 2020 All Schools Summary Report Available at: https://www.aamc.org/media/50081/download. Accessed July 8, 2022.

- *Start your extracurriculars early:* ADCOMs prefer longitudinal experiences, and early involvement in extracurriculars allows you to rise to leadership positions and pursue demonstrable awards and accomplishments. Volunteering—in particular—is best done this way, as ADCOMs generally prefer seeing a few hours of consistent volunteering over several years versus only cramming many hours into the summer before applying.
  - Research also benefits greatly from an early start. Much of success in research comes down to luck. Because of publication bias, positive significant findings are more likely to be published (compared to studies that fail to reject the null hypothesis, even if the original research question was well-posed and the methodology was sound).[12] It's difficult to predict *a priori* which research questions will yield significant, positive findings. As such, you maximize your odds of having publishable research by getting involved with research early and doing *many* projects over time. While publications are *not* necessary for admission to medical school, they are highly valued by some members of ADCOMs.
- *Your experiences are what you make of them:* If an experience seems like a waste of time, be creative about ways you can change your involvement. For example, most hospital volunteering can be exceedingly boring. Because volunteers tend not to have actionable medical training, their involvement—per the job description—can be limited to just clocking in, standing around for several hours, changing some bed sheets and refilling coffee, and then clocking out. Try to be mindful of your surroundings and make the best of your circumstances. Start interesting conversations with patients and staff. Go the extra mile when making a piece of toast for the patient—a perfect Maillard reaction with a picturesque tuft of butter will be noticed and can make a big difference to a patient who feels neglected.
- *Do something during your breaks, but also take the time to relax:* Summer and winter break are great opportunities to really dive into extracurriculars without the added stress of studying for classes. At the same time, take the time to relax! Once you enter the working world, these long carefree breaks become remnants of a distant past.
- *Study abroad if you can—if you want to:* Seeing how other people live around the world gives you an unrivaled perspective into the human condition. Your pre-medical career is likely the last opportunity you will have to pursue such an experience for a decade or longer. Unfortunately, it may be difficult to coordinate a study abroad experience amid pre-med course requirements and your extracurricular responsibilities.

## 3.4  Build Your Relationships and Mentorships

Refer to Chapter 2.4.4, Pillar 4: Social and Emotional Intelligence. While ADCOMs can get a very limited glimpse of your social skills on interview day, most of their assessment comes from your letters of recommendation. An ideal letter of recommendation convinces the ADCOM that you are able to work closely with someone for years while being honest, hard-working, and an overall pleasure to know. In addition, your letter writer has likely worked with many students in the past and can confidently say that you're in the upper echelon of students he/she has worked with.

Of course, this requires knowing and working closely with someone for years. As such, you should identify potential mentors as early as possible. Remember that you need 2 science and 1 non-science letter at minimum for your application. At the same time, we recognize that it can be difficult to make an impression on a science professor, especially when you're taking prerequisite courses among 500+ students—many of whom are also lining up at office hours to forge relationships. Thus, we recommend:

- At minimum, going to office hours and asking many (*reasonable, well-thought out, and relevant* questions during lecture. Do this regularly and make small-talk with the professors—get to know them as people!
- Consider taking multiple courses with the professor, especially if he/she teaches small upper-level courses.
- Consider doing research with the professor if you're genuinely interested in their work.
- Consider getting the professor involved with one of your extracurriculars.

---

[12] Song F, Parekh S, Hooper L. Dissemination and publication of research findings: an updated review of related biases. Health Technol Assess 2010;14(8):iii, ix–xi, 1–193. Available at: https://pubmed.ncbi.nlm.nih.gov/20181324/. Accessed July 8, 2022.

You should also introduce yourself to your pre-health office early, if applicable. Keep an eye out for emails and announcements about class-wide pre-health meetings.

We also recommend finding someone in medical school who can serve as a mentor. This is actually much easier than it sounds. In our experience, most medical students remember how daunting the pre-med experience was and are happy to help. Your prehealth or alumni office can probably get you in contact with an alumnus in medical school. Read more about mentorship in Chapter 19, Finding Mentors.

## 3.5  Keep an Open Mind and Remain Introspective

This expands on Chapter 2.4.4, Pillar 4: Social and Emotional Intelligence and Chapter 2.4.5, Pillar 5: Passion and Deep Achievement. While you should be comfortable saying "no" if you feel that you can't reasonably commit to something, be open to new experiences! Step outside your comfort zone. Your interests may evolve over time, and that's completely normal.

- *You may even discover that another, non-medical career path better aligns with your interests and values, and that's totally ok! Deeply pursue that other career and be honest with yourself about how you feel:* If you find yourself coming back to medicine, you will be able to tell the ADCOM that you explored alternative career paths that ultimately reaffirmed your passion for medicine. On the other hand, you may discover your true passion in life, which is a victory in itself.
- *Seek a realistic perspective on medicine:* ADCOMs value shadowing because applicants should update romanticized media depictions of medicine with an appreciation for the mundane, day-to-day experiences as a physician. Most physician shadowing experiences tend to be in relaxed outpatient private practice settings; this is *extremely* different from the stresses of inpatient hospital medicine, which will comprise the bulk of your training as a medical student and beyond. As such, we recommend trying to also shadow in an inpatient setting as well, as well as spending significant amounts of time with residents and attendings *on call* to gain an appreciation for the psychological impact of making serious medical decisions while exhausted.
  - Likewise, don't bias your shadowing with only "cool" experiences. For example, if you're shadowing vascular surgery, don't *just* stick around for the intense open abdominal aortic aneurysm repair. You should also keenly observe how the physician spends time on early morning rounding, documentation, postoperative follow-up, etc.
- *Consider keeping a personal journal:*[13] You should write about significant, transformative moments in your life, as the very act of writing out your thoughts and experiences will help you crystallize your personal story; this is also extremely useful for your application essays down the line. In addition, regular gratitude journaling has been shown to improve personal happiness and likelihood of helping others.[14]
- *Step outside of the medicine bubble whenever possible:* First and foremost, doctors are people. As a physician, you will work very closely with patients from all walks of life.[15] We recommend exposing yourself to a wide range of perspectives and lived experiences. Don't just hang out with other pre-meds; make friends with people unlike yourself to gain a deeper understanding of others' aspirations and struggles unrelated to medicine.
- *Leisure read about topics unrelated to medicine!:* Beyond expanding your intellectual horizons, leisure reading about non-medical topics will likely help you do well on the CARS section of the MCAT. In addition, ADCOM members love to ask applicants about their book interests (e.g., "What was the last book you read for fun?").
- *Continually reassess your interests and identity:* Inertia often keeps us stuck in commitments that are unfulfilling at best and actively soul-crushing at worst. Pre-medical students often find themselves

---

[13]  Much easier to do nowadays with smartphones that sync to the cloud and across devices.

[14]  Emmons RA, McCullough ME. Counting Blessings Versus Burdens: An Experimental Investigation of Gratitude and Subjective Well-Being in Daily Life. Journal of Personality and Social Psychology 2003;84(2):377–389. Available at: https://greatergood.berkeley.edu/pdfs/GratitudePDFs/6Emmons-BlessingsBurdens.pdf. Accessed July 8, 2022.

[15]  Considering the social determinants of health, most doctors tend to largely work with the disadvantaged, especially during their training. Additionally, because most medical school matriculants come from middle to upper-middle class households, most physicians end up working closely with people from very different backgrounds compared to their own upbringings.

juggling many different commitments. We recommend taking the time every semester to reassess whether each and every commitment is worth continuing or whether it's in your (and the commitment's) best interests for you to amicably part ways.

- For example, you may have decided to become an editor for your school newspaper when you were much more optimistic and enthusiastic. You now find yourself juggling many other commitments and don't feel that you're giving the newspaper the effort it deserves. It might be best for everyone involved if you stepped down and freed up the position to someone else more able to give the project the attention it deserves.

## 3.6 There Are No Guarantees

There's only so much you can personally do to maximize your personal odds of getting into medical school. At some point, it's out of your hands. Consider your academic performance, for example. While you can tremendously improve your odds of admission by giving your personal best and persevering over time, you are unable to change your genetics (which affect your ability to retain and apply information), your developmental history, and many aspects of your environment. While this may sound fatalistic, you can also nonjudgmentally accept it as a fact of reality and learn to roll with the punches. Try to look for the bright side in immediate setbacks; your failures should be reimagined as opportunities for personal growth. Take nothing for granted and strive to earnestly (and ethically) maximize your odds of success using the strategies put forth in this book.

### 3.6.1 Student Perspective: Mindfulness Meditation

Mindfulness meditation is an excellent tool for developing this Zen-like outlook to unexpected life events and unchangeable circumstances. In short, the practice trains you to pay very close attention to your subjective conscious experience in the here-and-now, to ultimately cultivate an intense but nonjudgmental awareness of your current state of mind. The goal is to achieve a baseline level of inner peace and contentment that is not significantly perturbed by external events. The author strongly recommends that all pre-medical students explore this practice, and he will continually suggest it as an effective intervention across the gamut of pre-med problems (particularly in Chapter 18, Self-Care and Wellness).

## 3.7 Summary

The 6 Pre-Med Pillars (academic excellence, selflessness, clinical experience, social/emotional intelligence, nonacademic excellence, and integrity) can be actionized into 6 principles to consider when making choices throughout your pre-medical career.

- Protect your GPA and integrity at almost any cost. The major caveats being threats to your physical or mental health, as well as doing things that are wholly unethical.
  - This is because these are incredibly difficult to salvage once they've taken hits.
- Aim to make the MCAT a one-and-done deal. Do not take it until you're at least averaging your target score under test-day conditions.
- Become an interesting person who can articulate a convincing, cohesive narrative that involves becoming a physician. Perhaps more importantly, have *demonstrable evidence* (e.g., letters of recommendation, awards) supporting this narrative.
- Start to build relationships and mentorships as early as possible.
- Keep an open mind to new opportunities and ways of thinking. Continually reassess your identity and interests throughout the journey.
- Accept the reality that although you can do a lot to maximize your odds of success, there are no guarantees in this journey.

# 4 The Types of Pre-Medical Students and Paths to Medical School

*Ray Funahashi and Joel Thomas*

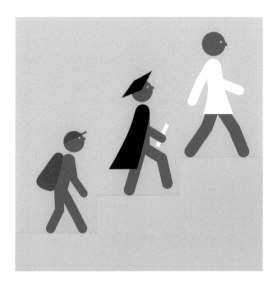

## 4.1 There Are Different Pathways to Medical School

US medical schools accept students from a wide variety of backgrounds, ages, and previous careers. Because of this, not only are there many different paths to becoming a medical school applicant, but also many strategies specific to each path.

Let's take a look at examples of three successful applicants who all decide to pursue medical school at different times:
1. High school student.
2. College student.
3. Post-baccalaureate student/career changing applicant.

## 4.2 The High School Student, Guaranteed Admissions Pathway

Keiran has wanted to become a doctor from a young age. He is inspired by his sports medicine doctor, and thinks he wants to go to medical school.
- He **volunteers** at the local hospital throughout high school to gain clinical experience to make an informed decision about working in healthcare.
- He also starts **shadowing** a physician in the clinic to learn more about what being a *doctor* is like. Shadowing means following a physician through their work day and observing them in the clinic or operating room. This requires arrangement with and permission from the doctor beforehand.
- He obtains a near-perfect GPA and excels on the SAT (or ACT).
- He also pursues his **personal interests and passions** and seeks to make an impact through **leadership roles.** From shadowing in sports medicine, he becomes interested in sports injury prevention. Because he saw that many of his friends were unfamiliar with common sports injuries and the ways to prevent them, he starts an educational program through his gym class to educate students about ways to stay safe while playing sports. He also becomes involved in **scientific research** by joining a lab at a nearby university studying the biological mechanisms involved in

concussions. He goes on to present his research at a science conference and publishes his results in an academic journal.

- He maintains excellent **mentorship relationships** with his teachers and receives glowing **recommendation letters.**
- In senior year of high school, he **applies to guaranteed admission programs (more in Chapter 7, Guaranteed Admission Programs and Early Assurance Programs) at medical schools.**
- From around August to January, he receives a few **interview invitations** from the medical schools he applied to. He makes travel and accommodation arrangements to each location.
- He **attends his interviews** at each school where he talks about his motivation for pursuing medicine and shares stories about his experiences and what he has learned. As a future physician, he would like to continue being an advocate for sports injury prevention.
- He receives acceptance, rejection, or wait-list letters and financial aid/scholarship offers from the schools. Luckily, Keiran receives letters of acceptance from several schools, and a few schools add him to their **wait-list.**[1]
- He completes **online financial aid forms** such as the FAFSA to qualify for financial aid and takes out loans to pay for college and medical school.
- Keiran **starts college with a place in medical school** in writing! Of course, this may be a conditional acceptance that is contingent on maintaining a particular GPA and/or obtaining a minimum MCAT score, depending on which program he enrolls in.

## 4.3 The High School Student, Traditional Pathway

Maria has wanted to become a doctor from a young age. She is inspired by her pediatrician and thinks she wants to go to medical school.

- Maria starts **shadowing** a physician in the clinic to learn more about what being a doctor is like. Shadowing means following a physician through their work day and observing them in the clinic or operating room. This requires arrangement with and permission from the doctor beforehand.
- She **graduates high school** and enters a 4-year undergraduate college to **earn a bachelor's degree.** She maintains **excellent grades** and volunteers for a local autism awareness and education nonprofit because she is passionate about the cause. Because Maria is especially interested in biology, she chooses this as her major.
- During her undergraduate years she **completes courses in science (biology, chemistry, organic chemistry, physics) and other required classes such as calculus, psychology, sociology, and English.**
- She also continues serving her community through **volunteering** at the autism nonprofit throughout undergrad.
- Maria continues to **pursue her personal interests and passions** and seeks to make an impact through **leadership roles.** From shadowing in pediatrics, she becomes interested in autism. Because she saw that many of her friends were unfamiliar with autism and the challenges autistic patients and their families face, she starts an Autism Outreach initiative on her campus where students can meet speakers on autism. She also becomes involved in **scientific research** by joining a lab on her campus studying the biological mechanisms involved in autism. She goes on to present her research at a science conference and publishes her results in an academic journal.
- Throughout undergrad, Maria develops an excellent professional reputation and **mentorship relationships** with her professors and receives glowing **recommendation letters.**
- She studies (several weeks to months) and **takes the MCAT exam** in her junior year and scores well.
- After finishing the spring semester of her junior year Maria **applies to medical schools** in June (beginning of official application season).
  - She submits her **primary online application**, academic transcripts, recommendation letters, and personal essay statement.
  - She receives and completes a **secondary online application**, completing more personal essays and paying additional fees from each school.

---

[1] If she is accepted off of a waiting list to another medical school, she may switch her enrollment as long as she has not already made her written commitment to a school. Read more in Chapter 36, Wait-List and Update Letters.

- From around August to January she receives a few **interview invitations** from the medical schools she applied to. She makes travel and accommodation arrangements to each location.
- She **attends her interviews** at each school where she talks about her motivation for pursuing medicine and shares stories about her experiences and what she has learned. As a future pediatric physician, Maria would like to continue being an advocate for autism and further research in autism.
- She **receives acceptance, rejection, or wait-list letters** and financial aid/scholarships offers from the schools. Luckily, Maria receives letters of acceptance from several schools, and a few schools add her to their **wait-list.**[2]
- Because Maria is a competitive applicant, she was invited to a **second look day** hosted by a few schools which have accepted her. This will help make her decision about where to commit to enrolling.[1]
- She completes **online financial aid forms** such as the FAFSA to qualify for financial aid and takes out loans to pay for medical school.
- Maria starts medical school!

## 4.4 The College Student, Early Assurance

Tommy is extremely motivated to become a physician. He feels that he already has a competitive application to medical school, as he already was active in research, volunteering, and clinical experience in high school and continues these activities in college. In addition, his SAT (or ACT) scores were extremely high. He identifies several schools he would be happy to attend through an early assurance program (more in Chapter 7, Guaranteed Admission Programs and Early Assurance Programs).

- He is currently enrolled in a 4-year undergraduate college to **earn a Bachelor's degree.** He has a near-perfect **GPA**, and his **SAT (or ACT)** score from high school was extremely high.
- He already has accumulated many hours of **clinical volunteering** and **physician shadowing**, much of which he acquired in high school and continued throughout college thus far.
- He has completed many of the **pre-med requirements** with excellent grades.
- Tommy has been surfing for most of his life, and he has actually won several competitions. He knows that this will distinguish him from other applicants.
- He has also been proactive about starting and maintaining relationships with professors and other mentors, and therefore receives glowing **recommendation letters.**
- With the help of his pre-medical office, he identifies several early assurance programs and applies to them in his sophomore year.
- From around August to January he receives a few **interview invitations** from the medical schools he applied to. He makes travel and accommodation arrangements to each location.
- He **attends his interviews** at each school where he talks about his motivation for pursuing medicine and shares stories about his experiences and what he has learned.
- He **receives acceptance, rejection, or wait-list letters** and financial aid/scholarships offers from the schools.
- Tommy finishes college with the peace of mind knowing that he's got an acceptance to medical school. Depending on which program he chooses, he may have to complete additional requirements such as maintaining a minimum GPA or obtaining a certain MCAT score.

## 4.5 The College Student (Sophomore)

John is interested in both English literature and science, so he used freshman year to explore those fields. Though he is currently an English major, he now feels certain about pursuing a career in medicine and wants to apply to medical school.

- John is currently enrolled in a 4-year undergraduate college to **earn a Bachelor's degree.** He has entertained the idea of becoming a physician at times, but wasn't committed to it at that time. He loves English literature and knows that medical schools don't require having a science major to apply. Therefore, he chooses to be an English literature major. He maintains **excellent grades** and plays rugby for the club team.

---

[2] If she is accepted off of a waiting list to another medical school, she may switch her enrollment as long as she has not already made her written commitment to a school. Read more in Chapter 36, Wait-List and Update Letters.

- He starts **shadowing** a physician in the clinic (after getting permission) to learn more about what being a doctor is like. He is surprised by how much he enjoys the experience. He establishes with the pre-med office and gets suggestions to enroll in the medical school pre-reqs.
- Even though John is an English major, he **completes courses in science (biology, chemistry, organic chemistry, physics) and other required classes such as calculus, psychology, sociology, and English.**
- John hasn't been **volunteering or participating in community service** up until this point. He wants to demonstrate that he is committed to being a person who is interested in serving others, and he also received suggestions from the pre-med office to volunteer to make himself more competitive to the ADCOM. Because his faith is important to him, he decides to dedicate himself to working with a faith-based service group on campus through the rest of undergrad. He also finds that he likes tutoring students in English literature.
- John also continues to **pursue his personal interests and passions** and seeks to make an impact through **leadership roles.** He eventually becomes a senior leader in his faith-based service group, helping to manage service projects by his senior year. He also is now co-captain on the rugby team and helps to lead practice sessions. Through his experience shadowing doctors at the hospital, he becomes interested in the role faith plays in the experience of patients in sickness and health. He publishes several essays on the role faith plays in modern medicine and for his senior thesis, examines the historical literature on this topic.
- Throughout undergrad, John develops an excellent professional reputation and **mentorships** with his professors and receives glowing **recommendation letters.**
- John studies several weeks for the MCAT, but he isn't consistently seeing the progress he wants. He meticulously researches alternative MCAT study strategies and resources online and discusses the recommendations with the pre-med office and his peers who already took the MCAT. Ultimately, he decides to enroll in an MCAT preparation course and supplements his studying with an online video series. To his relief, he sees improvement, and he ultimately **takes the MCAT exam** in his junior year and scores well.
- After finishing the spring semester of his junior year John **applies to medical schools** in June (beginning of official application season).
  - He submits his **primary online application**, academic transcripts, recommendation letters, and personal essay statement.
  - He receives and completes a **secondary online application**, completing more personal essays and paying additional fees from each school.
- From around August to January he receives a few **interview invitations** from the medical schools he applied to. He makes travel and accommodation arrangements to each location.
- He **attends his interviews** at each school where he talks about his motivation for pursuing medicine and shares stories about his experiences and what he has learned. As a future physician, John would like to incorporate aspects of his faith background to provide compassionate care to every patient, and continue to investigate the role faith plays in modern medicine.
- He **receives acceptance, rejection, or wait-list letters** and financial aid/scholarships offers from the schools. Luckily, John receives letters of acceptance from several schools, and a few schools add him to their **wait-list.** He completes **online financial aid forms** such as the FAFSA to qualify for financial aid and takes out loans to pay for medical school.
- John starts medical school!

## 4.6 The Re-Applicant

Neal had been interested in medical school since the beginning of freshman year of college and spent most of his time studying diligently to obtain a competitive GPA and MCAT score. He is deeply passionate about science and spent most of his free time conducting research in neuroscience. He also spent the summer before senior year volunteering at the local hospital.

- Neal is nearing the end of a 4-year undergraduate college to **earn a bachelor's degree.** He begins applying to medical school.
- While Neal obtained ~100 hours of volunteering experience over the summer, medical schools question him heavily on his longitudinal commitment to medicine, as his application overwhelmingly demonstrates a passion for science with a much weaker demonstrated interest in patient care.

- From around August to January he receives a few **interview invitations** from the medical schools he applied to. He makes travel and accommodation arrangements to each location.
- He **attends his interviews** at each school where he talks about his motivation for pursuing medicine and shares stories about his experiences and what he has learned. He is pressed on his apparent disinterest in volunteering and clinical medicine, given that he only has a summer's worth of clinical experience and is embarking on a lifelong career in medicine.
- He **is wait-listed and/or ultimately rejected** from *all* of the schools he applied to. He is extremely distraught, as he has spent thousands of hours and dollars over several years on the process of becoming a physician. At the same time, he refuses to give up so easily and reassesses the weaknesses in his application to have a successful reapplication cycle. He recognizes that while a "lost year" can be devastating, it is ultimately not the end of the world over the span of a lifetime as a physician. He commits to not making it a "lost year," and decides to take 2 years off to significantly improve his chances—otherwise he would have to start the application process next month, and hasn't had time to strengthen his candidacy yet.
- Neal **secures a full-time job** after graduating as an emergency department scribe. He gains hundreds of hours of direct, intense clinical experience and works with his pre-medical office from his alma mater to recraft a new medical school application addressing the weaknesses in his original application and how he is actively working to rectify them and to secure admission to medical school. His experiences deepen his interest in medicine, and he writes an improved personal statement that informs his interests more completely.
- Neal **applies again to medical school**, again interviewing at the schools that originally rejected him, as well as applying to 10 more schools. He passionately explains his commitment to medicine and how he went the extra mile to make up for his deficiencies in clinical experience and how he is still firmly committed to becoming a physician. He writes letters of interest for schools to which he did not receive an interview invitation, and receives two extra invites. He **receives acceptances** to multiple medical schools.
- Neal starts medical school!

## 4.7 Post-Undergraduate or Career Changing Applicant (31-Year-Old)

Lisa is a computer programmer who graduated from her state university nearly one decade ago. She helped care for her mom who was suffering from cancer, and after a lot of thinking and introspection, feels that a career in medicine is her calling. She wants to apply to medical school.

- Lisa already **earned a bachelor's degree in computer science.** Because she knows that medical schools don't require having a science major to apply, she knows she doesn't have to earn another bachelor's degree. But because she is missing many of the required (mostly science) courses needed for applying to medical school, she **enrolls in a post-baccalaureate pre-medical program** with an established reputation for successfully placing students in medical schools.[3]
- The program she joined can be completed in 1.5 years if full-time and 2 to 3 years if part-time. Because she can't afford to completely quit her job to study full-time, she opts to work part-time at her job and enrolls for the two-year part-time program. Her grades weren't that great in undergrad—GPA of 2.9, so she knows she still has to prove her academic ability by earning a high GPA in this program.
- She starts **shadowing** a physician in the clinic to learn more about what being a doctor is like.
- Following the post-bac program curriculum, she **completes courses in science (biology, chemistry, organic chemistry, physics) and other required classes such as psychology, sociology, and English.** Because she already had taken the advanced required math courses from being a computer science major, she was allowed to skip taking these classes.
- Lisa hasn't been **volunteering or participating in community service** up until this point. She wants to demonstrate that she is committed to being a person who is interested in serving others. Lisa knows how difficult it is to care for a patient dealing with terminal cancer from her experience with her mom. Because of this she decides she wants to volunteer in helping to care for patients at a local hospice. There she also volunteers her computer programming skills to help redesign the hospice website.
- Lisa continues to **pursue her personal interests and passions** and seeks to make an impact through **leadership roles.** She notices while working at the hospice that the patient's end-of-life care documentation is not easily accessible to caretakers. She starts a project to create software that can

---

[3] Read more in 2.10, Post-Bacs, Jobs, Gap Years and Additional Degrees.

help the hospice easily communicate patients' advanced directives to caretakers. In the process she learns more about the ethics and coverage policies of end-of-life care and begins reaching out to lawmakers to advocate for better policies on behalf of underserved hospice patients.

- Lisa already had an excellent professional reputation from working at her previous company. She also developed **mentorships** with her professors in the pre-medical program and receives glowing **recommendation letters.**
- Lisa studies (several weeks to months) and **takes the MCAT exam** and scores well.
- As she is finishing the final spring semester of her post-bac program, she **applies to medical schools** in June (beginning of official application season).
  - She submits her **primary online application**, academic transcripts, recommendation letters, and personal essay statement.
  - She receives and completes a **secondary online application**, completing more personal essays and paying additional fees from each school.
- From around August to January she receives a few **interview invitations** from the medical schools she applied to. She makes travel and accommodation arrangements to each location.
- She **attends her interviews** at each school where she talks about her motivation for pursuing medicine and shares stories about her experiences and what she has learned. After her mom's experience with cancer, Lisa decided she wanted to apply her technological knowledge in a clinical and medical setting and help future patients like her mother. As a future physician, Lisa would like to continue serving and advocating for better legislative and insurance policies for patients, especially for those who are underserved and/or terminally ill.
- She **receives acceptance, rejection, or wait-list letters** and financial aid/ scholarships offers from the schools. She completes **online financial aid forms** such as the FAFSA to qualify for financial aid and takes out loans to pay for medical school.
- Lisa starts medical school!

## 4.8  Your Pre-Med Journey

As you saw above, these applicants came from different backgrounds and had to prepare differently, but eventually converged in the application process. Now let's go over how you can get started on your own pre-med journey!

## 4.9  If You Are a High School Student...

Preparing for medical school as a high school student gives you a great head start to becoming a highly competitive applicant.

### 4.9.1  Step 1: Get Involved in Clinical Experience, Shadowing, and Research Opportunities

If your high school offers student healthcare exposure programs, definitely participate in these! It will allow you to get a head start on your physician shadowing,[4] and you can begin to build relationships with health professionals.

   Google search for high school summer research internships and programs. Gaining research experience while you are in high school will give you a great boost over the competition when looking for undergraduate research opportunities.

### 4.9.2  Step 2a: Consider Applying to a Guaranteed Admissions Program

If you're *extremely* confident that becoming a physician is the path for you, then you should consider applying to a guaranteed admissions program (more in Chapter 7, Guaranteed Admission Programs and Early Assurance Programs). These programs outline a very clear path to medical school with early reassurance if you can meet academic benchmarks.

---

[4] I.e., you can mention these in your medical school application to show longitudinal commitment.

Students in combined BS/MD programs are **Special Programs Applicants** who are admitted at the beginning of undergrad and have guaranteed admission to a connected medical school (with some qualifications). Sometimes these programs are "accelerated," meaning they have shortened bachelor's degree curriculums (i.e., 3 years instead of 4 years). This means you can obtain your MD degree earlier.

The downside of such a program is that you will be committed to a single medical school right off the bat, and that it moves at a very intense pace academically. You also might feel a bit "shortchanged" of the typical undergraduate experience. Still, these programs are well worth looking into.

### 4.9.3 Step 2b: Get into a Reputable College and Maintain a High GPA

The more common pathway to getting into medical school is applying at the end of—or after—college.

While in high school, you should prioritize your GPA and SAT/ACT. We generally recommend that you take and perform well in Advanced Placement (AP) classes, especially in the sciences.

It is also to your best advantage to get into the most competitive undergraduate college as possible. More competitive undergraduate institutions comparatively:
• Have better and more interesting extracurricular opportunities in research, internships, and clubs.
• Have more reputable academic professors whose recommendations carry more weight.
• Have a reputation and history of successfully placing their graduates into competitive medical schools.
• Will still work to your advantage if you decide not to pursue medical school.

For our purposes, a competitive undergraduate institution is roughly within the top 125 colleges listed in National Universities ranking in the US News & World Report. We don't recommend completing your premedical requirements at an institution outside of this range. Some top tier schools will rarely interview students applying from schools beyond this arbitrary range. This is presumably because there are so many competitive applicants already applying from the top 125 schools, where the base-level of academic rigor is fairly high. From the medical admissions committee's perspective, selecting applicants from these schools gives some quality and safety reassurance and it is also a way to avoid gambling on students who might have had it "easier" at less competitive undergraduate institutions.

In addition, while undergraduate prestige matters, it should *not* be the only factor you consider. Any accredited undergraduate institution will allow you to gain access to medical school. The cost of an undergraduate education has been rising dramatically, and thus we do *not* recommend paying an exorbitant amount of money for a prestigious undergraduate experience because you will likely also accumulate significant debt as a physician. Our ideal recommendation is an undergraduate institution that has a decent reputation (i.e., at least in the top 125 on US News) and is not prohibitively expensive. That said, different students will have different thresholds for "expensive." A price difference of $50,000 over 4 years to attend a school ranked #30 versus #60 may be a reasonable investment for some students, depending on their financial means. The value of a prestigious undergraduate experience is a highly personal decision, but our general recommendation is to avoid paying extreme differences for marginal improvements in prestige.

For perspective, the author of this chapter chose to attend his state school (ranked #88 on US News) for $7,000 per year in tuition over an undergraduate school ranked #5 on US News at $42,000 per year. He still got into a top 15 medical school and is attending a top 5 residency program. That said, others may think it reasonable to pay more for the more prestigious school and have additional peace of mind for medical school (and potentially career) aspirations. Keep in mind that it may be harder to obtain a high GPA at many higher-ranked schools because you will be competing against students with higher GPA and SAT/ACT scores going into college. This becomes especially relevant in classes graded on a curve. At the same time, there is tremendous individual variation across highly-ranked schools, as some are notorious for grade inflation (e.g., Harvard) compared to grade *deflation* at other prestigious schools (e.g., Princeton, Cornell).

## 4.10 If You Are a College Student...

### 4.10.1 Step 1: Evaluate your Institution and Course of Study

Consider if you are at an institution known to successfully place graduates into medical schools. Consider transferring if not—if and only if you feel that you're fighting an extreme uphill battle and that the quality of your education is seriously compromised.

If you are an undergraduate student who has decided to pursue medical school, first consider the institution you are studying at. Unfortunately, the top medical schools do seem to give applicants from well-known universities an advantage. They also tend to mostly invite students to interview from schools within the top 125 of the US World News and Report National University Rankings. If you currently do not attend a Top 125 ranked college, we strongly recommend searching for ways to improve your resume and to transfer to a Top 125 school if feasible (i.e., not prohibitively expensive). Though some critics may scoff at this advice, we believe being at a Top 125 (and yes, there are some exceptions above this range) institution will give you a better shot at any medical school in the United States, provided the rest of your application is solid. Although anecdotal, the authors of this book noticed an extreme paucity of applicants from outside of this ranking tier while interviewing. It is by no means impossible or improbable to overcome, and ranking colleges is by no means an entirely accurate gauge of quality (see Chapter 26, Medical School Rankings), but it's a disadvantage right from the start.

As we discussed above, being at a reputable institution has its advantages. If you cannot get into a competitive undergraduate institution or currently not attending one—fear not! In this case, one strategy is to be a non-science major (not taking any required pre-medical courses) initially at a less competitive college. You must maintain a high GPA regardless of your major. After a year, you may be able to transfer to a more competitive school. Your application to medical school will not bear the name of this institution and you will get the benefits of its reputation and resources.

Why do we recommend picking a non-science major if you are at a noncompetitive college? Two reasons. First, this will help you protect your GPA! Nothing will kill your chances of becoming a highly competitive applicant than a low science GPA. A low GPA is very hard to fix because even if you transfer and your GPA is "wiped clean" at your institution, medical schools will take into account your previous institution GPA into your cumulative average GPA.

Second, you will be disqualified from applying to many post-baccalaureate pre-medical programs if you have taken any pre-medical science courses already at any other institution! You will have to consider a special Master's program (SMP) instead, a generally longer and more expensive process.

Alternatively, you can complete a non-science major, graduate, and attend a reputable pre-medical post-baccalaureate program at a competitive university.

## 4.10.2  Step 2: Get into a Pre-Medical Program (If Your School Has One)

Traditionally, college students enroll in a **pre-medical program/listserv** at their undergrad school, though some schools do not have one. pre-medical programs are designed to prepare students for applying to medical school. Programs are headed by an advisor or director who is knowledgeable about the medical admissions process. They usually have an admissions and interview process and/or GPA requirements.

Once enrolled, the pre-medical program will assist you through academic advising, med school application guidance, and providing various resources.

### Just So You're Aware...

The expertise of pre-medical advisors and reputation of pre-medical programs vary widely. Program directors and advisors often have not gone to medical school, much less experienced the medical school admissions process. The medical school admissions process is constantly evolving, and even senior advisors such as doctors will not be able to give you the best advice unless they are directly and currently involved in admissions at medical schools. Accordingly, their advice should always be taken with a grain of salt. That being said, you want to stay in the good graces of these programs because they can seriously hinder your chances if they do not support you. More on this later.

You should do careful homework on pre-medical programs before enrolling in them. Web forums such as the Student Doctor Network (http://forums.studentdoctor.net) can be helpful for researching programs because you can read about other student experiences. That said, you should generally read these experiences with a grain of salt, as they typically disproportionately represent very positive or very negative experiences and therefore are not representative samples.

## 4.10.3 Step 3: Choose a Major. Yes, Any Major!

What major should you choose? People often debate whether a science major, such as biology or bio-chemistry, give you an advantage when applying to medical school. The bottom line is that you can major in *anything* as long as you complete the pre-reqs. We will discuss more in Chapter 8, School, Majors, and More, but major choice is a relatively unimportant variable to ADCOMs. Therefore, you should major in whatever is interesting to you and allows you to get a competitive GPA. Bonus points if this major opens job opportunities in the unfortunate case that you are not admitted into medical school or in case you ultimately decide on a different career path.

## 4.11 As You Near Undergraduate Graduation...

## 4.11.1 Decide Which Type of Medical School Applicant You Will Be

As an applicant, you will be grouped into **traditional, non-traditional, and special programs applicants.** The main differentiator is how much time you spend in and in between undergrad and medical school.

1. The **Traditional Applicant** is a "straight out of college" applicant who doesn't take any extra years in between undergrad and medical school (our example 1 applicant). The **Special Programs Applicant** is similar to this category because they are not taking any time off between undergrad and medical school.
2. The **Non-Traditional Applicant** is an applicant who doesn't apply to medical school straight out of undergrad (our example 3 applicant). Many of these applicants are **Post-bacs** (post-baccalaureate), meaning they already possess a bachelor's degree (in any field). Post-bacs are often enrolled in pre-med post-baccalaureate programs for completing academic requirements for applying to medical school.

## 4.12 If You Are a Non-Traditional Applicant...

If you already have an undergraduate degree before you apply to medical school, you are considered a non-traditional applicant.

**Step 1: Get into a Pre-Medical Post-baccalaureate Program, Get Another Degree, or Improve a Low GPA with a Special Master's Program** (All Discussed in Chapter 16, Gap Years, Employment, Graduate Degrees, and Post-Baccalaureate Fellowships).

If you already have any bachelor's degree from an accredited U.S. academic institution, you may apply to medical schools, provided you meet basic eligibility requirements and have already taken the MCAT exam and other science, math, and writing course prerequisites (more on this later). However, as you might be starting to realize, getting into medical school is far more involved than simply applying with prerequisite credentials.

**If you haven't yet taken any of the science prerequisite courses** to apply to medical school, we highly recommend applying to **post-baccalaureate (post-bac) pre-medical programs.** Post-bac programs allow you to enroll in a university and take a customized/predesigned course curriculum (full- or part-time) for completing the prerequisite classes necessary for applying to medical schools.

Post-bac programs are usually an extension of a university's pre-medical program. You will often get the same type of advisory and recommendations that the undergraduate students in the pre-medical program receive. Post-bac pre-med students and undergraduate pre-med students often end up taking the same requirement science classes at the school.

**If you have taken the science courses that are included in the prerequisites already in your past,** you have two options.

1. Apply to post-bac programs that allow you to only take the classes you are missing (or allow you to completely start over, including retaking those classes).
2. Re-enroll in college to finish taking the rest of the required classes. Between these two options, doing a post-bac program is preferred because they will be able to provide more guidance and some even have linkage programs to medical schools. However, many post-bacs will not accept students who have already taken part or all of the med school admissions prerequisite classes before.

**If you took all the prerequisite classes already during your undergrad degree,** you have three options.

1. If your grades are good, you can try contacting your alma mater's pre-medical program office and ask if they will support your application by writing a recommendation letter. You can proceed to start studying for the MCAT exam and focusing on completing other tasks necessary for preparing to apply to med school.
2. You can complete a graduate degree (likely a Master's), which will allow you to strengthen your credentials and connect with the pre-medical program at that institution (and rebrand your application with that school's name), which may support your application to medical school. While this does make you a more competitive applicant, it can be a costly option in both time and money.
3. If your grades are not good, you can try to rehabilitate your GPA and academic strength (as perceived by med schools) by completing a one-year SMP. These programs often simulate the initial basic science curriculums of medical schools and are academically very rigorous. It is designed to be challenging so you can prove your academic abilities. However, they can be costly to attend.

## What Is Considered a Bad GPA?

There are a range of acceptable grade-point averages (GPA) that differ according to each school. Generally speaking, if your GPA is in the 2's or lower, it's going to be significantly difficult to get into U.S. medical schools. This doesn't mean that it's impossible, but you will need to do serious GPA rehab via SMP programs and/or have a compelling case. More on this topic in later chapters.

### What Is the Advantage of Enrolling in Post-bac Programs?

Technically, any person who has completed the official prerequisites for medical school admissions is free to apply. However, given how competitive medical school admissions and potentially confusing the application process can be, it is a wise idea to enroll in these programs for guidance.

Regardless of how long you have been away from school, there are other benefits to "going back to school" to complete a pre-medical program before applying to medical school. Pre-medical programs may have contacts for shadowing physicians, as well as volunteer and research opportunities. Taking classes with science professors will help you obtain strong and up-to-date recommendation letters, especially to highlight your more recent academic abilities.

### Why Are Pre-med or Post-bac Pre-med Programs Important?

Generally speaking, if your school has a pre-medical program, you should consult a pre-med advisor as soon as possible to assess your specific situation and find out the requirements for gaining their support. Once enrolled, pre-medical advisors will help you plan out your coursework and give you generally helpful feedback on your activities and med school application. Pre-medical programs are run by a director and faculty advisors, who collectively form a **pre-medical committee**.

Besides advising you, when you submit your med school application, this pre-medical committee will write a **committee letter** for you, which medical school admissions offices generally prefer receiving in addition to individual recommendation letters. A committee letter is a composite letter that your pre-med advisor or director will compose using all of the individual letters from your letter writers. Sometimes the individual letters are also attached in a single document as an appendix in case schools wish to read them specifically. Because the quality of pre-med applicant candidates produced are a direct reflection on a pre-medical program's reputation, you will be prescreened before premed committees write their committee letter to medical schools. Prescreening may involve a panel interview from committee members, as well as a review of your resume, academic record, and motivation to pursue a career in medicine.

### Which Undergraduate School, Pre-Medical Program, and/or Post-baccalaureate Program Should You Choose?

Consider the time and cost of each program, but the general rule of thumb is that the best investment will come from attending a program or school that has a strong reputation for consistently getting students accepted into the medical schools you are targeting, year after year. Before applying to any program, always inquire where graduates of the program are landing consistently in recent years.

**What Are the Special Challenges of Being a Non-Traditional Applicant?**

As a non-traditional applicant you most likely will face different, additional challenges in medical school admission compared to traditional applicants. However, if you truly believe that a career in medicine is your calling, then you will find ways to persevere past these difficulties and get into medical school.

If you are set on switching careers and pursuing entrance to medical school, we recommend that you apply to a reputable pre-medical program and thoroughly study the rest of the book. You will have considerable catching up to do in completing the "unofficial requirements" to applying to medical school so you should read this book carefully.

You will have to convey a compelling reason to ADCOMs as to why you are leaving your career and pursuing medicine. In this respect you should take special note of Chapter 5, Building Your Narrative. We will work on emphasizing your difference from the majority of applicants as a major strength in your applications and med school interviews.

Don't let the "non-traditional" label trick you into feeling inferior to traditional applicants. Having experience outside of the conventional seamless track (from high school to college, then medical school) is an asset recognized by many medical schools.

## Does My Age Matter in Medical School Admissions?

We were unable to find any detailed research suggesting age discrimination in medical school and residency admissions. The only specific data we found was a direct survey sent to ADCOMs at 130 US MD programs about the the importance of specific applicant variables to acceptance. Applicant age was rated as "lowest importance", although it's unclear what exactly this means (i.e., are older or younger applicants preferred?)[5] That said, age discrimination favoring young applicants is a recognized feature of hiring in general.[6] Therefore, while we cannot point to solid evidence that it exists in medical school and residency admissions, we would not be surprised if it existed and manifested as a subconscious bias in admissions. In fact, several sources raise the possibility of age discrimination in medical school admissions.[7,8]

Consult the MSAR to see what the age ranges of matriculating students are to get a general sense of how receptive a school is to non-traditional applicants. Be cognizant that while a school may list the age range of matriculants as, say 22 to 32, this gives no information whether they accepted 99 students in the ages below 25 and one student that was age 32, for example. Don't necessarily give up your hopes on applying to a particular school solely because you lie outside of a school's age range. You can (anonymously) call the admission's office before applying and ask them how your age realistically affects your chance of acceptance. Just know that as more of your general qualities differ (in an undesirable way) from the average matriculant of a school, your chances of acceptance there correspondingly declines to some degree.

## 4.13 Summary

There are many different paths to medical school. Depending on where you are in the process, you might find that certain paths may be better than others.

---

5  Table 1: Using MCAT® Data in 2023 Medical Student Selection. Available at: https://www.aamc.org/system/files/2022-06/2023%20MCAT%20Data%20Selection%20Guide%20Online.pdf. Accessed July 8, 2022.

6  Hiring in the Age of Ageism. Available at: https://www.shrm.org/hr-today/news/hr-magazine/0218/pages/hiring-in-the-age-of-ageism.aspx. Accessed July 8, 2022.

7  Hilder DB. Med School Admissions Policy May Be Age-Discriminatory. Available at: https://www.thecrimson.com/article/1975/4/29/med-school-admissions-policy-may-be/. Accessed July 8, 2022.

8  Chatterjee A, Greif C, Witzburg R, Henault L, Goodell K, Paasche-Orlow MK. US Medical School Applicant Experiences of Bias on the Interview Trail. J Health Care Poor Underserved 2020;31(1):185–200. Available at: https://pubmed.ncbi.nlm.nih.gov/32037326/. Accessed July 8, 2022.

# 5 Building Your Narrative

*Chistian Morrill and Joel Thomas*

## 5.1 What Is a Narrative?

*"Don't ask yourself what the world needs. Ask yourself what makes you come alive, and go do that, because what the world needs is people who have come alive."*

— Howard Thurman

Perhaps the single most integral aspect of your application to medical school is be the narrative you present to the admissions committee. In its simplest form, a narrative answers the ADCOM's question of *"Why admit you to our medical school now?"*

Answering this question requires addressing three simpler questions: (1) "Who are you?" (2) "Why medicine?" and (3) "Why now?" Narratives neatly package the applicant's life story into a cohesive whole, and they are the main feature of personal statements and many school-specific essays. Your narrative is like the trunk of a tree; there is no detail of your application that does not branch from your narrative.

### 5.1.1 Who Are You?

Succinctly articulating who you are—especially in a manner appealing to the admissions committee—is an understandingly difficult task. Our primary self-image partially emerges from our subconscious views of ourselves. If you find it difficult to summarize your individuality, *relax*. You are in the clear majority. If, on the other hand, you're in the minority of individuals that have themselves figured out, take pause and consider what biases may be distorting your image of self.

Invariably, the process of preparing for and applying to medical school will elucidate aspects of your individuality. An essential, but overlooked, goal of secondary and undergraduate education is identity formation through exploration of talents, interests, and skills. This is why medical schools are interested in hearing how you spend your free time, why you chose your research projects, and why you chose the extracurricular/volunteering/shadowing activities you did. At baseline, you'll have up to 15 "Experiences and/or activities" in the American Medical College Application Service (AMCAS) application to cover the most meaningful aspects of your life before medical school. (See Chapter 30, Activities and Meaningful Experiences for more on AMCAS 15 activities.) Together with your personal statement, these activities provide a narrative of your growth, personality, and passion.

But this begs the question: *why do I need a narrative?* This is a complex topic explored by significant research in the social sciences and humanities. Some reasons include the following:

- Contextualizing your drives, desires, successes, and failures in a cohesive narrative structure appears to be correlated with personal well-being.[1,2]
- Modern medical practice increasingly recognizes the role of narrative identity in the therapeutic alliance.[3]
- Personal narratives allow ADCOM members to engage with *living, breathing human beings* when choosing among a sea of stats in an otherwise cold, calculated admissions process.[4]

---

[1] McAdams DP, McLean KC. Narrative Identity. Current Directions in Psychological Science. 22(3):233–238. Available at: https://journals.sagepub.com/doi/10.1177/0963721413475622. Accessed July 8, 2022.

[2] Tavernier R, Willoughby T. Adolescent turning points: the association between meaning-making and psychological well-being. Dev Psychol 2012;48(4):1058–68. Available at: https://pubmed.ncbi.nlm.nih.gov/22122472/. Accessed July 8, 2022.

[3] Charon R. Narrative Medicine: A Model for Empathy, Reflection, Profession, and Trust. JAMA 2001;286(15):1897–1902. Available at: https://doi.org/10.1001%2Fjama.286.15.1897. Accessed July 8, 2022.

[4] Kowarski I. 2 Med School Essays That Admissions Officers Loved. Available at: https://www.usnews.com/education/best-graduate-schools/top-medical-schools/articles/2017-06-12/2-medical-school-essays-that-admissions-officers-loved. Accessed July 8, 2022.

As such, consider how you *build* and *showcase* your narrative by choosing which activities you pursue. When choosing among opportunities in your pre-medical career, make conscious decisions that develop and enrich your narrative. Along the way, take the time to reflect on how you would communicate these choices and values in your eventual application to medical school.

**Try this:** Be an admissions committee (ADCOM) member for a day.

Congratulations! You were asked by the dean of admissions of a nearby medical school to join the ADCOM for a day. Today they are deciding which applicants to invite for interviews. You listen intently as another committee member reviews an applicant.

*Applicant: David Gonzalez*
*Hometown: Phoenix, AZ*
*Undergrad/Major: Phoenix College, Liberal Arts*

| | |
|---|---|
| *Activities:* | *2015–2018 Rick's Autobody Shop: Diesel Mechanic* |
| | *2014 NCAA Water Polo National Finalist* |
| | *2015–2018 Special Olympics Volunteer: Water Sports* |
| | *2015–2018 Cesar Chavez High School Assistant Swim Coach* |
| | *2016–2018 Resident Advisor* |
| | *2017 Indian Health Service Summer Intern* |
| | *2017 Poster Presentation: Insulin Availability among diabetic undocumented immigrants in Mericopa County, AZ.* |
| | *2018 Random House Literary Translator: Spanish* |

As a member of the ADCOM, what is your mental image of David? If selected, how do you feel David would contribute to the student body of his medical school? As a physician, how would David impact medicine and represent his medical school? Does David get out of his comfort zone? How has David shown personal initiative and leadership? How do you think David presented himself? What questions would you want to ask David if you were to meet him today? Should David be invited to interview?

## 5.1.2 Why Medicine?

Before addressing this question, we should understand the inquiry itself is actually two distinct questions. Why medicine? And, why *not* anything else? Medicine—despite being an extremely rewarding career—is wrought by an ever-increasing list of challenges that any applicant should be aware of. In addition to 7+years of delayed gratification as a trainee, physicians deal with ever-increasing bureaucracy, political uncertainty, increasing nonclinical demands, long working hours, technological evolution of practice, encroachment of their practice by midlevel providers, and increasingly complex patients who are understandably frustrated with the current healthcare system (more in Chapter 41, Real Talk on a Medical Career). The gravity of these challenges on physicians is clearly indicated in the current epidemic of physician burnout. Burnout is defined as exhaustion, depersonalization, and lack of efficacy, and it has been correlated with inferior patient care, higher medical error rate, increased physician turnover, substance abuse, and suicide.[5] It is now estimated that over 50% of

---

[5] Drummond D. Physician burnout: its origin, symptoms, and five main causes. *Fam Pract Manag* 2015; 22(5):42–47.

current physicians experience burnout.[6] In the face of this current climate, it is especially important that medical schools select students that know what they are getting themselves into. When reviewing applications ADCOM members look for both quality and quantity of experiences in exploring medicine. How does the applicant know he or she wants to go into medicine?

**Try this:** Be an ADCOM member for a day.

Compare and contrast the following applicants on their background knowledge and experiences of the medical field.

| Trisha | Riccardo | Prabhu |
|---|---|---|
| Shadowing experience: 90 hours over 3 years | Shadowing: 20 hours over 1 year | Shadowing: 300 hours over 19 months |
| Emergency Department Volunteer (3 years) | Both parents are physicians (Radiologist & Emergency Medicine) | Currently follows 6 TV medical dramas |
| Research Poster: Physician perspective on managed care plans | Loves to read physician-authors (Atul Gawande // Abraham Verghese // Pauline Chen) | EMT Certification |
| | CNA at assisted-living facility | |

Pause:
- Which applicants are likely to have realistic expectations of a career in medicine?
- Which applicants do you think understand the advantages/disadvantages of being a physician?

For many, the answer to "Why medicine?" comes as a natural application of their passions, goals, and personality to a field of medicine. This necessitates some order of self-awareness and exposure to the fields of medicine. What do you LOVE about medicine?
- *Why* does this applicant want to be a physician? Future goals?
- Would this applicant be successful in our program?
- Does this applicant "*fit*" in our program?
- Is the applicant emotionally healthy?

## 5.1.3 Why Now?

An underappreciated aspect of medical school is that it's quite difficult to stop once the ball starts rolling. By the time you've finished your first year, you've likely taken out $50,000 to $100,000 in loans, and you've invested a significant amount of time and energy into staying afloat. These are sunk costs,[7] however, and you're free to get off the ride if you wish. However, Newton's first law tends to hold true, in that most students will feel compelled to carry out with the journey, despite whatever doubts emerge.

As such, ADCOM members need to feel confident that *now* is the time for you to begin your journey to becoming a physician. Is there any major unfinished business in your life that you need to immediately address? Do you anticipate any significant changes in your life that would require substantial attention early in medical school? Are you emotionally prepared to handle the rigors of the years to come?

To reassure the ADCOM, you must be able to point to specific things that demonstrate that you are prepared to handle the upcoming challenges. Do you have an emotional support network that you can rely

---

[6] Shanafelt TD, Hasan O, Dyrbye LN, Sinsky C, Satele D, Sloan J, West CP. Changes in burnout and satisfaction with work-life balance in physicians and the general US working population between 2011 and 2014. *Mayo Clin Proc* 2015; 90(12):1600–1613.

[7] Sunk cost fallacy. Available at: https://www.behavioraleconomics.com/resources/mini-encyclopedia-of-be/sunk-cost-fallacy/. Accessed July 8, 2022.

on? How do you handle stressful situations such as interpersonal conflict?[8] Are you able to maintain external appearances, even when things get very stressful and hectic?[9]

You also need to convince the ADCOM that attending medical school is the next logical, natural step in your narrative. To that effect, you will need to articulate that while everything you have done already has been tremendously rewarding, the *only*[10] way to fully actualize your personal and professional aspirations is starting medical school. For example, you may say something in your personal statement along the lines of, "My experiences comforting children undergoing chemotherapy have been tremendously rewarding, but I desire to do more. Only a physician has the expertise to save a child from a life-threatening illness...."

Putting it all together, you must abide by this simple rule: never say anything without verifiable evidence. That is, you should "talk less" and "show more." If you're struggling with this, then you may need to gather more evidence. Depending on how big the deficit is and where you are in your pre-medical career, you may need to take some time off to cultivate meaningful experiences during a gap year. As an extreme example, an applicant with no clinical experience will absolutely need to take time off before applying to accumulate evidence of healthcare experience. In choosing additional activities, we recommend picking those that are continuations of other themes in your overall narrative. For example, if your narrative emphasizes an interest in sports, you may benefit from volunteering at a sports medicine clinic.

We will end this chapter with suggested techniques for building your narrative:

- **Narrative Sketch:** Simply list all activities you've done in college and identify methods of organizing them into different narratives. For example, multiple teaching experiences could be organized as a commitment to education, and you may emphasize the role of the physician as a teacher.[11]
  - Consider writing a 3- to 5-page autobiographical sketch. This will also be good practice for the essays you will be asked to write when submitting your primary and secondary applications. Your pre-med office may also require something similar.
  - Relate your experiences to core, unique aspects of your identity. Consider your family upbringing (e.g., how many siblings do you have? Who raised you growing up? How close are you with your extended relatives?), racial/ethnic background, socioeconomic status, geography, etc.
  - At every experience, you should consider at least some of the following: What motivated you to do it? What were your expectations heading in? How was it different? What did you learn? What are the insights you gained? How did it affect you as a person, your perspective, your beliefs, and the role of what medical training could play? What role can it play for your future? What is the theme and common thread that connects your experiences, or why you pursued them, or what insight you took away from them? How does this tie into your motivation to pursue medicine and reinforce your best qualities?
- **Tree diagram:** You (e.g., "John Smith") are the trunk of the diagram. The first, largest branches are your core personality traits, i.e., how your close friends and family would describe you. Those branches further split into activities and experiences corresponding to those traits, and you may have additional activities and experiences that "branched" from your earlier experiences. Your tree should be alive and flourishing; the most distant branches should continue to sprout as you explore new experiences. See the following example of a tree diagram (▶ Fig. 5.1):
  - **Trunk:** John Smith
  - **Core branch 1:** Creative
    - Branch: Guitarist.
    - Branch: Loves creative writing and takes several classes in it.
  - **Core branch 2:** Performative
    - Branch: Guitarist (ties in with the other branch).
    - Branch: Performs in drama club on campus.

---

[8] This is a common interview question that you may be asked directly by the ADCOM.

[9] Maxfield CM, Thorpe MP, Desser TS, et al. Bias in Radiology Resident Selection: Do We Discriminate Against the Obese and Unattractive? Acad Med 2019;94(11):1774–1780.Available at: https://www.ncbi.nlm.nih.gov/pubmed/31149924. Accessed July 8, 2022.

[10] Or "best" depending on the balance you want to strike between idealism and realism.

[11] After all, "doctor" comes from the Latin "docere"—"to teach."

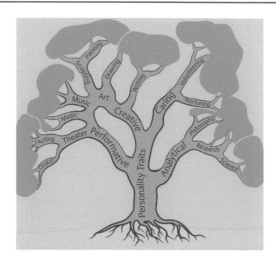

**Fig. 5.1**

- Core branch 3: Caring
  - Branch: Volunteers at a nursing home.
  - Branch: Volunteers at an animal shelter.
- Core branch 4: Analytical
  - Branch: Majors in philosophy.
  - Branch: Participates in biomedical research.
- *Avoid simply listing and rehashing your experiences (e.g., in personal statement), and avoid vague generalities and platitudes:* For example, "I love science, and I've always wanted a career that involves helping people. I did research because I like how medicine combines research and practical application. I like the intellectual challenge."
  - Instead, create a compelling streamlined narrative. Some effective examples include,
    - "Throughout my volunteer experiences with disabled children at camp, I saw patients as more than their disease, how they adapted, and how research was a source of hope and technology could vastly improve their quality of life."
    - "I saw how research is a source of hope for patients and tangibly affects their lives. I wanted to contribute to that, so I did XYZ."
  - Weaker motivations that shouldn't stand-alone include following your parents' footsteps and "I've always wanted to be a doctor from a young age."

## 5.2 Summary

You need to develop a narrative throughout your pre-medical career that's largely consistent with your experiences and interests. Your narrative should address the three questions: "Who are you?" "Why medicine?" and "Why now?" You will need demonstrable evidence to answer these questions (e.g., excellent letters of recommendation, longitudinal experiences, awards, etc.)

# 6 Common Pre-Med Diseases and How to Treat Them

*Joel Thomas*

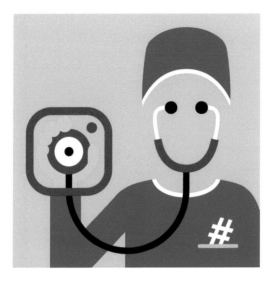

As you've probably realized by now, being pre-med can be stressful. It's critically important to develop healthy coping mechanisms, as your responsibility and workload will only continue to grow as you advance in your medical career. Along the way, you should take the time to really reflect on the identity you've cultivated. Who are you? What's truly important to you? If you don't allow time for introspection, you're at serious risk for developing one of the common pre-med "diseases."[1,2]

## 6.1 Pre-Medical Neurosis

### 6.1.1 Overview

Do you find yourself frantically analyzing every decision you make in terms of medical school admissions? Do you look like a deer in headlights when someone asks you, "What do you do for fun?" Do you have a picture of your future hopeful medical school as your computer background? If so, you might be suffering from *pre-medical neurosis.*

The patient with premedical neurosis operates on a one-track mind, placing virtually every decision in the context of medical school admissions. He or she lacks any personal interests cultivated for their own sake; every move is coldly calculated steps in advance to add valuable material to the American Medical College Application Service (AMCAS) application.

### 6.1.2 Risk Factors

#### Obsessive-Compulsive Personality Traits

Perfectionism. Orderliness. Carefully planning and controlling every detail of a project, even those that are arguably stylistic matters of taste. These personality traits are likely overrepresented among people

---

[1] By pre-med "diseases," we mean behavioral archetypes that we've invented. These should *not* be mistaken for actual mental illnesses, e.g., generalized anxiety disorder, panic disorder, delusional disorder, that should only be diagnosed and treated by a qualified medical professional.

[2] Please do not feel personally attacked if you feel that any of these descriptions hits too close to home. We are simply pointing out common thoughts and behaviors among pre-medical students that are easily correctable. Simply *recognizing* them in yourself is a big part of the process of changing!

who enter scientific careers. However, after a certain point, the time you spend on your work will yield significant diminishing returns and likely take a toll on your mental health.[3]

## Spending Too Much Time Surrounded by Other (Neurotic) Pre-meds

What did you and your friends talk about in the last week? If the answers revolve around "complaining about how unfair that organic chemistry test was," "complaining about that gunner, Jeff," or "how boring it is to volunteer by standing around all day at the hospital," you might want to consider branching out your friend group or being more proactive about new conversation topics.

### 6.1.3 Differential Diagnosis

### Normal Human Behavior

You might be thinking, "Wait a second. This whole book has been telling me that I have to juggle a million different priorities—GPA, MCAT, volunteering, research, clinical experience—at the same time, but now it's *also* telling me to take it easy?" It's true. Getting into medical school *does* require meticulous planning in advance, and most (if not all) of your major academic decisions should be made with consideration to medical school admissions. At the same time, it's important to be able to recognize which decisions are not worth losing sleep over. For guidance, we recommend talking to more experienced, successful pre-med students at your institution to get a better perspective on which decisions are worth microanalyzing.

We also recognize that the process can be extremely stressful, and sometimes it's incredibly therapeutic to just blow off steam with peers' going through the same experience. Misery loves company, after all. Just keep in mind that it's possible to overdo this; stewing in negativity runs the risk of warping your overall outlook toward the process,[4] and you run the risk of burning out at the beginning of your journey.

### Actual Psychiatric Conditions

Do you excessively worry about *virtually everything* in your life—including but not limited to your premedical career—to the point of causing functional impairment? You might have generalized anxiety disorder.

Have you lost all hope in the process of getting into medical school? Are you so demoralized that you suffer from poor overall self-esteem? Are you eating or sleeping too much or too little? Do you find that you're no longer able to enjoy the things that you used to do for fun? **Speak to a healthcare professional**. You might be suffering from a major depressive episode, which is very treatable and common. While it's normal (and regrettably even expected) to suffer bouts of depressed or anxious mood from time to time, it's *not* normal to have impairment in your personal, professional, or social life to the point that your sleep, appetite, and ability to enjoy life suffer.

If you're concerned about your mental health, recognize that you're not alone. Mental illness is increasingly common among college students. Moreover, many students feel that they're the only ones suffering because people are still hesitant to speak openly about it with their friends, despite the substantial progress in reducing stigma. Do not hesitate to see a professional, and consider taking one of the validated

---

[3] Hu KS, Chibnall JT, Slavin SJ. Maladaptive Perfectionism, Impostorism, and Cognitive Distortions: Threats to the Mental Health of Pre-clinical Medical Students. Academic Psychiatry 2019;43:381–385. Available at: https://link.springer.com/article/10.1007%2Fs40596-019-01031-z. Accessed July 8, 2022.

[4] 12 Cognitive Disorders in Academics. Available at: http://sarconline.sdes.ucf.edu/wp-content/uploads/sites/19/2017/07/12_COGNITIVE_DISTORTIONS_IN_ACADEMICS11.pdf. Accessed July 8, 2022.

tools for assessing depression,[5] generalized anxiety,[6] or PTSD[7] (which—regrettably—is more common among college students compared to the general population[8]).

## 6.1.4 Treatment

Spend some time with people on other career paths—you are much more than your medical school application. Get feedback from your close friends on how they perceive you: are you *always* talking about academics?

We also recommend setting aside dedicated time to fully engross yourself in a hobby or passion (if this is too hard to do at first, set aside the time at the end of the day once you've gotten a healthy amount of work done).

If you find your mental health taking a toll, we recommend—as a starting point—optimizing the low-hanging fruit for well-being. These include optimizing sleep hygiene, sticking to a regimen of healthy diet and exercise, practicing mindfulness meditation, and maintaining strong social relationships. Read more about maintaining and optimizing your mental health in Chapter 18, Self-Care and Wellness.

Keep in mind that **burnout** is a very real phenomenon, and there's a growing body of literature about its presence among medical professionals.[9] Realize that there's only so much productive work you can get done in any single day. Take regularly scheduled breaks between productive endeavors, as this will make you more productive in the long run,[10] even if you feel guilty in the moment.

Along this vein, it's common to hear about "work/life balance," but we believe that this perspective often leads to automatic, unhelpful associations of "work" as intrinsically painful and "life" as intrinsically rewarding. Instead, we encourage you to think about **work/life harmony.** Try to identify aspects of work that are intrinsically rewarding. For example, take pride in the time you spend on a Friday night in the library and how it will contribute to acing the organic chemistry exam and bringing your personal best. Relish in the fact that every successful study session you have strengthens your discipline and work capacity, eventually allowing you to thrive in more advanced academic environments. Monitor and track your progress—it's often incremental (e.g., your study sessions may gradually become longer over time), but taking a birds-eye view may allow you to better appreciate the fruits of your labor.

Lastly, recognize that *even though you will have to do a lot of work on your pre-medical journey, it does not necessarily have to be miserable or soul-crushing.* Your **mindset** has a tremendous impact on your premed experience, and you have the *choice* to either flourish or needlessly struggle depending on how you *choose* to frame your experience. Meditation practice is particularly useful for cognitive reframing,[11] and we, again, recommend regular meditation practice to minimize avoidable suffering during the pre-med journey.

## 6.2 Gunnerrhea

### 6.2.1 Overview

Gunnerrhea is the pathognomonic feature of "gunners": overtly and publicly ambitious pre-meds who take no issue with achieving their goals at the expense of their peers. You might be a gunner if you *boast*

---

[5] PHQ-9 (Patient Health Questionnaire-9). Available at: https://www.mdcalc.com/phq-9-patient-health-questionnaire-9. Accessed July 8, 2022.

[6] GAD-7 (General Anxiety Disorder-7). Available at: https://www.mdcalc.com/gad-7-general-anxiety-disorder-7. Accessed July 8, 2022.

[7] PTSD: National Center for PTSD. Available at: https://www.ptsd.va.gov/professional/assessment/screens/pc-ptsd.asp. Accessed July 8, 2022.

[8] Clemans TA. An Overview Of PostTraumatic Stress Disorder in the College Setting. Available at: https://www.mirecc.va.gov/visn19/docs/presentations/Overview_PTSD_College_Setting.pdf. Accessed July 8, 2022.

[9] Hansell MW, Ungerleider RM, Brooks CA, Knudson MP, Kirk JK, Ungerleider JD. Temporal Trends in Medical Student Burnout. Fam Med 2019;51(5):399–404. Available at: https://www.ncbi.nlm.nih.gov/pubmed/31081911. Accessed July 8, 2022.

[10] Ariga A, Lleras A. Brief and rare mental "breaks" keep you focused: Deactivation and reactivation of task goals preempt vigilance decrements. Cognition 2011;118(3):439–443. Available at: https://www.sciencedirect.com/science/article/pii/S0010027710002994?via%3Dihub. Accessed July 8, 2022.

[11] Scott E. How to Reframe Situations So They Create Less Stress. Available at: https://www.verywellmind.com/cognitive-reframing-for-stress-management-3144872. Accessed July 8, 2022.

about aiming for "X" school, program, or residency, *advertise* your MCAT score or GPA, or overtly *brown-nose to* superiors. Intent, however, is crucial. There's a difference between disclosing your MCAT or GPA score when genuinely inquiring about your competitiveness for medical school and shamelessly bringing it up with the intention of making others feel insecure.

*Gunnerrhea with severe features* presents as intentionally sabotaging others to gain a competitive advantage. Actual examples range from defaming other students via email chain to intentionally giving misleading information about upcoming tests and assignments.[12]

## 6.2.2 Risk Factors

### Antisocial or Narcissistic Personality Traits

Narcissistic personality traits include an exaggerated sense of self-importance, low levels of empathy, willingness to take advantage of others, and the desire for constant praise. Antisocial (not to be confused with asocial) personality traits include possessing a general disdain for others and frequently violating social norms and laws to achieve one's own ends. Individuals with *antisocial personality disorder* tend to be highly manipulative (and often charming), and treatment options are still suboptimal.[13] Realistically, if you display strong antisocial or narcissistic personality traits, medicine is not the best career for you; however, early adulthood is a time of identity formation, and you can still make tremendous changes in your behaviors and overall outlook toward life.

### Hypercompetitive Academic Environments

Research suggests that for poor performers, competitive environments increase the likelihood of cheating.[14] There is also evidence that moral reasoning (e.g., not cheating) changes in the context of chronic stress (e.g., academic pressure cooker environments).[15] Keep in mind that while lower GPA and MCAT scores can sometimes be excused if other application factors are favorable, professional/ethical violations on an application are taken extremely seriously.[16]

### Presence of Others with Gunnerrhea

Much like its gastrointestinal counterpart, gunnerrhea is highly contagious. For a variety of reasons, salient cheating in academic environments tends to lower the threshold for others to also cheat.[17] As the saying goes, "if you can't beat them, join them."

## 6.2.3 Differential Diagnosis

### Syndrome of Inappropriate Enthusiasm (SIE)

*SIE* (will be discussed shortly) and *pre-medical neurosis* share many features of gunnerrhea. However, there are subtle differences between these entities. While all three conditions are characterized by obsessive devotion to one's pre-medical career, SIE features outward expression of one's pre-med identity for the sake of external validation; in contrast, gunnerrhea motivates students to boast for the sake of undermining others' confidence (the two may coexist, however, as seen in *gunnerrhea with*

[12] https://www.goodcall.com/news/pre-med-culture-010987
[13] Partially because these individuals tend not to seek treatment because they don't believe anything is wrong with them.
[14] Schwieren C, Weichselbaumer D. Does competition enhance performance or cheating? A laboratory experiment. Available at: http://conference.iza.org/conference_files/TAM2007/weichselbaumer_d1168.pdf. Accessed July 8, 2022.
[15] Zhang L, Kong M, Li Z, Zhao X, Gao L. Chronic Stress and Moral Decision-Making: An Exploration With the CNI Model. Front Psychol 2018;9:1702. Available at: https://www.ncbi.nlm.nih.gov/pmc/articles/PMC6141736/. Accessed July 8, 2022.
[16] Facing Your Past: Disclosing Conduct Violations on Applications. Available at: https://www.cns.umass.edu/news-events/blog/facing-your-past-disclosing-conduct-violations-applications. Accessed July 8, 2022.
[17] Błachnio A, Weremko M. Academic Cheating is Contagious: the Influence of the Presence of Others on Honesty. A Study Report. International Journal of Applied Psychology 2011; 1(1): 14–19. Available at: http://article.sapub.org/10.5923.j.ijap.20110101.02.html. Accessed July 8, 2022.

*mixed features).* In addition, while patients with pre-medical neurosis tend to have depressed or anxious mood, students with SIE tend to have elevated mood. Prominent mood disturbances, however, are not a feature of gunnerrhea.

## 6.2.4 Treatment

Management of antisocial or narcissistic personality traits is beyond the scope of this book. The unfortunate reality is that many individuals who engage in these sorts of behaviors justify their actions to themselves and do not believe they need treatment. If you look back on your pre-medical career, however, and recognize a pattern of taking advantage of others for your own gain, then we *strongly* recommend speaking with a therapist.

Reframing cheating through cost-benefit analysis can also be helpful. There are very few "end-all" red flags for medical school admissions. **Academic dishonesty—e.g., getting caught cheating, plagiarizing, etc.—is one of the few.** Ask yourself if it's worth it to secure a few extra points on that lab report if a potential consequence is irreversibly damaging your career. Your prospects for back-up plans would also greatly suffer, as a documented history of academic dishonesty is universally seen as unacceptable by graduate programs and employers.

## 6.3 Syndrome of Inappropriate Enthusiasm (SIE)

### 6.3.1 Overview

As aforementioned, an individual with SIE has an excessive preoccupation with his or her premedical career and tends to (but not always) have elevated mood with feelings of grandiosity.

### 6.3.2 Risk Factors

#### Low Self-Esteem

While many students with SIE have elevated self-esteem fueled by the external validation of Instagram and Facebook likes, a subset of these patients suffer from poor self-esteem and thus feel the need to compensate by advertising their academic success. Similarly, lacking other noteworthy personality traits or skills is a significant risk factor. Interestingly, students with SIE tend *not* to be the premedical students with the greatest scores or accomplishments; presumably those students are self-secure enough in their achievements that they do not feel as much need to boast and receive validation.

#### Lack of Actual Exposure to Medicine

The student with SIE lives in a fantasy world of medicine, where doctors make pilgrimages to developing countries to single-handedly save entire villages. This beautifully naive view is noticeably devoid of the harsh realities of medical practice that contribute to physician burnout: seemingly intractable social issues (e.g., patients' lacking insurance or health literacy), bureaucratic and corporate takeover of medical practices, and defensive medicine practiced in fear of litigation, among others.[18]

### 6.3.3 Differential Diagnosis

#### Normal Social Media Culture

Some degree of bragging and sharing accomplishments is expected in our modern culture. However, if virtually all your social media posts revolve around medicine *and* are largely shared with the intent of seeking validation, you may be suffering from SIE.

---

[18] Patel RS, Bachu R, Adikey A, Malik M, Shah M. Factors Related to Physician Burnout and Its Consequences: A Review. Behav Sci (Basel) 2018;8(11):98. Available at: https://www.ncbi.nlm.nih.gov/pmc/articles/PMC6262585/. Accessed July 8, 2022.

## Gunnerrhea

Students with SIE and gunnerrhea both boldly advertise their pre-med status; however, whereas SIE features outward expression of one's pre-med identity to receive ego boosts; gunnerrhea is characterized by boasting to undermine competition. *Gunnerrhea* or *SIE with mixed features* presents with signs and symptoms of both conditions, with either gunnerrhea or SIE as the primary, more prominent condition.

## Pre-medical Neurosis

Again, while students with premedical neurosis tend to have depressed or anxious mood, students with SIE tend to have an elevated mood that is reinforced by their peers; however, a subtype of SIE may exist with depressed mood that's reactive to external validation. As with gunnerrhea, SIE may coexist or present as *SIE with mixed features* or *premedical neurosis with mixed features*.

### 6.3.4 Treatment

We recommend exploring clinical medicine across a variety of settings to gain a realistic understanding of what the career entails. While there is certainly opportunity to make tremendous differences in patients' lives, much of what you do will be mundane and arguably offer little benefit to patients. It's better to recognize this earlier when you still have time to process it (and potentially choose a different career path if reality doesn't align with your expectations), versus being blindsided by it for the first time during your clinical rotations.

We also recommend reflecting on and cultivating your personal interests outside of medicine. If your entire identity revolves around your career path, then obstacles or failures along that route run a real risk of derailing your self-esteem. Remember that you're a person first and a pre-med second.

## 6.4 Pre-medical Denial Syndrome[19]

### 6.4.1 Overview

You've wanted to become a doctor since you looked through your first microscope in eighth grade. You volunteer at the free clinic every weekend, do research in a cancer immunology lab, and take detailed, color-coded notes. You also have a 2.5 GPA. Your pre-med advisor has told you that your odds of getting into medical school are exceedingly low. *But it's not impossible—there's always someone that beats the odds.* If this sounds like you, you may be suffering from premedical denial syndrome.

### 6.4.2 Risk Factors

### Never Having Experienced Failure

For many pre-meds, failure does not seem to be an option. You're held to exceedingly high standards in terms of academics and extracurriculars, and the goalposts always appear to be moving. Many pre-meds are also used to excelling at whatever activity they pursue. In this context, receiving a failing grade in a course or earning a prohibitively low MCAT score may feel personally traumatizing. *Denial* is a defense mechanism against such threats whereby one refuses to accept the unpleasant reality of some painful situation.[20] For some, it is easier to live in delusion—to make your own reality—than to face harsh truths head-on.

### Lacking a Variety of Talents or Interests

Lacking a contingency or "back-up" plan in the event that medical school does not work out is a significant risk factor for premedical subtype delusional disorder. This is likely mediated by the denial defense

---

[19] Not to be confused with *delusional disorder*.

[20] Common Defense Mechanisms and Why They Work. Available at: https://psychcentral.com/lib/15-common-defense-mechanisms/. Accessed July 8, 2022.

mechanism, as it's much easier to accept the reality that attending medical school is out of the cards when you have alternative career paths you could see yourself happily pursuing.

### 6.4.3 Differential Diagnosis

#### Normal Human Behavior

While we believe that premedical students should have a realistic understanding of the average acceptance rates to medical school with respect to GPA, MCAT, and other variables, we also acknowledge that spectacular individuals can overcome spectacular odds. For example, academic dishonesty is a significant red flag that should discourage almost all applicants from applying to medical school. If, however, you could realistically see yourself taking several years between the incident—possibly working another career after graduation—to demonstrate a true change in character, then perhaps your "denial" was instead a carefully orchestrated plan to rise from the ashes.

### 6.4.4 Treatment

All premedical students should have a back-up plan (preferably several) in case medical school does not work out. Even if your GPA, MCAT, and extracurriculars are up-to-par with those of successful applicants, there is always the chance of falling through the cracks from bad luck (e.g., too many interviews on rainy days[21]). Interviewers also commonly ask applicants about their back-up plans to get a sense of which aspects of medicine are most appealing to them. Even if medicine is your true calling, you are probably multipotent: the same characteristics that drew you to medicine would probably allow you to thrive in a variety of different fields.

## 6.5 Senioritis

### 6.5.1 Overview

You've been giving your 110% for the past 3 + years. You've spent countless weekends in the library and missed out on too many parties to count. But it wasn't for nothing. Your final grades are in, and you've just hit the "submit" button on your medical school application. This is it: you can *finally* take it easy.

And just like that, you find yourself sleeping in every weekend, binge-watching whatever hit has debuted on your streaming service of choice. Your chosen medical schools vaguely state that your acceptance is contingent on satisfactory academic performance. As long as you don't fail anything, a few B's and C's here shouldn't be a big deal, right?

### 6.5.2 Risk Factors

*Significant academic achievement in high school (even worse with elementary/middle school).* Many pre-meds—particularly the successful ones—have a long history of academic excellence that may have begun as far back as elementary school. The risk of being burnt out with constant studying is directly proportional to the number of years spent on constant studying.

### 6.5.3 Differential Diagnosis

*Normal human behavior,* aka *subclinical senioritis.* Controlled senioritis can play a healthy (and hopefully fun!) role in your overall medical career. If your overall mood and ability to function in life are not significantly impaired, then you're probably on the right track. However, many pre-meds find meaning and satisfaction through tangible external accomplishments like high grades. Pay close attention to your mood throughout the process of senioritis. If you find your self-esteem slipping with your grades, consider either reassessing your value system or reigniting your passion for your work.

---

[21] Redelmeier DA, Baxter SD. Rainy weather and medical school admission interviews. CMAJ 2009;181(12):933. Available at: https://www.ncbi.nlm.nih.gov/pmc/articles/PMC2789141/. Accessed July 8, 2022.

*Actual psychiatric conditions:* Again, consider your overall mood, ability to experience pleasure from previously enjoyable activities, recurring thoughts (e.g., hopelessness, guilt, worthlessness) and neurovegetative symptoms such as sleep, appetite, concentration, and overall energy levels. When in doubt, seek expert opinion. The last thing you want to do is start medical school with poorly managed depression or anxiety.

### 6.5.4 Treatment

The management of senioritis is controversial. It's understandable to want to take a break (e.g., signing up for easier courses in your second half of senior year) after giving your best effort academically for 4+ years; your medical career is a marathon—not a sprint—and it's reasonable to catch your breath when safe to do so. Realistically, no medical school will rescind your acceptance over a minor GPA drop (e.g., cumulative GPA dipping from a 3.8 to a 3.7). However, we only recommend doing this if you have a precise understanding of your academic potential. Can you realistically predict how much your grades will drop if you cut down your studying to 70 to 80%? Can you ensure that you only get B's and (ideally no more than one) C's in your classes rather than D's and F's? If you don't feel that you can comfortably make these forecasts, then we advise continuing your current academic trajectory. You'll still have the summer to let your brain relax.

You should also recognize that only 40% of applicants to medical school gain acceptance to at least one school; if you don't get in this year, your senior year grades will *absolutely* matter for your reapplication. In addition, if you find yourself on the wait-list at your schools of interest, it may help your application to update schools with strong grades in upper-level senior-year courses.

If you've already gained acceptance to a medical school, however, our recommendations are laxer. The first year of medical school will bring on an unprecedented level of academic stress, and we recommend taking a controlled breather so you can start medical school with full force.

## 6.6 Summary

Pre-medical neurosis, gunnerrhea, syndrome of inappropriate enthusiasm, pre-medical denial syndrome, and senioritis are common but treatable conditions. Know the risk factors and presentations of these entities to guard your body and spirit.

# Section II

## Succeeding as a Pre-Medical Student

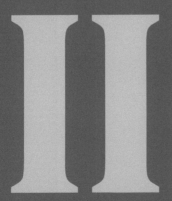

# 7 Guaranteed Admission Programs and Early Assurance Programs

*Samyuktha Melachuri, Chinweoke Osigwe, Eva Roy, and Joel Thomas*

In this chapter, we will discuss programs that offer early guaranteed admission to medical schools. Broadly, these include *combined bachelors/doctorate programs* and *early assurance programs*.

## 7.1 Combined Bachelors/Doctorate Programs

### 7.1.1 What Are Bachelors/Doctorate Programs?

Combined Bachelors/Doctorate programs, also known as guaranteed admission programs (GAP) are combined programs that accept students from high school into both college and medical school in either a guaranteed or conditional manner at the same time. These programs offer a variety of undergrad degrees (e.g., BA, BS) combined with either an MD or DO. *Important Note: These programs are almost entirely for students in high school currently about to apply for college and who know they want to pursue a medical career. If that isn't you—feel free to skip this chapter!*

They are one of the most competitive college admissions processes, but hopefully this chapter can give you some insight into whether these programs would be best for you, and if so, how to approach this process.

### 7.1.2 The Good and the Bad

Like any path to medical school, GAP programs have their advantages and disadvantages. This section should be able to answer the question, "Are these programs for me?"

## Pros

- **Saves Time:** The benefit of a GAP program is that it can reduce time as some programs are 6 or 7 years instead of the traditional 8 years.
- **Reduces Stress:** A huge weight is lifted off your shoulders knowing that you have been accepted to medical school. It relieves the stress of applying during your senior year of college or after taking some gap years.
- **Allows free time:** With the stress of applying to medical school gone, you have the time to truly explore your hobbies, interests, and passions. You can spend your free time the way you want instead of what you think an ADCOM wants.
- **Skipping the Medical College Admission Test** (MCAT): Some programs allow you to bypass the MCAT completely, one of the most difficult parts of the admissions process.

## Cons

- **Binding:** Some programs are binding, so once you commit to a program, you cannot apply to other medical schools or you will lose your seat.
- **Residency:** Many programs exist in lower ranked undergraduate colleges and medical schools, which could potentially affect your residency a few years down the line.
- Many programs only offer conditional acceptance, which means that you may be dismissed from the program if you don't obtain a certain grade point average (GPA), MCAT, or other requirements in your undergraduate years in the program. *Make sure you know what—if any—requirements there are for conditional acceptance at your programs of interest before you apply.*

## 7.2 If GAP Programs Are for You

### 7.2.1 What to Do in High School?

If you know you want to be a doctor in high school, a GAP program may be the right path for you. The earlier you can come to this decision, the better. Essentially everything you would do in college to apply for medical school, you should try to do in high school. As such, your GPA and standardized tests (Scholastic Assessment Test/American College Testing [SAT/ACT]) are *critically* important. Beyond that, the four main components are volunteering, research, shadowing, and extracurriculars.

## Grades and Standardized Test Scores

Your high school GPA and SATs/ACTs are critically important. The median GPA and SAT/ACT varies across programs, but many successful applicants have perfect or near-perfect scores.[1] These quantitative measurements are used as screening tools to get into these competitive programs. If you are thinking about applying to one of these programs, take the highest level science classes offered such as Advanced Placement (AP) Biology, AP Chemistry, AP Physics, Human Anatomy, and Organic Chemistry. If your school doesn't offer AP, take the hardest science courses available such as International Baccalaureate (IB) courses or courses at your local community college. In addition, your standardized test scores are an important benchmark for gaining an interview to one of these programs.

## Clinical Experience

GAP programs want to see that you have a realistic perspective on patient care. This can be obtained through paid jobs (e.g., working as an emergency medical technician (EMT) or emergency room scribe) or through volunteer experiences (e.g., at a hospital, pharmacy, or free clinic). While employment has the obvious benefit of getting paid, it often requires a great time commitment and is generally more competitive to obtain compared to volunteering.

Volunteering in a hospital is a great way to gain exposure to clinical infrastructure, the different specialties, and interaction with patients. Go check out your local hospital and see what the volunteering department offers. Most hospitals have a wide variety of jobs such as helping at the front desk, filing charts, gift shop worker, flower delivery, and helping patients into and out of the hospital. That said, ADCOMs will want *direct patient exposure*, and many of the available volunteering opportunities at a hospital will not meet this requirement. Therefore, our recommendation is to find a position that has you—at the very least—in the same room as living, breathing patients. In addition, you should be aware that some programs will require a specific number of hours at minimum. Go check out Chapter 14, Volunteering for more ideas!

## Research

If you have access, research is another great thing to do in high school. This can be from small science fair projects to doing an internship at an academic institution. If you are too busy during the school year, a great way to do research is in the summer. These are often paid and set you up with a mentor, which makes life much easier than trying to find a mentor willing to take a high school student. Doing research is always beneficial as you gain experience and may have the opportunity to present a poster or oral presentation. *This leads to an important note that summers are a great time to do medically related activities.* Doing research or a medically related camp are excellent ways to involve yourself in the field and show that you are truly interested in medicine. That said, research mentors tend to have humble expectations for research from high school students. Don't be discouraged if you're not producing high-quality publications in major journals. At this stage in the game, the quantity of time spent doing research and letters of recommendation likely matter more than raw scientific output. For more information on how to approach a PI or find research opportunities, check out Chapter 15, Research.

## Shadowing

Another important component to show that you are committed to medicine would be to shadow! This is the best way to see what the daily life of a doctor consists of. You can shadow a variety of specialties or

---

[1] How Does The BS/MD Admissions Process Differ From Traditional Admissions? Available at: https://www.forbes.com/sites/kristenmoon/2019/09/04/how-does-the-bsmd-admissions-process-differ-from-traditional-admissions/. Accessed July 8, 2022.

stick with one doctor that you really like. If you find someone that takes the time to explain what you are seeing, stick with them. I would make sure to keep track of everyone you are shadowing and details from that day so this will be easier when applying. Check out Chapter 13, Shadowing for more info.

## High School Clubs

Getting involved with your own high school clubs is an important way to show leadership skills. There is no need to join every club, but focus on a few that you truly enjoy and want to spend time with. Putting effort into one or two clubs and then becoming more involved with those is the best route for showing commitment. If there are any medically related clubs, go ahead and get involved. However, do not limit yourself to just medically related clubs. Pursue whatever you are passionate about, such as sports, band, theater, etc. If you are interested in something and there is no club, go ahead and start one! Colleges and medical schools love to see students take initiative. Check out Chapter 11, Extracurriculars for additional inspiration!

No matter what you do, just show that you are passionate and committed to medicine. Since you are so young, the best way to show interest in medicine is that you have explored medicine. This is best done through shadowing, volunteering in hospitals, and medically related experiences such as camps or internships. It is hard to know what you want to do in high school especially when you are 15 or 16. However, if you are possibly thinking about a career in medicine, high school is a great time to explore the field of medicine and see if this is the right path for you and if it is then apply to BS/MD programs!

## 7.2.2  How Do GAP Admissions Work?

Are you wondering how this admission process works? For starters, different programs have slightly different application processes, but they can be categorized into four groups.
1. Apply via the common application. Once you indicate interest in the specific BS/MD program, the supplemental section will show up in the Common App itself or a separate application will be emailed to you.
2. Apply to the undergraduate school and receive admission, then you can apply to the associated medical school. Sometimes this is guided by the program facilitators, other times it is completely your responsibility.
3. Apply to both the undergraduate institution and medical school at the same time.
4. Submit grades and scores, then they will filter the applicants by only sending the supplemental application to students with scores above a threshold.

Once all supplementals reach the medical school admissions, the process is similar. A small proportion of the applicants are offered interviews, the type of which can vary upon school. This is typical to the traditional admissions process, which will be discussed in an upcoming chapter. However, the major differentiating factor is passion and dedication for medicine. The admissions committee is looking for students who will be committed to this school and path for the next 6 to 8 years. There are a limited number of seats, so it is crucial to fill them with the best suitable students for both medicine and the values of the school.

## How to Apply?

To apply to GAP programs, you'll start with completing the common application and applying to your schools of choice. Then, you'll have an additional, program-specific application that will be your application to the GAP. Please be aware of the deadlines for these programs. Some deadlines are as early as October 15th of the application cycle, so plan your application process accordingly. You can expect the following components in the application process. High school transcripts need to be submitted. Send each school your previous standardized test scores including AP/IB and SAT/ACT scores. Many programs also require SAT subject tests: usually Math 2 and at least one science subject test.

Like any college application, these programs want letters of recommendation. Make sure these recommendations come from teachers, counselors, employers, or anyone else who can speak to your potential for these programs. Some programs require specific class teachers or mentors to provide these letters. In addition to the common application essays, programs will have supplemental essays asking about your interest in medicine. There will also be a section for you to fill in your high school medical and nonmedical activities or you can attach your resume/CV.

## Essays

We will briefly touch on essays here, but there is a later chapter devoted to essays that you should refer to (Chapter 31, Personal Statement). Essays are a chance to give the admissions committee insight into your application beyond just grades and scores. You do not need to convey that you are applying to a GAP program in your common application essay, an essay all high school students write that is sent to most of the colleges to which they apply. In fact, it shouldn't. Most, if not all GAP programs will ask the question "why do you want to be a doctor" in some way within the application process. Keep in mind when writing your essays to keep them compelling but moderate in length— 650 words maximum.

## Interviews

We will also touch on interviews in this section; however, there is an entire chapter covering it later on (Chapter 34, Interviews). If you have gotten to this part of the application process, congratulations! Not many students make it this far. That being said, this is one of the most crucial parts of your application process. An Admissions Committee is trying to verify if you are genuine as your essays seem and if you really want to be a doctor. These are all pretty big questions that need to be answered in a small time frame. Different schools have different interviewing methods, which we shall discuss in an upcoming chapter. The interview is to truly see if you are mature enough as a senior in high school to make a decision and commitment this large about your future. Interviews are typically from January to April and decisions are released from March to May.

## Once You Are Accepted!

To maintain your seat in the medical school, usually there are some requirements. Most usually require the maintenance of a GPA greater than 3.6 (or something similar). You can find more information in the table of programs at the end of the chapter. Some also want their students to take the MCAT and get a certain score. The year before your matriculation into medical school, the medical school admissions committee reviews your progress in undergrad and makes sure you are fit to join the medical school class.

## 7.2.3  What Is Undergrad Like as a Combined Bachelors/Doctorate Student?

So you've decided to pursue a GAP program at your chosen college. You have put in a lot of time and effort to get here, and now you're at the fun part. Going to college is an amazing privilege, and we're excited for you to start this new journey. As a GAP student, you have the freedom to expand your horizons and explore new possibilities while you're in undergrad. You are starting college with something that many people covet: you have a potential idea of where you want your life to go and a medical school admission. Your plan doesn't have to be set in stone, but your current sense of direction will be helpful for mapping out your next 2 to 4 years. So, let's get drawing.

You are going into school with two big things in mind. One, you're a new pre-medical college student. Second, you're a new GAP student. Both of those things elicit a lot of new freedoms, but they also come with a handful of requirements that must be addressed. Most, if not all, GAP programs offer *conditional* acceptance into their respective medical school. Every school will have their own exact list of requirements and benchmarks, so make sure you are familiar with it. Your program director or your program's website would be good resources to help you figure that out. Here we'll discuss some of the requirements you may come across and how you could tackle them as a GAP undergrad.

## MCAT

One of the main benchmarks that your school will dictate is whether or not you are required to take the Medical College Admission Test, or MCAT. The MCAT is a tedious, expensive exam, so knowing whether or not you need to take the test is key. If your school doesn't require you to take the MCAT, that's a great benefit. However, if your school does require it, plan in advance on when to take it and how to prepare for it. Chapter 17, Crushing the MCAT discusses common resources used to help prepare for the MCAT.

## GPA

Another benchmark that your school will likely set for you is a minimum GPA requirement. Whether you're in undergrad for 2 years or 4 years, you will be taking classes with other undergraduate students in a variety of disciplines. Each course will give you a grade at the end of the semester, and that letter grade will be associated with a number on a scale from 0.0 to 4.0, similarly to how your grades in high school worked. You will have an overall GPA for your classes and GPA for just your science classes. Your school may require you to keep both of them above anywhere from around a 3.0 to a 3.8. Your school may check up on your grades each semester or they may just check your graduating cumulative GPA. In either case, though, keeping your grades at the level your school requires is essential and failing to keep your GPA within this range may result in losing your guaranteed admission.

   Although the high GPA may seem daunting, you have so much more time in college to be able to study. Second, you were selected from a competitive group to join a GAP program, and that means you have serious potential. Your GAP directors wouldn't have given you a highly coveted spot in a selective program if they didn't believe in your ability to succeed at your given institution. Take their faith and run with it. You got this, and refer to Chapter 10, Obtaining a Solid GPA for additional guidance!

### 7.2.4  Length of Program

As with any school program, GAP programs are often different lengths. Some programs will last 8 years, with 4 years of medical school and 4 full years of undergrad. However, some programs are only 6 or 7 years, with 4 years of med school and an abbreviated 2 or 3 years of college. With an expedited program, you will likely spend a lot of time focusing on your science coursework. You have all of the typical pre-med classes to cover in less time, so you'll have to be quite focused and might have to plan ahead how you'll arrange your schedule. In fact, some programs may require you to take summer and/or winter courses!

   In contrast, if you attend a full-length 8-year program, you will likely have more freedom to deviate from your medical interests and enrich yourself in other disciplines. You will probably take two to three science courses each semester, leaving you with at least two open non-science courses to do what you want with. This is an excellent time to explore your other interests! Whichever type of program you decide to pursue, there are pros and cons, but both will set you up with skills that will help you become a better doctor.

### 7.2.5  The Fun Stuff: Unique GAP Student Opportunities

Now that you have an idea of some things you'll have to keep in mind with your program, let's talk about some of the unique opportunities you'll have as a GAP student. We can break these down into medically-related and non-medically-related opportunities. You know that you're interested in medicine, so undergrad is a time to enrich that, but you are also in college, so this is a time to enrich *yourself* as well. Both are relevant and important, and strengthening both aspects will make you into your best doctor.

   Getting hands-on medical experiences is one of the best ways to learn more about medicine and all the different fields it offers. A great way to experience this as an undergrad is through shadowing. You can learn a lot about a particular specialty through shadowing. Engaging in shadowing at some point in your undergrad career will be very valuable. Your GAP program may have a shadowing setup for you in a variety of specialties or you may have an advisor/director who can help you pursue these opportunities. Your program may also introduce you to upperclassmen, who may be able to give you some suggestions of places that they like to shadow. Reach out and see what you can find that interests you.

As important as medically-related opportunities are, your undergrad years are also a time for fun. There is a reason that people say "college is the best four years of your life." There won't be many other times in your life where you can just dive head-first into your most diverse or eclectic passions. In addition, as a future doctor there is so much more to learn than just the basic sciences, and your passions may teach you some super valuable life lessons that will carry over into being a physician. Luckily, GAP students have even more freedom to learn because they don't have to spend time applying to medical school. You will have chunks of time that your peers don't, and that time is ripe for exploration. Let's talk about some ways that GAP students make the most of their non-science time.

For the more pragmatic GAP students, academic freedom in GAP programs could mean taking classes that teach them about the social, psychological, and cultural aspects of medicine. Taking classes in different disciplines such as sociology, anthropology, and psychology expose you to new things that you won't learn in your science classes. Social science courses like these might teach you a lot about your future patients. Your patients will be coming from a variety of cultural, racial, and socioeconomic backgrounds, so learning more about diversity and tolerance is key to becoming a kind and caring physician. Take advantage of your academic freedom by taking courses that enrich your cultural competencies.

If you can swing it, studying abroad is an excellent way to expand your cultural competencies. Your non-GAP classmates might have a hard time fitting in study abroad due to rigorous or lab-dependent course schedules, but as a GAP student your program may allow you the flexibility to make study abroad feasible. Study abroad is an important educational experience for a future physician to have. Experiencing new cultural dynamics while abroad will help you connect with diverse patient populations once you're back home. And, as previously mentioned, cultural competence is a pivotal skill for everybody living in our globalized world. Relish your GAP freedoms and find a way to study abroad.

## 7.2.6  Final Thoughts

Overall, GAP programs are a great path for people who know they want to pursue a career in medicine. We all have different reasons for choosing to go into medicine, but if you know that as a high schooler this is the path for you, then apply! It is a big decision to commit to medical school as a high schooler, but in the long run it is worth it.

Becoming a doctor is a long journey and making that process easier in any way is beneficial in the long term. If you cannot see yourself doing anything else as a career, start exploring in high school whether it be shadowing, research, or volunteering. The application process can be a bit tedious and intimidating, but it will be worth it in the end. As someone who has gone through the process, I can say that it was one of the best decisions I have made. These programs are here to take the huge weight of getting into medical school off your shoulders and help you focus on what you truly want to do in college, not what you have to do to get into medical school. If this all sounds appealing, then start early and apply. We have attached a table of some of the available programs to provide examples of what's available 2021 (▶ Table 7.1). *This table is NOT inclusive of all the programs that are out there.* Therefore, we encourage you to reach out to your high school guidance counselor about the specific programs available in your geographic area.

Additional programs to consider, among others, include ones at:
- Albany Medical College (Albany, NY).
- CUNY Sophie Davis (New York, NY).
- Cooper Medical School of Rowan University (Camden, NJ).
- Florida Atlantic University (Boca Raton, FL).
- George Washington University (Washington, DC).
- Hofstra University (Uniondale, NY).
- Howard University (Washington, DC).
- Indiana University (Evansville, IN).
- Lake Erie College of Osteopathic Medicine (Erie, PA).
- Marshall University (Huntington, WV).
- Medical College of Georgia (Augusta, GA).
- Mercer University (Macon, GA).
- Saint Louis University (Saint Louis, MO).

**Table 7.1** Guaranteed admission programs 2021

| Program | Undergraduate | Medical school | Length of program | Requirements to apply | Requirements to matriculate | MCAT |
|---|---|---|---|---|---|---|
| Baylor[2] Medical Track Program | Baylor University | Baylor College of Medicine | 8 y | 3.7 GPA (or top 5% of class), ACT 32 or SAT 1430 | 3.5 cumulative GPA, 3.6 Science GPA | Yes, at least in 501–507 range |
| Boston University Liberal Arts/Medical Education Program | Boston University | Boston University School of Medicine | 7 y | None | 3.2 cumulative GPA, 3.2 Science GPA | Yes, Score at least in 80th percentile |
| Brown Program in Liberal Medical Education (PLME) | Brown University | Warren Alpert Medical School of Brown University | 8 y | None | None | No |
| Case Western Pre Professional Scholars Program (PPSP) | Case Western Reserve University | Case Western Reserve University School of Medicine | 8 y | | 3.63 cumulative GPA, 3.63 science GPA | No; if you choose to take it, you must get at least the 94th percentile, however. |
| Drexel Early Assurance Program | Drexel University | Drexel University School of Medicine | 8 y | 3.5 GPA and 1420 SAT or 31 ACT | 3.6 cumulative GPA, 3.6 science GPA | Yes, at least a 513 with no subsection score less than 127 |
| Rutgers, Health Careers Program Combined BS/MD Program | Montclair State University | New Jersey Medical School at Rutgers University | 8 y | Must be from a "financially and educationally disadvantaged background", New Jersey resident, class rank in the top 10%, "B" average or higher GPA (including science GPA), SAT 1100 (with 550 in each section) | "B" science GPA, 3.4 cumulative GPA, research project | Yes—must get "competitive scores" |
| Rutgers University New Jersey Medical School, School of Arts & Sciences-Newark | Rutgers University-Newark School of Arts & Sciences | New Jersey Medical School at Rutgers University | 7 y | 1400 SAT or 32 ACT | Required summer research internship, 3.5 GPA | No |

(Continued)

**Table 7.1** (*Continued*) Guaranteed admission programs 2021

| Program | Undergraduate | Medical school | Length of program | Requirements to apply | Requirements to matriculate | MCAT |
|---|---|---|---|---|---|---|
| Sidney Kimmel Medical College, College of Medicine at Thomas Jefferson University | Penn State | | 7 y (no required summers) | SAT or ACT are optional for 2022 and 2023; previously, the requirement was a 1470 SAT or 32 ACT | 3.5 GPA | Yes—508 with a minimum of 127 in all sections except CARS, which has a minimum of 126 |
| University of Cincinnati-Connections Dual Admissions Program | University of Cincinnati | University of Cincinnati | 8 y | 1300 SAT or 29 ACT | 3.5 GPA and 3.5 science GPA | Yes |
| University of Missouri-Kansas City School of Medicine's B.A./M.D. program | University of Missouri-Kansas City | University of Missouri-Kansas City | 6 y | 1160 SAT or 24 ACT (superscore accepted) | 3.0 GPA | No |
| University of Pittsburgh Guaranteed Admission Program (GAP) | University of Pittsburgh | University of Pittsburgh School of Medicine | 8 y | 3.75 cumulative GPA, 3.75 Science GPA, SAT of 1490 or ACT of 34, as well as clinical experience, leadership, research, and community service | Minimum MCAT requirement if no SAT or ACT scores | Yes (if you are admitted without SAT or ACT) |
| University of Rochester Early Medical Scholars | University of Rochester | University of Rochester | 8 y | None | 3.4 GPA/science GPA in freshman year, 3.5 in sophomore year, and 3.6 during junior and senior years | No |

Abbreviations ACT, American College Testing; GPA, grade point average; MCAT, Medical College Admission Test; SAT, Scholastic Assessment Test.

- Stony Brook University (Stony Brook, NY).
- SUNY Downstate (Brooklyn, NY).
- Temple University (Philadelphia, PA).
- University of Colorado (Aurora, CO).
- University of Connecticut (Farmington, CT).
- University of New Mexico (Albuquerque, NM).
- University of Nevada Reno (Reno, NV).
- University of Alabama (Birmingham, AL).
- University of Oklahoma (Oklahoma City, OK).
- University of South Alabama (Mobile, AL).
- University of Florida (Gainesville, FL).
- University of Toledo (Toledo, OH).
- Wayne State University (Detroit, MI).

## 7.3 Early Assurance Programs

BS/MD programs are to be distinguished from *early assurance programs*, which are programs that accept college students (e.g., freshman and sophomores) before the normal application cycle. Early assurance programs often accept students before they take the MCAT, although many require that the student gets a minimum MCAT score before matriculating. These programs can provide a peace of mind to college students by allowing them to avoid the stress and expenses of applying to (and interviewing at) many more programs down the line. In addition, many students will feel free to explore extracurriculars and experiences that may have been harder to pursue as a traditional pre-med, given the time constraints of studying for the MCAT, pressures of striving for perfect grades (versus reaching the minimum requirements for conditional acceptance), and aggressively pursuing more "traditional" extracurriculars. That said, some of these programs commit you to the school you are admitted to, leaving you unable to apply to other medical schools down the line.

Early assurance programs generally evaluate the same metrics as regular admissions, (i.e., GPA, extracurriculars, and letters of recommendation). Some require SAT/ACT scores to standardize academic metrics across applicants.

There are many different early assurance programs, and many are restricted to undergraduates of specific schools. *Therefore, we encourage you to ask your prehealth advisor (or upperclassmen at your school) about which ones are available to you.* Here is a list of some (but not all) medical schools with early assurance programs. We encourage you to use it to do more research on early assurance programs in your geographic region that may be available to you, as the details about GPA, MCAT, SAT/ACT, and binding versus nonbinding differ greatly among programs.

- Albany Medical College (Albany, NY).
- A.T. Still College of Osteopathic Medicine (Kirksville, MO).
- Boston University (Boston, MA).
- Brody School of Medicine (Greenville, NC).
- California Northstate University College of Medicine (Elk Grove, CA).
- Dartmouth School of Medicine (Hanover, NH).
- Drexel University (Philadelphia, PA).
- Georgetown University (Washington DC).
- George Washington School of Medicine (Washington DC).
- Hofstra School of Medicine (Hempstead, NY).
- Icahn School of Medicine, Mount Sinai (New York, NY).
- Jefferson Medical College (Philadelphia, PA).
- Michigan State University College of Human Medicine (East Lansing, MI).
- Northwestern University (Chicago, IL).
- Penn State (Hershey, PA).
- Rutgers Robert Wood Johnson (Piscataway, NJ).
- SUNY Upstate (Syracuse, NY).
- Temple University (Philadelphia, PA).
- Tufts University (Boston, MA).

- Tulane University (New Orleans, LA).
- SUNY Buffalo (Buffalo, NY).
- University of California Riverside (Riverside, CA).
- University of Chicago Loyola (Maywood, IL).
- University of Cincinnati (Cincinnati, OH).
- University of Florida (Gainesville, FL).
- University of Kentucky (Lexington, KY).
- University of Miami (Miami, FL).
- University of Pennsylvania (Philadelphia, PA).
- University of Rochester (Rochester, NY).
- University of South Carolina Greenville (Greenville, SC).
- University of Texas Rio Grande Valley (Edinburg, TX).
- University of Toledo (Toledo, OH).
- Virginia Commonwealth University (Richmond, VA).
- Wake Forest University (Winston-Salem, NC).
- Wright State University (Dayton, OH).

## 7.4 Summary

Guaranteed admission programs and early assurance programs may be great fits for certain applicants, and everyone considering a medical career should be aware of these programs. Many of them still have conditional requirements for admission to medical school, however, and several programs are at lower-ranked medical schools and hospital systems, which may impact your career down the line. Some allow you to get your medical degree earlier, although this is often at the cost of an accelerated, more stressful educational pace.

# 8 Schools, Majors, and More

*Christian Morrill and Joel Thomas*

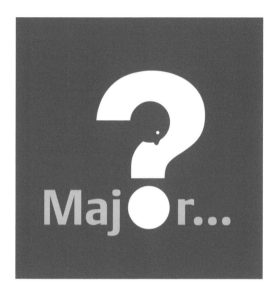

## 8.1 Choosing an Undergraduate School or Pre-med Program

As in choosing a medical school or a career in medicine, the factors that guide your decision to attend a certain undergraduate program should be unique to your individual interests and career aspirations. Do you want to be close to home? Which colleges have the majors you're most interested in? Maybe you want to go to your parent's alma mater?

Strictly speaking, you can obtain your undergraduate education from any accredited 4-year university and gain admission to a medical school. That said, it's worth stating that while there are more similarities between US MD medical programs than there are differences, not all medical schools are created equal. So you'll want to attend the undergraduate institution that is best for *you*—both in terms of getting into the best medical school for you and your personal development as a well-rounded individual. These general principles can help you decide on the best undergraduate school for you.

## 8.2 High-Yield Advice

### 8.2.1 Excellence Breeds Excellence

The strongest predictor for success is previous success. Therefore, if you are aiming for top medical schools, consider attending a US News Top 125 undergraduate school. As mentioned earlier, prestigious private medical schools greatly value attendance at a prestigious private undergraduate school. That said, we do *not* necessarily recommend attending a dramatically more expensive "prestigious" school for a mild-to-moderate increase in "prestige" over other available options. The college you ultimately choose will depend on a variety of factors, including price, prestige, geographic location, unique opportunities, and other intangible factors; in the end, you will have to make an educated decision on incomplete information and make the best of your available resources.

## 8.2.2  Student Perspectives on Undergraduate Prestige

**Joel Thomas:** I attended SUNY Binghamton, a public undergraduate university ranked #88 on US News for no debt compared to taking out ~$160,000 in loans to attend the University of Chicago, ranked between #4 and #10 (depending on the year) on US News. I graduated from the University of Pittsburgh School of Medicine, a top 15 medical school on US News and matched to the Mallinckrodt Institute of Radiology at Washington University in St. Louis, a top 5 residency program (per Doximity) in a competitive specialty and have absolutely no regrets about my educational choices. At the same time, I could see an argument for attending the more expensive, prestigious school in retrospect; perhaps I would have participated in a broader range of educational experiences that led me down a different career path altogether (e.g., academia, finance). It's important to remember that even if you're absolutely committed to becoming a physician at the beginning of college, you should keep an open mind and expose yourself to a broad array of experiences to minimize the odds of missing out on an alternative career path that would be more fulfilling. There's no clear right answer to what I should have done in retrospect, but convincing arguments can be made for either choice.

It's also important to note that while more prestigious schools often have more generous need-based aid and scholarships, many middle- to upper-middle class students find themselves in the unfortunate position where their family makes just enough money to be excluded from need-based aid but doesn't make enough to cover the sticker cost. This is exactly what happened to me during college admissions, and it was the major deciding factor for my undergraduate school choice.

**Ray Funahashi:** If you want to give yourself the best chance to attend a top-tier medical school, I strongly believe in choosing a school that is at least known nationally. I worked for a couple of years at a top-tier medical school. They posted the schools represented in admissions interviews on a daily basis. Not a single time did I see a university which I had not heard of before represented. I attended a regional state university that is not known outside of my state and if I could do it over again I would choose a more reputable university.

Yes, there is a cost to consider, as less prestigious universities may have cheaper tuition, but the top universities often make up for this with more opportunities for financial aid and scholarships.

There is definite value in attending a well-known university, including better study abroad opportunities and alumni network. There is also a major difference in opportunities to get involved in research, projects, and link to internships. Research funding somewhat parallels university rankings. So even though my university was moderate-sized we had an undersized research faculty. At my university, as pre-med students, we had to fight over the limited research assistant positions and opportunities. Keep in mind, research is a key extracurricular for top-tier medical schools.

There is also a perception that prestigious universities are more academically rigorous. True or not, this bias exists.

All this is not to say that you have no shot at a top-tier medical school if you attend a lower ranked undergrad. It just means you may have to do subjectively more to impress admissions committees. Attending a reputable undergrad only makes opening the door to medical school slightly easier. It is far from a guarantee for admission into a top-tier medical school. But for you as a pre-med, it has the combined additive effect of helping you get "better" research, "cooler" extracurriculars, more reputable recommendation letter writers, and the school name and alumni.

If you are struggling to determine whether or not to attend a lesser-known undergraduate school, the grand litmus test is to ask the pre-med office of the school where students have matriculated in the last 5 years. If none have attended the top-tier schools, and you aim to attend those programs, I would reconsider choosing that undergraduate school. You could also consider not taking any pre-med requirements at your undergrad of choice, and afterward attend a reputable pre-med post-bac program (at a reputable university) to complete your pre-med requirements also. These programs often do get students admitted to top-tier programs but they can also be expensive. This method is very roundabout, and it would just save cost and time to attend the best undergrad you can to begin with.

If you're already almost finished with your undergraduate work or if attending a more competitive undergraduate program is not feasible, then consider attending summer internships or completing graduate work at these universities. Of course, it's true that there's likely a strong selection effect in terms of the effect of attending prestigious institutions. That is, top universities were not entirely *causally* responsible for their students' success in medical school admissions, as these students would likely also do well at other universities. Nonetheless, simply attending a Top 125 undergraduate school likely carries intrinsic weight in your application (e.g., through signaling effects[1]), which persists even after controlling for standardized individual performance variables, (e.g., Medical College Admission Test (MCAT) score).

## 8.2.3 Medical Alumni

Regardless of where you attend, you should *always* ask for a history of how many of the program's graduates successfully matriculated into medical schools and where they currently attend. Medical schools will view you as a representative applicant from the school where you last graduated from. If the medical school has NEVER matriculated students from your undergraduate program, they may—at best—view you as a wild card and be more exacting in their evaluation of you or—at worst—simply decline to interview you, especially if you're a borderline applicant.

## 8.2.4 Prehealth Advisors

Does your university have a prehealth advisor? If so, what is the advisor's experience? At best, advisors can be extremely efficient and effective, providing you with nuanced information about the specific courses and opportunities available at your institution. On the other hand, they may be confusing and full of generic and unhelpful—or worse—inconsistent and inaccurate information. The best way to determine this is by reaching out to current (and former) pre-medical students at the university and ask for honest opinions of the prehealth advising. Another option is to look for graduate matriculation into medical school, 4-year pre-med timelines, and general advising either in-person or online. Be wary if they can't supply you with specific numbers or plans.

## 8.2.5 Prehealth Clubs

Explore what extracurricular organizations exist relevant to prehealth and pre-med students at the university. Reach out to the organization presidents and ask them for the previous year's impact reports, activities, and programs. Usually, greater interest and organization for pre-med will equate to better opportunities to get prepared for medical school outside academia. Also be mindful of whether members of these organizations gained acceptance to medical school.

## 8.2.6 Opportunities for Exposure

Getting into medical school requires lots of involvement outside of academia. Physician shadowing, community service, leadership, and patient exposure require opportunities in the community surrounding your university and extracurricular clubs. For instance, in many areas opportunities for physician shadowing are extremely limited and restricted by red tape. In other areas, there is ample need for phlebotomists, certified nursing assistants (CNAs), and emergency medical technicians (EMTs) where properly trained pre-med students can gain experience caring for patients and working in medical teams. It is well worth your time to research such opportunities (either through the university or surrounding community) before selecting your undergraduate university. You can do this by inquiring current pre-med students at your university, doing a quick job search for introductory-level healthcare positions in the area, or talking to pre-medical advisors.

---

[1] Bostwick V. Signaling in higher education: The effect of access to elite colleges on choice of major. Available at: https://onlinelibrary.wiley.com/doi/abs/10.1111/ecin.12340. Accessed July 8, 2022.

## 8.3 What Major Should I Choose?

The short answer here is that there isn't a preferred pre-medical major. This is a comforting fact if you decided on medicine later in life. In fact, medical schools are very clear that interested applicants should major in whatever discipline they desire. However, your selection of your undergraduate major will undoubtedly color your pre-medical experience and preparation for medical school, and should therefore be considered carefully.

### 8.3.1 By the Numbers

Data on pre-medical undergraduate majors and matriculation into medical school is compiled by the American Association of Medical Colleges for each year. The majority of pre-medical students who matriculated into medical school in 2021 pursued a major in biological sciences (58.1%). However, pre-meds majoring in biological sciences had lower acceptance rates to MD schools than humanities, math and statistics, and physical science majors (▶ Table 8.1). Among applicants for the 2021 to 2022 medical school class, math and statistics majors achieved the highest MCAT average of 515 followed by physical sciences (514) and humanities (513).

Don't choose your major blindly via statistics because there is likely significant selection bias complicating the results. We hypothesize that students applying to medical school with majors in mathematics and humanities are just *qualitatively different* as a group. That is, there are likely significant differences in baseline interests and ability that may contribute to differences in admissions success. Major alone is unlikely to explain differences in admissions success.

Keep in mind that if you're—say—majoring in philosophy, then you would have to do some extra planning to go out of your way to take a year of physics, organic chemistry, and other classes to finish your application requisite classes. This won't necessarily lengthen how long it takes to get your degree, but will consume most of your elective coursework time. If not properly planned for, this can add time and cost to your undergraduate experience.

The following are admissions data for applicants and matriculants to US MD schools by major (▶ Tables 8.1 and 8.2). These statistics should demonstrate that successful matriculation into medical school can be obtained from essentially any major.

That said, for a variety of reasons (e.g., diversity of educational experiences), some medical schools seem to be working to increase the number of students with "non-traditional majors" (e.g., social sciences, humanities, + /− physical sciences and mathematics) matriculating at their school. While the proportion of

**Table 8.1** Acceptance rates by major, MD programs

| Major | Acceptance rate |
|---|---|
| Biological sciences | 36.0%[a] |
| Humanities | 44.1% |
| Math and statistics | 40.4% |
| Other | 33.5% |
| Physical sciences | 42.5% |
| Social sciences | 34.9% |
| Specialized health sciences | 35.2% |
| All matriculants | 36.3% |

[a] Note that this is extremely similar to the acceptance rate for "all matriculants," which is unsurprising, given that it's the single largest group of applicants. The acceptance rate for other types of majors do not appear to be dramatically different from that of "all matriculants." As such, we doubt that individual majors has a dramatic effect on overall matriculation rate.

Table 8.2 MCAT and GPAs for applicants and matriculants to US MD-granting medical schools by primary undergraduate major, 2021–2022

| Applicants | MCAT CPBS | | MCAT CARS | | MCAT BBLS | | MCAT PSBB | | Total MCAT | | GPA science | | GPA nonscience | | GPA total | | Total Applicants |
|---|---|---|---|---|---|---|---|---|---|---|---|---|---|---|---|---|---|
| | Mean | SD | Mean | SD | Mean | SD | Mean | SD | Mean | SD | Mean | SD | Mean | SD | Mean | SD | |
| Biological sciences | 126.3 | 2.8 | 125.6 | 2.7 | 126.8 | 2.8 | 127.2 | 2.8 | 505.9 | 9.5 | 3.50 | 0.42 | 3.76 | 0.27 | 3.60 | 0.34 | 36,520 |
| Humanities | 126.6 | 2.8 | 126.9 | 2.6 | 126.9 | 2.7 | 127.8 | 2.6 | 508.2 | 9.2 | 3.44 | 0.46 | 3.72 | 0.30 | 3.59 | 0.34 | 1,927 |
| Math and statistics | 127.9 | 2.7 | 126.7 | 2.9 | 127.6 | 2.9 | 128.0 | 2.8 | 510.2 | 9.9 | 3.55 | 0.42 | 3.70 | 0.30 | 3.60 | 0.35 | 399 |
| Other | 125.9 | 2.9 | 125.5 | 2.8 | 126.3 | 2.9 | 127.0 | 2.9 | 504.7 | 10.0 | 3.47 | 0.45 | 3.73 | 0.29 | 3.59 | 0.35 | 10,070 |
| Physical sciences | 127.6 | 2.7 | 126.4 | 2.7 | 127.4 | 2.7 | 127.7 | 2.7 | 509.1 | 9.2 | 3.56 | 0.40 | 3.71 | 0.30 | 3.62 | 0.33 | 5,201 |
| Social sciences | 125.7 | 2.9 | 125.9 | 2.8 | 126.1 | 2.9 | 127.5 | 2.8 | 505.2 | 9.9 | 3.37 | 0.49 | 3.65 | 0.33 | 3.52 | 0.36 | 5,652 |
| Specialized health sciences | 125.4 | 3.0 | 125.2 | 2.8 | 125.8 | 3.0 | 126.7 | 3.0 | 503.2 | 10.4 | 3.44 | 0.46 | 3.73 | 0.28 | 3.59 | 0.33 | 2,674 |
| *All applicants* | *126.3* | *2.9* | *125.7* | *2.8* | *126.7* | *2.8* | *127.3* | *2.8* | *505.9* | *9.7* | *3.48* | *0.44* | *3.74* | *0.28* | *3.59* | *0.34* | *62,443* |
| Matriculants | MCAT CPBS | | MCAT CARS | | MCAT BBLS | | MCAT PSBB | | Total MCAT | | GPA science | | GPA nonscience | | GPA total | | Total Matriculants |
| | Mean | SD | Mean | SD | Mean | SD | Mean | SD | Mean | SD | Mean | SD | Mean | SD | Mean | SD | |
| Biological sciences | 127.8 | 2.2 | 126.8 | 2.3 | 128.3 | 2.0 | 128.7 | 2.0 | 511.7 | 6.6 | 3.68 | 0.31 | 3.84 | 0.20 | 3.74 | 0.25 | 13,158 |
| Humanities | 127.9 | 2.1 | 127.9 | 2.1 | 128.1 | 2.1 | 129.1 | 1.8 | 513.0 | 6.1 | 3.61 | 0.33 | 3.81 | 0.22 | 3.71 | 0.25 | 849 |

(Continued)

**Table 8.2** *(Continued)* MCAT and GPAs for applicants and matriculants to US MD-granting medical schools by primary undergraduate major, 2021–2022

| Applicants | MCAT CPBS | | MCAT CARS | | MCAT BBLS | | MCAT PSBB | | Total MCAT | | GPA science | | GPA nonscience | | GPA total | | Total Applicants |
|---|---|---|---|---|---|---|---|---|---|---|---|---|---|---|---|---|---|
| | Mean | SD | Mean | SD | Mean | SD | Mean | SD | Mean | SD | Mean | SD | Mean | SD | Mean | SD | |
| Math and statistics | 129.0 | 2.1 | 127.6 | 2.3 | 128.9 | 2.2 | 129.3 | 2.0 | 514.9 | 7.0 | 3.68 | 0.35 | 3.79 | 0.24 | 3.72 | 0.29 | 161 |
| Other | 127.6 | 2.2 | 126.9 | 2.3 | 128.0 | 2.1 | 128.8 | 2.0 | 511.3 | 6.6 | 3.66 | 0.32 | 3.83 | 0.20 | 3.75 | 0.23 | 3,374 |
| Physical sciences | 128.7 | 2.1 | 127.3 | 2.3 | 128.5 | 2.1 | 128.9 | 2.0 | 513.5 | 6.7 | 3.71 | 0.29 | 3.79 | 0.24 | 3.74 | 0.25 | 2,208 |
| Social sciences | 127.4 | 2.2 | 127.3 | 2.3 | 127.8 | 2.1 | 129.1 | 1.9 | 511.7 | 6.5 | 3.60 | 0.34 | 3.77 | 0.25 | 3.69 | 0.26 | 1,974 |
| Specialized health sciences | 127.4 | 2.3 | 126.8 | 2.3 | 127.8 | 2.1 | 128.7 | 2.0 | 510.7 | 6.8 | 3.65 | 0.31 | 3.83 | 0.20 | 3.75 | 0.23 | 942 |
| *All matriculants* | *127.9* | *2.2* | *127.0* | *2.3* | *128.2* | *2.1* | *128.8* | *2.0* | *511.9* | *6.6* | *3.67* | *0.31* | *3.83* | *0.21* | *3.74* | *0.25* | *22,666* |

Abbreviations: BBLS, biological and biochemical foundations of living systems; CARS, critical analysis and reasoning skills; CPBS, chemical and physical foundations of biological systems; GPA, grade point average; MCAT, Medical College Admission Test; PSBB, psychological, social, and biological foundations of behavior.

Source: https://www.aamc.org/system/files/2021–10/2021_FACTS_Table_A-17_1.pdf.

Notes: MCAT scores and GPAs are displayed by mean and standard deviation (SD). The means and SDs of MCAT scores are calculated based on data from applicants who applied with MCAT scores (each year, approximately 2% of individuals apply without MCAT scores). Specifically, 60,334 applicants and 21,942 matriculants in 2021 were included in the calculations. Only the most recent MCAT score is used for individuals who took the exam more than once. The means and SDs of UGPA are calculated based on applicants with available GPA data. Specifically, 62,140 applicants and 22,483 matriculants in 2021 were included in the calculations. Each academic year includes applicants and matriculants that applied to enter medical school in the fall of the given year. For example, academic year 2021–2022 represents the applicants and matriculants that applied to enter medical school during the 2021 application cycle.

Please email datarequest@aamc.org if you need further assistance or have additional inquiries.

majors that are traditional (biological sciences) versus non-traditional varies between different medical schools, the proportion of non-traditional majors has been approaching nearly 50% of the student body at certain schools. So how does one choose between a traditional and non-traditional major (or both)?

One thing to keep in mind is that it is very hard to generalize—not all non-traditional or traditional majors are created equal; the constraints, demands, responsibilities, and opportunities are uniquely different between a degree in English literature, philosophy, and anthropology. The same can be said about biology and chemistry, and can even be said about the same biology major at two different colleges, and even the same biology major at the same college experienced by two different individuals. So, the advice in this section should not be taken as law, but only as general guidelines.

## 8.3.2 Pros of "Traditional" Majors

- It's mostly like the first 2 years of medical school: Courses taken in the first year of medical school can be some of the hardest, and many of them can be at least partially prepared for by taking their undergraduate equivalents. Some examples are genetics, biochem, microbiology, anatomy and physiology, neuroscience, immunology, psychology, and parts of general biology and chemistry. While anyone in any major can often take most of these courses, there is something to be said for being able to take all of them, something that is possible in biology or human biology major. Not only do some (albeit, a minority of) medical schools require some of these courses, but also excelling in them is an excellent way to show that you do not struggle with the type of material covered in medical school, even though the material is generally covered over a much longer time in undergrad.
- MCAT prep: Preparing for the MCAT is difficult and expensive, and it's one of the most important aspects of your application. Many successful students will have taken prep courses, and there never appears to be an ideal time to study. Also, many students do not immediately take the MCAT after finishing the basic medical pre-reqs. Instead, many end up waiting—often through circumstance—until years after completing the pre-reqs: when much of the information has been forgotten. A notable benefit of pursuing a traditional biology degree is that much of the pertinent scientific info on the MCAT gets repeated in numerous bio classes. DNA replication, for example, is covered in cell biology, molecular genetics, and biochemistry, and so on. You would have several shots at some of the more difficult concepts too, getting a chance to salvage (to a degree) a subpar grade obtained in a lower level science class.
- Easier transition to medical school: Medical school is a rough transition for many people. For example, the author of this section had an adjustment period getting used to the constant memorization of many facts of medical school, compared to the deep, conceptual thinking about one to five topics per week per class encountered in his philosophy major.[2,3]

## 8.3.3 Pros of "Non-Traditional Majors"

- Wider lifetime exposure to "mental models":
  - As suggested earlier, while seeing medical school material in college provides some advantage to relearning the same material in medical school, there is an opportunity cost to missing out on nonmedical material during this time. Most physicians will forget the specifics of material not immediately relevant to their field of practice. In contrast, many physicians will likely remember *general* conceptual principles and "mental models" from other fields encountered in college. By "mental models", we mean general conceptual frameworks and ways of thinking that allow you to understand and appreciate things across different disciplines. Examples of mental models include "economies of scale," "tragedy of the commons," "Veblen goods," "representativeness heuristic", and other topics from various disciplines that allow you to better appreciate the subtle contexts and interactions in your life that you otherwise might not have appreciated.
- Potential advantage for medical school admissions:
  - As stated earlier, a non-traditional major—all things being equal—likely does not confer a significant advantage to medical school admissions. However, pursuing non-traditional extracurricular opportunities

---

[2] Admittedly, this transition period only took a few weeks, and some degree of it was likely felt by all of his classmates, regardless of college major.

[3] The other authors think the above statement is ridiculous.

(e.g., political advocacy organizations, research in humanities) may provide intellectual/educational *diversity* that allows you to distinguish yourself from other applicants come application cycle.

## 8.4 Guiding Principles for Mapping Out Your Curriculum

### 8.4.1 What Are Your Passions Outside of Medicine?

Pursuing a career in medicine means you literally have a lifetime of learning the human body and biological sciences ahead of you. College is one of the best and last opportunities to dedicate significant time and attention to something interesting outside of medicine. This is a point that is difficult to appreciate until one has spent years engrossed in medicine, and the authors strongly encourage readers to spend time pursuing passions outside of medicine when they are easily able to do so.

**Admissions Highlight**

Popular interview questions during medical school applications include "What would you do if you couldn't do medicine?" and "What are your interests outside of medicine?" A non-traditional major such as Outdoor Product Design serves as strong evidence for an applicant that "loves rock climbing, camping, mountain biking" and "[if I couldn't do medicine I] would love to design better rescue devices for alpine climbing." In this regard, the applicant's major choice supports the applicant's narrative in a very significant way.

### 8.4.2 What Will Prepare You the Most?

In contrast to Principle 1, learning about the human body is HARD and there is so much information to learn that it will take you a lifetime. As such, anything you can do to study this material in college will make you that much more prepared to cover this material in medical school. While all schools expect you to be competent in the pre-medical requisite courses (biology, chemistry, physics, humanities, etc.), some majors allow you to dive deeper into human physiology and pathology than others. For example, neuroscience majors are arguably the most well-prepared students when it comes to medical school neurology classes. Showing competency in the areas of biological/chemical sciences will demonstrate your likelihood to be successful in medical school.

At the same time, one should consider the opportunity cost of studying—say—neuroscience versus sociology in college. At the end of the day, medical education is sufficiently standardized and streamlined that all graduates will have the requisite understanding of medical science to succeed as a physician. Moreover, all physicians engage in lifelong learning pertinent to their specific fields and largely forget the specifics of wholly unrelated medical topics. As such, we can also appreciate the argument for learning the *general concepts* of other seemingly unrelated fields (e.g., sociology, philosophy, computer science) to develop a lifelong repository of mental models[4]/conceptual schema versus pursuing a marginal advantage to studying more in-depth medical topics (e.g., by taking anatomy and physiology in college).

### 8.4.3 Challenge Yourself (Within Reason!)

Medical schools are looking for individuals with a sustained pattern of success in individuals that continually challenge themselves. That said, what is "challenging" varies from individual to individual depending on individual competencies in academic domains. For example, a curriculum in critical theory may be more challenging to a natural mathematician compared to a curriculum in engineering physics (and vice versa for the literature aficionado). As such, we recommend pursuing a major that aligns with both your interests *and* strengths (vs. picking something that seems "objectively" easy or difficult). While doing this, you should aim to challenge yourself in a way that ideally allows you to produce something that's tangible and impressive *without* compromising your GPA. A common example of this is an independent research project that yields a presentation or publication.

---

[4] The Great Mental Models: General Thinking Concepts. Available at: https://www.goodreads.com/book/show/44245196-the-great-mental-models. Accessed July 8, 2022.

**Admissions Highlight**

Many majors lend themselves to very different challenges that range in difficulty according to the individual. For example, calculating the static load distribution of the Golden Gate bridge—while entertaining for the engineering student—is a nightmare to the English major. However, conveying the meaning of the load distribution of the Golden Gate Bridge if left to the engineering major may be utter nonsense to the general population. We all have strengths and weaknesses, the ideal applicant is mindful of their own strengths and weaknesses and are proactive in their own development.

## 8.4.4 Skill Development

More than a degree, you should leave college with a skill set that will benefit you not only in your medical career but in multiple aspects of your life. As such, we recommend making an effort to pursue legitimate skills like statistical literacy, computer programming, foreign languages, and persuasive writing if feasible (i.e., without tanking your GPA).

**Admissions Highlight**

Each year, more qualified pre-medical applicants apply to US medical schools than there are seats available. This means that not every qualified pre-medical student will make it into medical school every year. So how then do admission committees select their students?

Out of the qualified applicant pool, admission committees "build" their classes by selecting students that will complement the overall learning of student body through their interests, experiences, and skill sets. Your classmate who majored in sociology may have experience helping refugees gain citizenship will likely add experience and expertise to your refugee clinic. A classmate that majored in statistics can help you design your research and analyze the data. The classmate who was a technical writing major can help you write that grant you've been too afraid to apply for.

## 8.4.5 College Faculty

The school, college, and department you choose to do your major with can make an innumerable impact on your success in college. In fact, the 2014 Gallup-Purdue Index found that a mentor who encouraged your goals and dreams was found to more than double the odds of being engaged at work beyond graduation for college students.[5] While large departments will typically have more resources (research, faculty, special programs, scholarships, etc.) you may be one student out of hundreds in classes where it's impossible for the professor to know each student and competition is more severe. On the other hand, smaller departments often have less funding and auxiliary programs but with smaller class sizes and therefore have more opportunities for mentorship and interaction with professors. Big or small, you should consider the departmental history of mentoring students for any major you consider.

**Admissions Highlight**

A crucial point of your medical school application will be your letters of recommendation. At least one (if not more) letter of recommendation should be from a college professor that taught you or with whom you conducted research with. Such letters of recommendation serve as "third party" assessments of your character, work ethic, and interest in medicine. Having a longitudinal relationship with a professor that can speak to these traits over the course of your college career is the gold standard.

---

[5] Great Jobs Great Lives The 2014 Gallup Purdue Index Report. Available at: https://www.gallup.com/file/services/176768/The_2014_Gallup-Purdue_Index_Report.pdf. Accessed July 8, 2022.

### 8.4.6  Don't Burn Yourself Out

You should be challenging yourself during your undergraduate years but don't feel like you need to do everything. **Be aware that whatever you choose will mean giving up something on the other side and it's impossible to do everything.** You can work to mitigate these weaknesses through extracurriculars, adding a minor, or dedicating a gap year toward these pursuits.

## 8.5  Summary

Choosing an undergraduate school and course of study is a highly personal decision. All things equal, your best bet is choosing a highly ranked institution that offers you great social support, gets its alumni into medical schools of their choosing, and has ample opportunities for relevant and interesting extracurriculars. Ideally it will not be prohibitively expensive. Your major choice largely doesn't matter; pick something that genuinely interests you and allows you to get a high GPA.

# 9 Timing, Class Structure, and Personal Schedules

*Phillip Wagner and Joel Thomas*

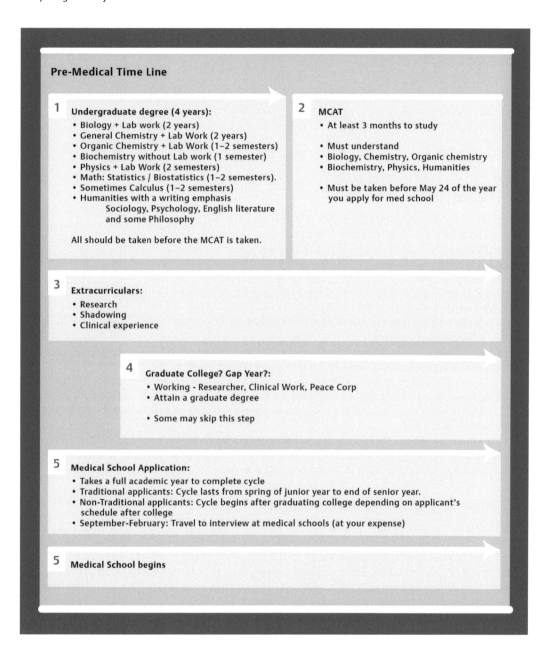

**Pre-Medical Time Line**

**1 Undergraduate degree (4 years):**
- Biology + Lab work (2 years)
- General Chemistry + Lab Work (2 years)
- Organic Chemistry + Lab Work (1–2 semesters)
- Biochemistry without Lab work (1 semester)
- Physics + Lab Work (2 semesters)
- Math: Statistics / Biostatistics (1–2 semesters).
- Sometimes Calculus (1–2 semesters)
- Humanities with a writing emphasis
    Sociology, Psychology, English literature
    and some Philosophy

All should be taken before the MCAT is taken.

**2 MCAT**
- At least 3 months to study

- Must understand
- Biology, Chemistry, Organic chemistry
- Biochemistry, Physics, Humanities

- Must be taken before May 24 of the year
  you apply for med school

**3 Extracurriculars:**
- Research
- Shadowing
- Clinical experience

**4 Graduate College? Gap Year?:**
- Working - Researcher, Clinical Work, Peace Corp
- Attain a graduate degree

- Some may skip this step

**5 Medical School Application:**
- Takes a full academic year to complete cycle
- Traditional applicants: Cycle lasts from spring of junior year to end of senior year.
- Non-Traditional applicants: Cycle begins after graduating college depending on applicant's
  schedule after college
- September-February: Travel to interview at medical schools (at your expense)

**5 Medical School begins**

Now let's go over course planning for medical school applications in more detail.

In general, US medical schools take a "holistic" approach, considering more than academic scores and numbers to evaluate applicants. They also consider your applicant "type" when constructing the incoming class (as described in Chapter 5, Building Your Narrative). That said, the two most important factors for applying to medical schools are still your cumulative undergraduate (and graduate, to a lesser extent) grade point average (GPA), and your Medical College Admission Test (MCAT) score.

**Table 9.1** Completion of requirements (courses, MCAT, extracurriculars)

| What you are doing | How you are doing it |
| --- | --- |
| Coursework for 4-year Bachelor's degree (any major) | "Reputable" 4-year US college (recommended) or transferring to 4-year US college to finish degree |
| Coursework for prerequisites | Reputable 4-year US college or reputable post-bac pre-medical program |
| MCAT | Dedicated study time after finishing most or all of your science class requirements (recommended) or part-time study over a longer period |
| Shadowing physicians | In hospitals, clinics, private practices, or operating rooms |
| Extracurricular activities | Meaningful pursuits such as hobbies, jobs, research, volunteer experiences |

## 9.1 Prerequisite Classes[1]

Medical schools generally require that applicants have taken the following classes:
- **Biology** with accompanying laboratory work (two semesters worth).
- **General Chemistry** with accompanying laboratory work (two semesters worth).
- **Organic Chemistry** with accompanying laboratory work (one to two semesters worth).
- **Biochemistry** *without* accompanying laboratory work (one semester worth).
- **Physics** with accompanying laboratory work (two semesters worth; does not have to be calculus-based).
- **Math** (usually Statistics/Biostatistics → one to two semesters worth, with possibly one or two semesters worth of Calculus).
- **Humanities classes** with writing emphases (more than two semesters worth; Sociology, Psychology, and English literature classes or some Philosophy classes may meet this criteria).

Of course, it is always possible that a specific school has different requirements. As such, we encourage you to check the websites of individual schools you are interested in to make sure that you don't miss any requirements (▶ Table 9.1).

Here is a brief overview of the application cycle to medical school and what you'll be doing (▶ Table 9.2). The timeframe of application to acceptance can take up to 1 year, running from June to about May of the following year, and this is referred to as the application cycle (more in Chapter 20, The Big Picture).

## 9.2 Interview and Admissions Process

Medical schools have Admission Committees composed of Dean of Admissions, additional faculty, and sometimes select medical students. This committee meets on a frequent basis to review candidates and vote on admission or rejection of an applicant.
- Members of this committee have access to your primary (AMCAS/AACOMAS) and secondary application information. Some members will only have access to certain parts of your application, such as essays, for example.
- Each school will differ in its process of reviewing applicants; however, one example could be this sequence:
  - Schools receive completed applications (primary and secondary applications combined).
  - A numerical cutoff limit may be used to reduce the number of qualified applications (e.g., 3.3 GPA and above and 508 MCAT and above).
  - Essays and "resume" and activities portions of the application are reviewed by committee members.
  - Application is rated by members in several categories (e.g., Interest in medicine: 8, Cultural competency: 7, Leadership: 6, Volunteer experience: 10, Research experience: 5).

---

[1] As stated before, these requirements have changed over time. This is the general curriculum meeting requirements at most schools, but we recommend double-checking with individual schools and your prehealth office.

**Table 9.2** Actual application timeline (assuming your coursework is done)

| Month | What you are doing | How you are doing it |
|---|---|---|
| April | Recommendation letters | Ask in person, then follow with formal email request |
| April-May | Personal statement | Multiple drafts, edits, and reviewed by advisors, medical students, residents, and/or physicians |
| May | Transcript | Request all colleges you have attended to send official paper transcripts to AMCAS or AACOM |
| February-May | MCAT | Study for MCAT and take the exam at an official test center |
| May/June | AMCAS or AACOMAS or TMDSAS (Texas schools only) | Online portal opens in May |
| June | Secondary essays and application | Schools will send you email requests to complete additional essays and pay additional fees online |
| Between September and March | Interviews | Schools will send you email interview invitations to schedule through an online portal. Interviews are held typically at the school and in-person |
| Between February and May | Second looks | Schools will invite you to come visit again on their Second Look Day, where you will meet other accepted students and be wooed by faculty and students to choose their school |
| July or August | Matriculation: Your first day of medical school | Usually you will have an orientation day(s) and then classes will begin |

- Committee members will decide on which applicants to extend interview invitations to.
- Applicants complete their in-person interviews with assigned faculty member and sometimes current-student interviewers.
- Interviewers rate the applicants on various categories.
- A ranking schema (specific to each school) adds up values and ranks applicants in numerical order of desirability.
- Letters of acceptance are emailed and mailed out to applicants.
- Applicants will accept or reject admissions offers.

## 9.3 Class Structure: Common Pitfalls in Scheduling

Depending on what you plan to major in, your concerns in class scheduling will be different. However, there is no reason to get complicated. We have only one rule you should follow: protect your GPA and integrity. The best way to do that is avoid some of the more common pitfalls with scheduling, such as the ones described below.

### 9.3.1 Overloading Your Scheduling

Your course-load, or the combined measure of how many credits you take per semester in context of the difficulty level of classes you are taking, is often mentioned on forums and medical admissions guides. One piece of advice I had come across several times is to stack credits or difficult classes in one semester to impress medical school admissions.

You might think that you're smarter than the average student, and you might be right. However, the risk/benefit profile probably does not work out in your favor. Ask yourself, what happens if you do well?

## Pros

If you do well, med schools can see that you can take on extra work and excel.

## Cons

Your GPA will be at risk of falling. Or—maybe—the person that reviews your application for each medical school, a person with hundreds of applications to review, may not take the time to realize that the semester credit load was more than the average student. What if your GPA was lowered from a 3.5 to a 3.45 when you took an extra 4 credits? That slight decrease in GPA would make it so you would be eliminated from the applicant pool at many different schools. What if your GPA fell from 3.75 to 3.7? You just went from average in the applicant pool to below average in quite possibly the most important factor in a strong application.

There is speculative, minimal upside. Maybe someone will crunch the numbers and realize you did more, but the downside—risking the most important aspect of your application: your GPA—is far larger. The pro gives a positive spin to a weaker application; the con can be the difference between getting into medical school and not. In our opinion this is a tactic with too small of a benefit/risk ratio. Not only does it hold little weight in the grand context of your application, but also you risk compromising your GPA. Remember, academic credentials are mostly large initial, computer-based filters. Your time and effort will be much better spent working toward deep achievement in your extracurriculars.

## 9.3.2 Too Many Science Classes with Labs

Science classes with labs are generally 4 credit hours, and medical schools often require the lab portion of the class be completed. One of the biggest myths is that a four-credit class with a lab is (1) the same amount of work as a four-credit course in another discipline and (2) only 33% more work (one credit more) than the three-credit science class without the lab. One-credit labs are time consuming (e.g., requiring 10 + page lab reports weekly), and can be almost as much work as the entire three-credit science course. They can double your work. So if you are following reasonable credit guidelines, e.g., 16 credits with four of those credits being the lab for four science classes, then you can quickly find yourself overwhelmed, something that will put your GPA at risk.

## Solution

Try to keep to only two classes with associated labs per semester.

## 9.3.3 Trying to Schedule for Maximum Quality of Life

One of the favorite student schedules—especially for commuters or those that live off campus—is the one that gives business days off. Common iterations, just due to the way classes generally work, are to load your classes on only Tuesdays or Thursdays, or conversely, Mondays, Wednesdays, and Fridays. While this can make life simpler for you early on, it tends to complicate life later in the semester and put you at risk for harming your GPA.

First, all your assignments tend to be due at the same time. This is especially important during midterms, weeks before holidays or breaks, and finals. If you have even the slightest touch of procrastination in your identity, this can be a death blow to your semester. You can cruise along for weeks before midterms, managing well, until you realize all your assignments are due on the same day. You can get away with this scheduling, but ask yourself: are you always perfectly organized? Do you ever procrastinate?

Likewise, all of your tests tend to be at the same time. You may think that you have the mental endurance to take three finals on the same day. You might be right, but you will likely not do as well as if you had three finals over 3 days. Your transcript, and your medical school application, have no spots to indicate: "give this person a break; they took all these finals on the same day."

You will also have limited flexibility. Everyone gets sick. Everyone has relatives that get sick, or worse. Many people have times when their family needs them. Virtually everyone has one of these things happen during the 4 years in school. When you are under the weather, or have to travel for a funeral, or anything you wouldn't want to miss, it is much easier to recover from missing the two classes you had on Monday, than missing the five classes you had on Monday.

You may also run into letter of recommendation issues. To get them, you have to impress your teachers. To do that, you have to be present, active, and at least pretending to be interested in class. You should be talking to your teachers afterwards, being seen, etc. Ask yourself: will being in class from 7 a.m. to 5 p.m. on a Tuesday make you very likely to look alert, be alert, or be at your best when that last class of the day starts? If you will, can you imagine doing that every time? Split up your classes into a reasonable schedule to be more likely to impress people.

### 9.3.4 Scheduling Class Times You Know Will not Work for You

Don't schedule 7 a.m. classes if you know you are one of those people that cannot function well in the morning. You will have to not only be there, but be involved, discuss, and take tests then.

### Taking Classes You Aren't Prepared for

Pre-reqs exist for a reason, but many professors will waive them if a student is passionate. Just try to avoid this and go through the steps if you are passionate. The pre-req system is also not perfect, and getting into a 400-level PoliSci course may not require any introductory PoliSci classes. Once there, it might not be until the midterm, until it's too late to drop the course, that you are in over your head. Take the easier classes, get the easier grade, and then push yourself to take the harder ones.

### Multiple Majors and Minors

If you can keep a stellar GPA while doing this, then go for it. Although it won't really impress schools much on its own, it can be a plus if it is part of your compelling narrative.

## 9.4 What Happens if I Do Poorly in a Course?

It depends on how poorly you did:
- If you received a D or an F in any pre-req, *you must retake it*. MD schools will see every grade you have ever received in a college course, so they will still see the original grade. Nonetheless, demonstrating that you actually learned the material the second time significantly helps your application.
- If you received a C or higher, we don't recommend retaking the course. We do, however, advise you to take time to relearn and conceptually understand the material well to ace the MCAT down the line. We also recommend taking upper level courses in the same subject to demonstrate that you were able to do better the second time.

## 9.5 What Do I Do with My Vacations? (e.g., Summer Break)

First and foremost, you should relax. Seriously—being pre-med can be exhausting, and it's important to give yourself time to unwind so you can hit the academic year with full force. At the same time, you should aim to be productive in *some* capacity during your breaks. Many students will use this time to conduct scientific research full-time to maximize their odds at getting presentations and publications down the line. We also recommend internships, educational experiences abroad, in-depth clinical experiences, and intensive MCAT prep if you're at that stage of the journey.

## 9.6 Personal Schedule—Why You Need One, and Why You'll Probably Enjoy It

It should be clear by now that being a successful pre-med requires juggling a seemingly endless list of commitments.

Creating and sticking to a schedule can make this herculean task manageable and—I daresay—*fun*. You might be groaning that we're trying to turn you into a mindless automaton who's a slave to the schedule. We get it. There's a sense of limitless possibility and freedom to being unfettered by your Google Calendar.

This sense is an illusion. Yes, creating and sticking to a schedule will limit the amount of time you spend procrastinating and chasing quick dopamine hits (e.g., browsing social media). At the same time, you will have the freedom to spend your scheduled leisure times *fully disengaged* from your responsibilities because you'll be enjoying your off-time guilt-free, without that uncompleted assignment looming over you.

You should also anticipate that not everyone will stick to his/her schedule 100%. That's just life—unexpected stuff happens all the time. Simply creating a schedule and committing to it even 50% of the time, however, gives you a tremendous leg-up over your unorganized self, and you will amaze yourself with your capacity for achievement—both as a pre-med and a person.

Use whatever resource allows you to stick to your schedule (e.g., Calendar app with phone reminders). Optimal schedules will vary tremendously depending on the students' needs, but we recommend the following general principles:

- For college students, create/update your schedule every academic term, as it will change dramatically with different class times. For other students, we recommend reassessing your schedule every month or so.
- Avoid multitasking. The psychological research is now clear that for cognitively demanding tasks, humans simply *cannot* multitask well. You will achieve worse results when you try to multitask anything requiring focused attention.[2] As such, we emphasize doing **deep work** whenever possible (more in Chapter 10, Obtaining a Solid GPA) and avoiding fragmenting your attention for *both work and leisure*.
- Break down large, intimidating tasks into small, concrete steps and give yourself a scheduled block of time for each small step. For example, "study everything for the final" and "write this 20-page paper" should be broken down into "I will give myself 2 hours to do all the practice problems for chapters 1–4" and "I will spend 1 hour writing the outline for the paper," respectively.
- Maximize your "idle time." Need to do 500 Anki cards today? You'd probably shock yourself with how many you'd get done on the bus instead of mindlessly checking Facebook in the same period of time.
- Enter the non-negotiable, "fixed time" items into your schedule first because you will have to work around them for the more flexible items.
  - Sleep is non-negotiable. Promote good sleep hygiene by scheduling in roughly the same times for falling asleep and waking up that allow 7–9 hours of sleep nightly. Allow yourself 30 minutes to 1 hour before falling asleep to mentally and physically unwind (e.g., no highly mentally stimulating activities, minimal screen time).
  - Mandatory school stuff (e.g., labs, mandatory lectures, small-group sessions) is mandatory.
  - Self-care is non-negotiable. Give yourself enough time in the morning/evening to shower, brush your teeth, clean your living space, dress nicely, etc.
- Identify essential tasks that allow flexibility in scheduling. Note that some tasks are better suited for *long periods of **deep** (i.e., undistracted, focused) **work***, whereas other tasks can be done in short periods around the deep work periods.[3]
  - **Exercise** needs to be *scheduled*, and you need to have a *plan* for your workouts. Don't rely on yourself to just exercise "whenever and however you can" because it *will* fall to the wayside. It can typically be done in 1- to 1.5-hour bursts. Popular times include immediately upon waking, after a long study session, or around noon to give energy for the afternoon slump.
  - **Meditation** (if you practice it) can typically be done as a 5- to 20-minute flexible block *literally* anywhere.
  - **Clinical experience/shadowing.** Plan to spend a long block or two (3–6 h) every week.
  - **Research** typically falls in this category—just be sure to allow yourself several hours at a time if needed.
  - **Studying** obviously needs to be done daily. Schedule this in 2- to 4-hour blocks using the Pomodoro technique (as per Chapter 10, Obtaining a Solid GPA).
  - **Relationships** need to be preserved. At least weekly, schedule protected time to meet up and call friends and family. Give your loved ones *focused attention*. Do not fragment your time by trying to study or catch up on social media.

---

[2] Crenshaw D. The myth of multitasking: How "doing it all" gets nothing done. Jossey-Bass; 2008. Available at: https://psycnet.apa.org/record/2008-13076-000. Accessed July 8, 2022. Cherry K. How Multitasking Affects Productivity and Brain Health. Available at: https://www.verywellmind.com/multitasking-2795003. Accessed July 8, 2022.

[3] These are not all things that every student is expected to do—just suggestions for scheduling!

- **Miscellaneous life requests:** Car break down? Find time in your schedule to go to the shop. Need groceries? Put in a time in your schedule.
- Reassess how things are working every few days or so. Are you finding that transit time (e.g., to the gym) is longer than you expected? Adjust accordingly.
- Give yourself protected daily time for **leisure**! Seriously! It's ok to put the hard brakes on working at 7 to 8 p.m. and let yourself just listen to music, surf the Web, and read books until you go to bed. Call friends and family! Not *everything* in your day needs to be completely micromanaged, and the beauty of scheduling is that you still have a remarkable degree of freedom *within* your scheduled blocks of time. We strongly advise you to avoid working during your protected leisure time to avoid burnout: you don't want to "maximize" productivity each and every day if it means burning out and losing productivity—as well as your well-being—over the long run.

## 9.7 Summary

All medical schools require completion of specific undergraduate courses; we recommend planning out your undergraduate course schedule in advance to accommodate these requirements. In addition, you should make yourself familiar with the big-picture timelines for applying to medical school. We discuss several strategies and considerations in this chapter for optimizing your schedule, both in terms of the big-picture (i.e., your overall pre-medical career) and the day-to-day timelines of being a pre-medical student.

# 10 Obtaining a Solid GPA

*Eva Roy and Joel Thomas*

It can be easy to get carried away with the seemingly endless extracurricular expectations as a pre-med. However, your grade point average (GPA) is critical in applying to medical school. Exceptional extracurricular activities will not make up for a poor GPA,[1] as GPAs are often a screening tool used to rule out applicants. MD Admissions Committees (ADCOMs) typically want to see a GPA of 3.5 or greater.[2] Based on admissions statistics for DO schools, we recommend aiming for a 3.2 to 3.3 at minimum.[3]

In addition, for most students, college is much harder than high school. Therefore, we urge you to be extremely cautious and mindful of what works for you in the first few weeks of your first semester[4] to make sure you don't tank your GPA from the get-go. In order to do this well, you need to *track* your progress (e.g., grades on quizzes and assignments), *trial* a new intervention (e.g., flashcard apps) for an adequate period of time (e.g., a few weeks), *reassess* your progress from baseline, and adjust accordingly over time as you repeat the **"track-trial-reassess" cycle**.

## 10.1 Tips for Succeeding in Your Classes

### 10.1.1 Don't Cram

In college, it can be easy to put off studying until right before the exam. There is no one telling you to study and there may be very little homework or required assignments. However, when there are only two to three exams for the whole course, performance on each exam really matters. Review content from each lecture sometime after the lecture and before the next lecture. Typically classes meet two to three times a week, so there should be time in between classes to review the content. We strongly recommend taking at least part of a day each weekend to review the material in the course thus far, with particular emphasis on developing a *cumulative understanding* of the material. This is because examiners love to test cumulative understanding of the course concepts across multiple topics on final exams! We also want to reassure you that it's ok to miss a few days here or there, or to have some suboptimal study days. Consistency is key—as long as you're spending *some* focused time reviewing the course material on most days, you will be putting yourself at a tremendous advantage compared to your peers. It also will pay off in the long run, as you will develop your work capacity and "grit,"[5] i.e., the capacity to relentlessly persevere over long periods of time—a crucial predictor of success across multiple disciplines.

This advice applies to finals and midterms, as well. You might be tempted to cram for these because they're rare events in the semester. The truth is that optimal sleep matters *the most* for these days because you will be taking long, high-stakes tests that require optimal working memory. Do *not* compromise your performance by cramming and getting less sleep.

### 10.1.2 Prioritize Active, Undistracted Studying

It's incredibly easy to delude yourself into thinking that sitting at the library for hours every day while bemoaning your lack of a social life means that you're fulfilling your pre-med duties. Doubly so if you're alternating between surfing the Internet, responding to text messages and emails, and passively re-reading and highlighting your notes.

The truth is that it's not enough to study *hard* (i.e., spending a lot of time or many hours dedicated to work). You need to learn how to spend long periods of time engaged in **deep work**,[6] or high-quality

---

[1] Or significant disciplinary violations!

[2] Kowarski I. What College GPA Is Needed for Med School? Available at: https://www.usnews.com/education/best-graduate-schools/top-medical-schools/articles/2018-10-02/how-high-of-a-college-gpa-is-necessary-to-get-into-medical-school. Accessed July 8, 2022.

[3] 2020 AACOMAS Profile Applicant and Matriculant Report. Available at: https://www.aacom.org/docs/default-source/data-and-trends/2020-aacomas-applicant-matriculant-profile-summary-report.pdf?sfvrsn=d870497_20. Accessed July 8, 2022.

[4] And ideally all throughout your academic career!

[5] GRIT. Available at: https://angeladuckworth.com/grit-book/. Accessed July 8, 2022.

[6] Newport C. *Deep work*: *rules for focused success in a distracted world*. New York; Boston: Grand Central Publishing.

engagement with cognitively demanding tasks with *minimal distractions*. Part of this involves *identifying* your distractions. Chances are these will include your phone and Internet surfing. One strategy the author strongly recommends is the Pomodoro extension/app,[7] which divides your time into periods of work versus leisure (e.g., 25 min of deep work with 5 min of a break). Divide your study blocks into several 25-minute work/5-minute break sessions, and give yourself a 20-minute long break every 2 hours or so. Over time, you will find that you will be able to further tweak the ratio of work to study (e.g., 35 min of work to 5 min break). The app will also block distracting websites during the work time and grant access to them during your break time. In addition, we recommend setting your phone to airplane mode during study sessions; if you feel the need to check texts/emails, do so sporadically every few break sessions. **Meditation**—a practice we consistently recommend throughout this book—will also improve your ability to do deep work, as there is now significant literature demonstrating that even *brief meditation practice* increases one's capacity for focused attention and executive functioning (e.g., choosing to avoid distractions and impulsive behavior).[8]

While all students should focus on deep work, each learner should figure out which *active learning* strategy works best for him/her. We distinguish active learning from the *passive learning* strategies that most of us have used throughout high school, (e.g., re-reading notes, summarizing material, and highlighting lecture content). Passive learning requires little effort, and it's easy to delude ourselves into thinking that we're being productive because we can spend hours doing it. Modern learning research, however, suggests that passive learning is probably *not* the best use of our time.[9] *Therefore, we recommend minimizing time spent on passively re-reading notes, highlighting, and rewatching lecture material.*

In contrast, **active learning** methods can help solidify the material, and most research in learning theory suggests that active study methods are a much more efficient use of time compared to passive learning. Some examples include summarizing content in your own words, spaced repetition (e.g., Anki, Quizlet), and doing practice questions to test your learning.[10] Group studying such as quizzing each other or drawing out and explaining diagrams can be beneficial as well, especially if you're able to explain and elaborate on concepts out loud to your peers.[11] For additional examples of implementing evidence-based active learning strategies, we defer to this excellent article by MedSchoolInsiders, "7 Evidence-based study strategies (& how to use each)."[12]

We also recommend that any serious academic review the free "Learning how to learn" curriculum on Coursera,[13] as the modern information economy greatly values the ability to learn and apply new material on-the-fly, compared to the outdated emphasis on memorizing and regurgitating information. Since most of us have access on our smartphones to cutting-edge encyclopedias and calculators, our ability to research, synthesize, and utilize new information becomes far more desirable. Ultimately, learning how to learn is important not only for obtaining a solid GPA, but also for a future of many more exams and being an educated, functioning member of modern society.

---

[7] Marinara: Pomodoro® Assistant. Available at: https://chrome.google.com/webstore/detail/marinara-pomodoro%C2%AE-assist/lojgmehidjdhhbmpjfamhpkpodfcodef?hl=en. Accessed July 8, 2022; Be Focused—Focus Timer. Available at: https://apps.apple.com/us/app/be-focused-focus-timer/id973134470?mt=12. Accessed July 8, 2022; Jun S. Tomato Clock. Available at: https://addons.mozilla.org/en-US/firefox/addon/tomato-clock/. Accessed July 8, 2022.

[8] Zeidan F, Johnson SK, Diamond BJ, David Z, Goolkasian P. Mindfulness meditation improves cognition: evidence of brief mental training. Conscious Cogn 2010;19(2):597–605. Available at: https://pubmed.ncbi.nlm.nih.gov/20363650/. Accessed July 8, 2022.

[9] Student News. Available at: https://studentnews.manchester.ac.uk/2021/04/29/highlighting-doesnt-work-heres-what-does/. Accessed July 8, 2022.

[10] We particularly recommend spaced repetition (e.g., Anki), as it is a highly popular strategy for studying in medical school and beyond. For additional information about how to best make use of Anki, we defer to this excellent article by MedSchoolInsiders: https://medschoolinsiders.com/medical-student/anki-flashcard-best-practices-how-to-create-good-cards/

[11] A&S Academic Advising and Coaching. Available at: https://www.colorado.edu/artssciences-advising/resource-library/life-skills/the-feynman-technique-in-academic-coaching. Accessed July 8, 2022.

[12] 7 Evidence-Based Study Strategies (& How to Use Each). Available at: https://medschoolinsiders.com/study-strategies/7-evidence-based-study-strategies-how-to-use-each/. Accessed July 8, 2022.

[13] Learning How to Learn: Powerful mental tools to help you master tough subjects. Available at: https://www.coursera.org/learn/learning-how-to-learn. Accessed July 8, 2022.

### 10.1.3 Master Both Understanding and Memorizing

Memorization gets a bad rap nowadays. It seems silly to "waste time" memorizing things that can be easily looked up with the smartphone in your pocket. That said, success in high-level biomedical sciences requires both strong conceptual understanding *and* brute-force memorization. This is very different from many other disciplines and greatly contributes to the learning curve in medical school. General chemistry, physics, and most introductory college mathematics and humanities courses tend to emphasize conceptual understanding with relatively little brute memorization. In contrast, most high school and lower-level college biology[14] courses will force you to memorize enormous amounts of information without requiring heavy critical thinking. Your college organic chemistry course will likely be the first class you encounter in college that requires you to master both cognitive domains. Top students tend to both build on their strong conceptual understanding of chemistry from general chemistry *and* memorize the seemingly endless lists of reaction mechanisms.

Balancing understanding and memorization is a skillset we encourage you to continually develop throughout your academic career. When presented with a new body of information to learn, we encourage you to use *metacognition* (i.e., thinking about your thinking) to disengage and think, "Is this something that I can understand in some conceptual way to *help* me memorize it?" For example, you will be expected to remember enormous lists of side effects for various medications in medical school. One approach to doing so would be to simply memorize everything without any context and to use spaced repetition to continually strengthen your mental associations. Another approach is creating a logical association between the *mechanism* of the drug and the side effects. While this method requires greater "activation energy" or upfront investment when sitting down to learn the material for the first time, it greatly reduces the mental effort required to *recall* the information down the line. For courses with enormous volumes of information that *also* require higher-level conceptual understanding, making the recall process easier is invaluable.

Likewise, whenever you use spaced repetition techniques (e.g., Anki), make sure that you *conceptually understand* the material presented on the flashcards before caching them in your mental association bucket. It's one thing to memorize that the body tends to become more alkaline when it loses fluid, but it's another thing to tie this to the mechanism of the renin-angiotensin system at the kidney so that you can reason your way through the association if you have trouble remembering it from brute force alone down the line. Likewise, it's also easy to deceive yourself into believing that you *understand* the material on the back of the flashcard and its association to the front when—in reality—you simply memorized the association. Be honest with yourself and mark the card as "wrong" if you couldn't flesh out the association cold.

We also encourage you to create mental webs of understanding when doing flashcards; everything in science is connected, and your conceptual understanding grows tremendously when you are able to find connections between seemingly unrelated topics.[15]

### 10.1.4 Manage Your Time with Technology

Make a list of all the exams and important due dates for the semester as soon as you get each syllabus at the beginning of the semester. Immediately enter them into your electronic schedule (e.g., Google Calendar) with appropriate reminders (e.g., several days to a week in advance for major assignments and exams). This way you can figure out when you need to start studying for each exam or start working on a project or paper. This also ensures that you don't find out you have a big assignment due the next day. Planning can be helpful in not feeling super stressed or overwhelmed when there is a week that you may have multiple exams and assignments due.

### 10.1.5 Understand Your Optimal Study Space(s)

Some people love studying at home, but that may not work if you have loud or unpredictable roommates. The library or other buildings on campus with study spaces are always a great option. If you like silence,

---

[14] And other science courses without heavy quantitative components, e.g., psychology, earth science, etc.

[15] This is also the type of thinking that Medical College Admission Test (MCAT) writers *love* to test, so do yourself a favor and get into the habit of doing it!

find quiet-only floors in the library. If you like to discuss topics with your peers, book small group rooms that allow you to draw on the whiteboard. If you get distracted by people walking by, cubicles may be the best option. If you want to get off campus, local coffee shops can be a nice change of environment. If you find that you're unable to sit still for long periods of time and study, don't be afraid to get up and change your scenery as often as needed. Find a spot(s) that can allow you to be productive for several hours at a time and makes you happy!

## 10.1.6 Reach Out for Help as Early as You Think You Need It

If you are not happy with how you are doing, then reach out for help! The earlier you reach out, the better for you and your grades. There are quite a few options. Your professor is always a great resource and should have office hours available. Always attend at least one office hour session. Establishing a relationship with your professor can be beneficial for showing that you care, as well as obtaining letters of recommendations, future classes, or research. If that feels too intimidating, then teaching assistants (TAs) are an excellent option as well, as they most likely took the class not too long ago.[16] It's also completely acceptable to show up to office hours without knowing exactly what you need help with; experienced teachers tend to be great at identifying the specific gaps in your understanding. In addition, many universities have academic resource centers with tutors for difficult courses such as organic chemistry, biology, physics. Also, reaching out to a friend who is in the same class to discuss content or how they are approaching the class can be helpful. The Internet (e.g., reddit.com/r/premed, Student Doctor Network, MedSchoolInsiders, etc.) also has abundant resources. All of these are important subjects to learn well as they appear again for your MCAT.

## 10.1.7 Don't Schedule Too Many Difficult Classes Together

The workload of pre-med core requirements can add up. Our advice is to not take all the notoriously difficult classes in the same semester. This will just lead to an extremely stressful semester with underperformance in most likely all the classes. If possible, take no more than two difficult science classes a semester. A great word of advice is to look at Ratemyprofessors.com[17] and see what people say about your professors. Take some time and do your research to make sure you have the best professors you can. If your schedule seems impossible, take summer and winter classes. Sometimes summer classes can be a great option to take time and focus on one or two classes. Also, do remember that at application time, your BCPM GPA will be specifically looked at. The BCPM GPA includes all biology, chemistry, physics, and math courses taken. Spend time and do well in these courses as they are specifically looked at. **Taking a lower credit semester (but no fewer than 12 credits per semester) and doing well is much better than an 18-credit course load with mediocre grades.**[18]

## 10.1.8 Consider Third-Party Materials

Sometimes, the course material can be presented in a way that can be really confusing. This is when outside resources can come in and save the day. Khan Academy is an excellent free tool that has hundreds of short videos going over a wide range of concepts. Organic chemistry as a second language is also a helpful tool. As always, reach out to peers, your professors, and the Internet to find the most up-to-date and useful resources.

That said, it can be easy to fall into the trap of resource overload, wherein you find yourself overwhelmed by the sheer amount of available resources and feel that you need to sample all of them to do

---

[16] That said, we generally recommend going to a professor over a TA whenever possible, as the former allows you to work toward a meaningful letter of recommendation at the same time.

[17] With a grain of salt, of course. Like most reviews, those on Ratemyprofessor are subject to reporting bias and will disproportionately show highly positive or highly negative reviews. The average student who thought the class was "ok" probably would not go out of his/her way to write a review online.

[18] If possible, take as many credits "on paper" to achieve ~16 credits per term (or whatever the average number of credits is per student). You don't want to give the impression that you're slacking. We recommend taking easy A's or pass/fail courses (e.g., doing research for credit, getting credits for a job by converting it to an academic internship, teaching assistant, etc.) to bolster your credit hours/semester if possible.

your best. In reality, there's likely diminishing returns with resources in most subjects at the undergraduate level. We generally recommend sticking to one high-quality resource and making the most of it in combination with your course material.

## 10.1.9 Take a Break!

There may be an added pressure when applying to medical school of needing an extremely high GPA. This may make you feel like you have to study at all hours of day. However, we want to emphasize it is ok and encouraged to take a break. Studying for 12 hours a day without a break can be exhausting on the mind and body. Regular breaks have been shown to help increase productivity![19]

## 10.2 So What if I Have a Low GPA?

If you have a low GPA one semester, it is generally ok as long as overall your GPA is still high by application time. In addition, a reasonably low GPA in the first semester of college is acceptable as long as you demonstrate an upward trend in GPA since then and your overall GPA by application season is competitive. Nonetheless, we want to again emphasize that you absolutely can end your chances of becoming a physician by performing poorly enough in your first semester of college. Conversely, it reflects poorly if you did really well and then start declining over time. Do not fret, you do not need a 4.0 to get into medical school. Just do your best and work hard each semester. Shoot for the moon and land among stars, as they say.

If you have graduated college with a low GPA, you can consider a post-baccalaureate program (more in Chapter 16, Gap Years, Employment, Graduate Degrees, and Post-Baccalaureate Fellowships). This is a 1- to 2-year program that can help improve your GPA and chances of getting into a medical school.

We want to *again* emphasize just how important your GPA is to applying to medical school. Your GPA is a proxy for both your work capacity over time and baseline academic aptitude. It is a measurement of 4 years of dedicated hard work. Medical schools want to see strong GPAs because medicine is one of the only careers that requires rigorous engagement with academics (i.e., "book smarts") over the *entirety of one's life*. Work hard in your classes and it will pay off in your GPA, application time, and the future when you take the MCAT—as well as when you are a practicing physician who is expected to quickly understand and apply new academic material (e.g., the new JAMA or NEJM study and its impact on your day-to-day practice). Developing strong study skills is important now and will help you for the rest of your career.

## 10.3 Summary

People have different study strategies, but some are especially evidence-based and will likely serve you exceptionally well in medical school and beyond. We recommend avoiding cramming and focusing on consistent, daily studying over time. We also recommend active, undistracted study (i.e., deep work using spaced repetition or practice problems, vs. low-effort re-reading/highlight notes); emphasizing both memorization and conceptual understanding; using technology to optimize your output; finding and creating your ideal study environment(s); avoiding scheduling too many difficult classes together; reaching out for help as early as possible; being open-minded about third-party materials; and taking breaks as needed.

---

[19] Ariga A, Lleras A. Brief and rare mental "breaks" keep you focused: Deactivation and reactivation of task goals preempt vigilance decrements. Cognition 2011;118(3):439-443 Available at: https://www.sciencedirect.com/science/article/pii/S00100277710002994?via%3Dihub. Accessed July 8, 2022.

# 11 Extracurriculars

*Eva Roy and Joel Thomas*

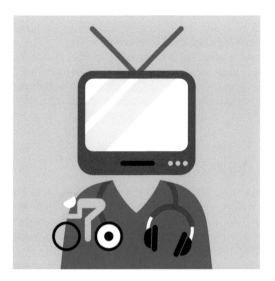

Extracurricular activity is a catch-all category for everything outside of your academics, test scores, and letters of recommendation. When pre-meds and medical school admissions refer to someone's "extracurriculars," they are referring to not only the person's hobbies and semiprofessional/professional pursuits, but also to their research, community service, clinical exposure, and leadership experiences. The American Medical College Application Service (AMCAS) application includes the following list of potential categories for extracurriculars in the "Work and Activities" section:

1. Artistic Endeavors.
2. Community Service/Volunteer—Medical/Clinical.
3. Community Service/Volunteer—Not Medical/Clinical.
4. Conferences Attended.
5. Extracurricular Activities.
6. Hobbies.
7. Honors/Awards/Recognitions.
8. Intercollegiate Athletics.
9. Leadership—Not Listed Elsewhere.
10. Military Service.
11. Other.[1]
12. Paid Employment—Medical/Clinical.
13. Paid Employment—Not Medical/Clinical.
14. Physician Shadowing/Clinical Observation.
15. Presentations/Posters.
16. Publications.
17. Research/Lab.
18. Teaching/Tutoring/Teaching Assistant.

Thus, while a pre-med applicant with **strong numbers** has a high grade point average (GPA) and Medial College Admission Test (MCAT) score, an applicant with **strong extracurriculars** has a strong background/experience in two or more of the categories in research, community service, clinical experience, and leadership.

---

[1] Note that with this "Other" designation, your extracurriculars could literally include anything.

Ideally, you want to be an applicant who has strong numbers *and* strong extracurriculars. The majority of students who get into top medical schools have strong numbers and virtually everyone there has very strong extracurriculars. We will again, however, emphasize that for the vast majority of applicants, strong extracurriculars will *not* make up for a weak GPA and MCAT. As such, if you feel that you are unable to commit to your extracurricular demands, you should gracefully disengage and refocus your efforts on academics. You will always have time to add additional extracurriculars to your application (e.g., vacations, gap year(s)), but poor academics are dramatically harder to salvage.

The totality of your extracurriculars helps paint a picture that stands out from the crowd of applicants and so it is a big piece of your pre-med preparation. In the following chapters (12, Clinical Experiences; 13, Shadowing; 14, Volunteering; and 15, Research), we will discuss in greater detail specific categories of extracurriculars that are *de facto* requirements for admission. In the remainder of this chapter, we will focus on extracurriculars in general, with greater emphasis on activities not covered in those chapters.

## 11.1  So What Can You Do?

With classes, research, volunteering, and shadowing, you probably think there is absolutely no time left to do any extracurriculars. As a pre-med student, there are a lot of things that you have to balance. That is why it is important to get involved with activities that you truly enjoy; otherwise, it will be hard to stay committed when your time is short (which is to say—often). Most schools have an activities fair during orientation week, where you may be tempted to sign up for 10 different clubs. Although the fair can be slightly overwhelming, it is a great way to see what your college offers and what you might be interested in.

### 11.1.1  Medically Related Clubs

There are a variety of clubs that you can get involved in. You might be inclined to get involved with a medically related club as you want to pursue a career in medicine. There are the classic American Medical Student Association (AMSA) or Pre-Medical Organization for Minority Students (POMS). These types of clubs truly can be hit or miss. Some chapters might provide you with great resources about what professors to take for classes and older students as mentors while others might not be that helpful and can lead to you constantly comparing yourself to other members. **Please remember that you definitely do not have to join any of these medically related clubs.** If you find that they will be beneficial for you, then go ahead! But there is no rule that if you are not in one, you are not interested in medicine.

### 11.1.2  Non-Medically Related Clubs

Since most of your other activities are medically related, this is the time for you to truly show what you are passionate about. Go ahead and join the Harry Potter Club or Salsa Club! Medical schools prefer to see that you are in fewer clubs and you stick with them, rather than being a member of 10 different clubs. If you truly enjoy something, then you are more likely to continue going to meetings even when school is busy or the meeting is on a Sunday night at 9 p.m. before an exam. If you are truly passionate about what you are doing, you will be able to speak about it enthusiastically in interviews.

### 11.1.3  Sports

There are so many different options to pursue. If you were a high school athlete and would like to continue that, join an intramural or club sport team. If you were a debate super star in high school, join your school's speech and debate team. If you played an instrument in high school, join the marching band or symphonic orchestra. These types of clubs foster a sense of community and can be a great way to make lifelong friends. Don't be afraid to join something because you think it will take up too much time. Unfortunately, your free time only decreases once you are in medical school or residency, so now is truly the time to spend your free time the way you want to!

## 11.1.4  Sororities, Fraternities, and Professional Societies

Another category you might be thinking of are sororities, fraternities, and professional medical fraternities. If you want to get involved with Greek life, then go ahead. *Just be aware that some people (e.g., Admissions Committee (ADCOM)) hold negative stereotypes about Greek life. As such, be extremely mindful of doing anything that could be perceived (e.g., on social media) as illegal or unethical as a member of Greek life (e.g., hazing, risky underage drinking).* In addition, "pledging" a fraternity is associated with decreases in GPA, likely due to the significant psychological and time demands.[2]

At the same time, fraternities often fundraise significant amounts for charities by virtue of their prominent role in the social scene on campus. As such, responsible participation in Greek life can be a great way to gain leadership and volunteer experience that makes a genuine, tangible impact on campus and beyond. Also, medical fraternities can be a great way to gain connections and hear about opportunities for research or other cool medically related things going on at your university.

You will also most likely hear about honor societies. There is no need to join every one that you get invited to. Instead, take time to see the requirements of each and how prestigious they are. For example, one of the most well-known honors academic societies is Phi Beta Kappa as it is the oldest one in the United States. That said, we feel that you most likely will not gain much by joining an honor society beyond putting it on your resume (unless you are unusually active within the society).

## 11.1.5  Explore Your Passions

College can be a great time to explore clubs or activities that your high school did not offer. This can be the time to discover a passion that you might not even know you have had. For example, there are a ton of different dance teams ranging from Bollywood to hip hop or jazz. Sometimes you need stress relief from all your pre-med classes, and extracurriculars can provide that! If your college does not offer a club that you were hoping to join, then you can even start it. Starting a club is a great way to show initiative and leadership on your medical school application.

Along this line, do not limit yourself to just clubs. If you want to dedicate your free time to building an app or starting a nonprofit, go for it! Showing that you are well rounded and unique can be advantageous when it comes application time, so do not be afraid to stray from the typical pre-med path. There are no stringent guidelines that you have to join an *x* amount of clubs. Spend your limited free time the way you want to. Just don't waste it.

## 11.1.6  Other Leadership Opportunities

If you are worried about leadership positions or are not interested in joining any clubs, then a great opportunity is mentoring or tutoring. Tutoring shows that not only did you excel in that course material, but you can also communicate it and teach it to your peers. In addition, being a teaching assistant (TA) for a class is an excellent opportunity to gain connections to faculty at your school and can help down the lane for letters of recommendation.

## 11.1.7  Non-Traditional Extracurriculars

Extracurriculars don't have to be related to your university. For example, extracurricular activities can also include jobs. There are many medically related options such as working as a scribe in a hospital or a patient care tech. These can both provide valuable experiences and be great talking points during your interview and application. In addition, your university may have paid jobs working in the medical school library or office of undergraduate research. Also, your job doesn't have to be medically related. It could be teaching a workout class or being a barista at your local coffee shop. As long as you are happy doing it and learn from the experience, that's what matters.

We really do encourage you to be creative with your extracurriculars. Seriously, think of the things that *genuinely make you happy*—that you actually spend your free time on—and brainstorm ways to turn these

---

[2] Even WE, Smith A. Greek Life, Academics, and Earnings. Available at: https://papers.ssrn.com/sol3/papers.cfm? abstract_id=3257025. Accessed July 8, 2022.

into achievement-focused extracurriculars that you can sell to medical schools. Do you like to sing in your free time? Join or start a music group. Do you like video games? Play competitively or consider spearheading a program that uses video games as therapy for hospitalized children. Again, if you are genuinely passionate about what you do, you will be much more likely to excel in it and to gain transformative insights along the process.

## 11.2 What Are Medical Schools Looking For?

Medical schools want to see commitment, passion, and leadership. These are all qualities that will lead to a compassionate well-rounded physician. The journey to becoming a doctor is a long road. ADCOMs want to see that you are someone who is able to commit to what you put yourself into. You can show commitment by staying involved in a club or activity for all 4 years of college. It looks better to be in a few clubs for a longer period of time than just being in a ton of clubs for 1 year here and there.

The passion will come through when you talk about it in your interview or your application. At the same time, consistent journaling—*as we've recommended several times in this book already*—will make it significantly easier to generate deep insights about your experiences for applications and interviews. We recommend periodically checking in (e.g., at the end of each semester) on your longitudinal extracurricular experiences by reflecting on what you accomplished, what you wish you had accomplished, what you plan to do next semester, and how you felt overall with the extracurricular activity.

We also recommend against stretching yourself out by joining so many clubs that you are only involved with each of them minimally. When it comes to application time, you won't be able to talk about them in length. By dedicating yourself to only a few extracurriculars, you can achieve so much more.

The passion ties into the 6 pillars of an applicant we discussed earlier. Medical schools want to see passion and deep achievement. These attributes can be seen from your level of commitment to your extracurriculars. The more you put into your extracurriculars, the more you will get out. This is the one part of the application that you have the freedom to show who you (i.e., developing your narrative) truly are beyond the numbers. Your outstanding extracurricular activities could be the turning point to pick you versus someone who has the same numbers as you.

Finally, leadership can take form in a variety of ways. Associate Dean of Admissions at the David Geffen School of Medicine at UCLA, Dr. Theodore Hall explains, "We're looking for students who want to become leaders in academic, community, research, and policy areas. Leadership experience could come from being mentors or teachers, officers in student organizations or research PIs or coauthors. Leadership takes different forms."[3] The leadership skills you gain from your extracurriculars can be important indicators of your future career path.

There are so many extracurriculars to choose from, so choose wisely. Assistant Dean of Admissions at the University of Michigan Medical School, Steven Gay says, "Let us know who you are, and put yourself in the best light you can. We want to know what is important to you and what you are passionate about."[4] The extracurriculars you choose reflect on your core values and can show so much about you to the application committee. The decisions you make reflect on what you value and what is important to you.

At the end of the day, extracurriculars are something that you should *want* to do! You should not feel forced to do anything. There are so many different options to choose from. Do not think that you have to do every medically related club your college offers. There is no formula on what are the right extracurriculars to get into medical school. Remember, this is a part of the application that can really set you apart and make you memorable from other applicants. So truly take time and consider what you are passionate about and join those clubs!

## 11.3 Summary

Great academics alone are unlikely to get you into medical school; you need interesting extracurriculars to add multidimensionality to your application. Fortunately, the sky's the limit in terms of your extracurricular options. Virtually anything that interests you can be pursued as an extracurricular activity that can strengthen your medical school application and allow you to grow as a person.

---

[3] UCLA. Available at: https://medschool.ucla.edu/body.cfm?id=1158&action=detail&ref=971. Accessed July 8, 2022.

[4] 8 Ways to Make Your Medical School Application Shine. Available at: https://labblog.uofmhealth.org/med-u/8-ways-to-make-your-medical-school-application-shine. Accessed July 8, 2022.

# 12 Clinical Experiences

*Phillip Wagner and Joel Thomas*

Aside from your grades, test scores, and research, medical schools care about your experiences. All of your jobs, volunteer positions, clubs, and shadowing fit into the "experience" category, which Admissions Committees (ADCOMs) will make you classify into clinical or nonclinical experiences.

Clinical experiences entail exposure to direct patient care. It's a broad category, comprising a wide array of options. The types of clinical experiences can be grouped into some general categories, including shadowing, medical employment, and medical volunteering. The following chapters describe each of these in detail. What's important to take away is the following[1]:

- 73% of medical schools "highly recommend or require" applicants to have clinical experience when they apply.
- 87% of medical schools believe applicants without clinical experience put themselves at a disadvantage.

While it's technically possible to get admitted to medical school without clinical experience, our opinion is that even a "pointed" applicant would be wise to have *some* clinical experience on their resume, as the vast majority of medical schools treat it as a likely (but not definite) red flag to lack clinical experience. We therefore suggest having at least one significant (ideally longitudinal) clinical experience that is in keeping with your narrative for why you would make an excellent doctor, even if your application suggests community service, the humanities, bench research, or something else is your primary strength.

Of all the things you can control in your application process, one of the things you cannot directly control is who interviews you and what their values are. Consider that even at those 13% of medical schools that do not feel a lack of clinical experiences hurts you, you will still be interviewed by individuals with their own biases and opinions. The truth is that despite what criteria interviewers are asked to rate a candidate on, if they themselves feel a wealth of clinical experience is necessary to be a doctor, they might penalize you for it. Even more likely is that it may be difficult for an interviewer to sell your case for admission to the committee if your story is "I always wanted to be a doctor," and yet you have never bothered to shadow, volunteer, work, or do research in a clinical environment that would indicate you know what you are getting yourself into. It's a fair question to ask yourself, as well, before you travel down a very arduous path; if you have never done those things, do you *actually* know you want to be a doctor?[2]

One last caveat: Not all schools have perfect overlap in how they classify clinical experiences. If you are disproportionately interested in admission to a specific medical school, it will pay off to figure out what they consider "Clinical Experience." It would be quite unfortunate to believe that your shadowing counted, only to find out later that your preferred institution reviewed your application, counted it as a nonclinical experience, and is one of a majority of schools that feels this puts you at a disadvantage. So, if a particular school really matters to you, then you should make sure you know what they specifically are looking for.

Some things to consider:

- Many clinical experiences will have logistical obstacles to overcome before you are able to start. For example, many healthcare settings require being thoroughly vaccinated before setting foot in a clinical environment. To be on the safe side, consider getting up-to-date on the following vaccination schedule that the Association of American Medical Colleges (AAMC) puts forth for medical students: https://www.aamc.org/system/files/c/2/440110-immunizationform.pdf
- If your undergraduate institution has many pre-medical students, you may be competing with them for time slots at the most popular, well-known clinical experience opportunities. As a result, you may find yourself gritting your teeth during your weekly hours at Clinical Site X that was unpopular among your peers for a variety of reasons (e.g., staff basically treat you like a ghost, rude patients, etc.). If you find yourself in this scenario, we recommend reaching out to upperclassmen, your prehealth office, the Internet, and *local healthcare professionals* for the insider scoop on "hidden gem" clinical experiences.

---

[1] Clinical Experiences Survey Summary. Available at: https://www.aamc.org/media/23336/download. Accessed July 8, 2022.

[2] Of course, we later point out in Chapter 41, Real Talk on a Medical Career that you probably will never get a realistic perspective on many of the grievances of practicing medicine until you're actually deep into medical training, when it's functionally too late to turn back.

- Be wary of medical mission trips. These have recently become very controversial due to cultural issues of "voluntourism."[3,4] Simply put, many well-intentioned organizations coordinate short-term medical missions to developing countries with the intention of providing medical care that is otherwise scarce in that country. However, emerging research suggests that this has unintended consequences for the local communities and that many of these trips allow participants to perform procedures that they otherwise would not be qualified to perform in their home countries.[5] At the same time, we recognize that the opportunity to engage in medical care abroad can be a transformative experience to those interested in international health. As such, we recommend doing extensive research on the particular organization you are considering working with to make sure that they abide by strict ethical guidelines before engaging in international medical work—especially when you don't have any specific medical qualifications yourself.

## 12.1 Summary

We explore each of the possible types of clinical experiences in depth in the following chapters. The most important points to remember:
- Have at least one significant, meaningful, and prolonged clinical experience, but generally more if possible.
- Not having a clinical experience puts you at a disadvantage regarding the vast majority of medical schools.
- Most applicants have clinical experiences, so if you do not, *you will stand out in a bad way.*

---

[3] Sullivan HR. Voluntourism. Available at: https://journalofethics.ama-assn.org/article/voluntourism/2019-09. Accessed July 8, 2022.

[4] 7 Reasons Why Your Two Week Trip to Haiti Doesn't Matter (An Update). Available at: https://medium.com/@cryptor-egs/7-reasons-why-your-two-week-trip-to-haiti-doesnt-matter-an-update-a9a934ef3c8b. Accessed July 8, 2022.

[5] The justification presumably being that scarcity makes it acceptable. After all, some might argue that a suboptimal screening pap smear that identifies precancerous changes is preferable to no screening exam that leads to full-blown invasive cancer down the line.

# 13 Shadowing

*Philip Wagner*

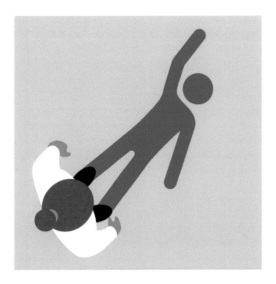

## 13.1 What Is Shadowing?

In the context of medical school admissions, shadowing is the act of literally following a doctor around during the course of their day—seeing what they experience, enjoy, and endure. It is seeing a day in the life of a doctor by being the shadow behind them.

## 13.2 Why Is It Important?

Like other clinical experiences, it shows that:
- *You are actually interested enough in medicine to try to see what it is like to be a doctor, and you still want to move forward despite the drudgeries*; Admissions Committees (ADCOMs) want to know—among other things—that what you know about medicine isn't solely informed by what you see on TV. You can even use shadowing to see if you are really interested in medicine as a career. Moreover, you have spent enough time experiencing the realities of a typical day as a physician. You understand that—at the end of the day—it's *simply a job* in many respects, much like being an accountant or a cashier. The days are not jam-packed with exciting, life-altering decisions. Instead, much of what you will do is mundane secretarial work (e.g., extensive documentation, playing phone tag with secretaries and hospital operators) that's necessary to uphold the medicolegal framework of modern medicine. And yet, you *still* want to become a physician—suggesting a more mature, developed passion for medicine.
- *You have some insight regarding avenues for improvement within the medical system:* You are aware of some of the benefits as well as some of the flaws. ADCOMs ideally would like to produce physicians who actively work toward improving the *systems* of medical care. Applicants who can intelligently discuss shortcomings of the current system, (e.g., in their personal statement, secondary essays, and medical school interviews) will stand at an advantage.
- *You read their prerequisites:* Some schools require shadowing to even review an application and consider you. Getting into medical school can be very much a numbers game, and ruling out certain schools—especially local, state, or Doctor of Osteopathic Medicine (DO) schools who tend more often to require shadowing—is not a risk some of you will want to take.

Other than helping your application, shadowing has some very real benefits as well:

- *It's relatively easy to do.* Unlike other ways of gaining clinical experience, shadowing is usually free, flexible to schedule, and generally a minimal commitment activity.
- *It can help develop your interest in medicine further.* It is incredibly common for an applicant to gain interest in a specific medical field or specialty by shadowing a doctor in that field. Likewise, it's incredibly common for an applicant to rule out a specialty that he/she was originally interested in after spending enough time understanding the day-to-day realities of that specialty.

## 13.3 How Are These Shadowing Experiences Weighed by Admissions Committees?

Every school's ADCOM weighs certain experiences differently. Shadowing is no different. And just like research or community service, some schools even require that you engage in some shadowing to even be eligible for admission. However, like any other experience, you can almost guarantee that your experiences will also be weighed regarding how long you shadowed, how in-depth your experience was, and what you took away from those experiences as assessed by what you said during the interview or wrote in your application.

Remember, quality is more important than quantity. Instead of shadowing eight different doctors for 5 hours each, it may be more beneficial to try for more hours with fewer doctors.

The question of "How much shadowing do you need to do?" comes up frequently. The answer is disappointingly vague, not terribly evidence-based, and specific to both the institutions to which you apply and what your strengths and weaknesses as an applicant are. Recommendations normally follow some anecdotal evidence. "I did [insert x number of hours] of shadowing, and I got in." However, there is not great data on what is a sensible yet competitive number.

Some schools require it, and some don't. However, the differences do not end there. Even at the same institution, some of your interviewers will value shadowing very differently, and there is a wide spectrum. We have colleagues who do not care if you have shadowed at all, but also have colleagues who think it is as important as wearing business attire to the medical school interview—it's an essential checkbox for them. The trouble for you is that you don't know which of these types of people is going to interview you—and medical schools don't screen their interviewers by their opinions on shadowing. Be aware, however, that *95% of matriculating MD students participated in physician shadowing in 2020.*[1]

For this reason and the others listed above, we strongly recommend engaging in at least 100 hours of shadowing across at least three different providers, with at least one being a primary care physician (e.g., family medicine, outpatient internal medicine, or general pediatrics). If you plan to apply to DO schools, you should have at least 50 hours of shadowing an osteopathic physician (even better if he/she uses osteopathic manipulative treatment).[2]

## 13.4 Nuts and Bolts of Shadowing

### 13.4.1 First Contact

Getting shadowing experience generally is not hard, especially if you live near a hospital. Here are some different ways to go about this:

- **Reach out:** Setting up a shadowing experience can be as simple as calling a doctor's office, telling them that you are interested in going to medical school, and asking if you can shadow. You can also email the doctor; many doctors have official email addresses listed on their hospital's website. Attaching your resume to the email to share a little about yourself can increase your success rate.
- **Use your network:** Family, friends, research mentors, and, especially, your pre-medical advisor, etc. Simply ask them if they know any physicians or anyone who works in healthcare who could introduce you to a physician. Cold-calling or emailing practicing physicians can be fairly inefficient—sometimes knowing someone (especially a pre-med advisor or a personal contact in healthcare) can really boost your efficiency.

---

[1] (AAMC 2020 Matriculating Student Questionnaire), https://www.aamc.org/media/50081/download
[2] To locate osteopathic physicians in your area, you can use the helpful database search at http://www.osteopathic.org/

- **Go through more standardized methods:** Bigger hospitals often have channels for going about shadowing. Like applying to volunteer, they require an application to be filled out, and it may take a few weeks to get placed with a doctor. However, these programs may have minimum or maximum hour requirements of which you may want to make a note. Some are significant time commitments, and may even require payment to participate, which means they are not open to everyone. However, if you are able to convey that they were significant clinical experiences for you, they can pay big dividends in application strength.

### 13.4.2 Meeting the Doctor

Dress nicely as if for a job interview when you finally sit down to meet with the doctor. Bring another copy of your resume. Let them know you are hoping to go to medical school and interested in learning more about becoming a doctor. Be cordial and also ask a few questions about medicine, being a physician, and practicing their specialty. This way even if the doctor ends up declining your request to shadow, you gained at least a little insight. Politely ask for shadowing opportunity possibilities and then get started! Ask for just a few preliminary sessions. Don't ask to do once a week right off the bat, for example. You will see why next.

### 13.4.3 The Quest for The One

Now that you have scheduled shadowing with one physician, go find several more physicians to shadow. Try to get at least three different physicians to shadow initially. Then, after going to one or two sessions with each doctor, pick and go with the doctor who you had the best connection with *and* has time to talk to you. Doing so brings several benefits: You learn more from the experience, get opportunities to ask questions and receive answers, and you may potentially develop a good relationship with the physician which in turn may result in a recommendation letter from him or her.

Now, of course, the overall goal of shadowing is to observe things about medicine and what physicians do; not necessarily to get a recommendation letter. But getting a recommendation letter from a physician can only help you, not hurt you. So if you can get one, you should. And obviously the better your rapport and interactions with the doctor is, the stronger your recommendation letter will potentially be!

Not all physicians will agree to write you a recommendation letter, however, just because you shadowed them. They will say they won't have much to write about you since you just sat there like a fly on the wall. If you shadow a physician who won't or can't interact much with you, they are right. That is why shadowing a surgeon in the OR—while it may be awesome to observe—won't yield a better recommendation letter than shadowing a family physician who takes the time to talk to you, has lunch with you, etc. You can still shadow in the OR for example, but don't expect a recommendation letter to come from doing that. Start shadowing physicians with whom you can potentially develop great relationships with (e.g., by asking intelligent, insightful questions about their lives and careers). Then you can move onto other specialties of medicine also if you desire. After this you have shadowing experiences with at least a few different physicians and at least one who can say some great things about you for your application. Win!

One word about selecting physicians based on their backgrounds: Just because a physician is an alumni of a certain medical school doesn't necessarily give you any advantage in applying to that school if you receive a recommendation letter from him or her. However, if the physician is currently a *faculty member* at a medical center or hospital strongly affiliated with the particular medical school or actually a faculty member of the medical school, this may give you a slight boost when applying to that same medical school—if the physician writes a very strong letter that is. However in my opinion, finding a physician you can connect well with regardless of their background or affiliation pays larger dividends.

## 13.5 Shadowing Basics

Your shadowing experience will largely be what you make of it. Physicians are busy people, and even though your mentor may be eager to engage you with the vagaries of their practice, they will likely be more focused on the demanding tasks of doctoring. As such, you should try to ask thoughtful questions about what you witness. Ideally, you'll have done *some* background reading on what to expect so you can ask informed questions. For example, "I read that there's still no good agreement on the *best* treatment option for this patient's condition. Why did you recommend X vs. Y?" That said, there's no need to over-burden yourself with deep, detailed research on the specifics of your mentor's field. Your mentor will likely be impressed by any demonstration of interest in what they do.

In addition, we recommend that you bring and write in a journal. Record all your impressions, thoughts, and observations either between patient encounters or right after you finish shadowing. Especially write down what you thought initially about something, but realized was different after observing. These kinds of minilessons make good material incorporating into your narrative, application essays, and interviews (e.g., "Tell me about a meaningful shadowing experience/patient encounter"). Try to write stories and anecdotes. These will serve as excellent material to use when it comes time to write your personal statement and secondary essays. It could also become useful for your school interviews.

Business casual attire is appropriate for shadowing, unless the doctor or an attendant at the office speci-fies otherwise. You can always google "business casual" if you are unsure what business casual entails. If you are shadowing in the operating room, you may or may not be asked to change into scrubs. If there's a possibility of shadowing in the operating room, you should bring a pair of shoes you'd feel comfortable standing in for several hours.

Be extra polite and friendly. Do not address the doctor by his or her first name unless he or she explic-itly gives you permission or ask you to do so.

Be enthusiastic. Use your common sense and best judgment to modulate your affect and disposition (e.g., don't be grinning ear-to-ear when a patient breaks down into tears).

Ask thoughtful questions, and even prepare a few ahead of time if you want. In general, ask the physi-cian *judgment/value*-based questions, versus factual questions that you can easily Google. Consider asking why the physician chose this particular field of medicine and this particular practice type. What other fields did they consider? What do they enjoy the most and least about their day? How does they antici-pate their practice—and medicine more broadly—changing in the next few years? Would they do it all again? If so, would they do anything differently? What were the best decisions they made along their career?

Don't expect to learn or understand much *medical* decision-making. This will come with years of medical training, and no physician will expect you to understand the intricacies of clinical judgment while shadow-ing. Instead, focus on what the physician spends *most* of his/her time doing. Paperwork? Emails? Common medical conditions that are not particularly exciting? Try to put yourself in the physician's shoes and antici-pate how you would *feel* doing such things over and over again for decades. Keep in mind, however, that your values and preferences will change tremendously over the course of your life. What may seem boring now may seem comforting years down the line. Likewise, what may seem exciting in the moment may eventually become stressful (e.g., when your family's livelihood may be impacted by a malpractice suit).

To protect patient privacy, before beginning to shadow, you may be asked to sign a Health Insurance Portability and Accountability Act (HIPAA) form agreeing not to disclose patient information.

If you are observing during a doctor's clinical visit with a patient, the doctor often will inform and ask permission from the patient for you to stay in the examination room. Most patients are fine with you staying in the room, but don't take it personally if a patient feels uncomfortable or says no to you observ-ing. If you are in the room try to be discreet and out of the doctor and patient's way. Don't interrupt the doctor or talk to the patient unless you are asked to join the conversation. Be a fly on the wall. Smile.

Eventually things may get a little more casual as you and the doctor get to know each other; however, always maintain professional conduct and respect for patients.

After each shadowing session don't forget to thank the doctor for his or her time and for the opportu-nity. Make sure you also send a thank you email after the first session, and definitely after your very final session.

Keep in mind—if you feel like you are not developing a great relationship with the doctor after a few sessions, it's probably time to move on and find a doctor who you can better connect with. Use your gut instinct.

On your last day of shadowing remember to politely ask for a recommendation letter in person. Contact them immediately with your recommendation letter materials while you are fresh on their mind. **Use social cues—don't ask for a recommendation letter if you haven't established some sort of relationship.**

## 13.6 How Does Shadowing Develop Your Narrative?

Let's examine an example as to how shadowing helps develop an applicant's narrative.

*Kevin is a neuroscience major: grade point average (GPA) 3.3, no research experience, and has the Medical College Admission Test (MCAT) scheduled for 3 months from now. He has very little clinical experience, having only volunteered at a hospital emergency department for 3 months.*

- *Forty hours with a family practice Doctor of Osteopathic Medicine (DO) in an outpatient clinic.*
- *Forty hours in an outpatient neurology headache clinic.*
- *Forty hours following an inpatient neurologist on the stroke service.*

So, let's analyze these choices. One hundred and twenty hours is a good amount of time spent shadowing, higher than almost any medical school, DO or MD, requires. The student got an impressive breadth of experience in such a short time, and managed to further specify their interest. While neuroscience got them interested in medicine initially, they have experienced what the life of both an inpatient and outpatient neurologist can look like, and further solidified their interest in not just medicine, but a specific type of medicine. This fits an easy narrative for the admissions committee, telling a logical and clear story, and helps the candidate in all the ways listed above, plus a few ways specific to the candidate's situation.

The candidate has a 3.3 GPA, and an unknown MCAT score, as well as no research. This student could very well get into an MD program, but is not a very competitive applicant, so admission is not assured. This candidate should therefore also be considering DO schools. Shadowing a primary care doctor not only got the patient some experience and knowledge (including outpatient internal medicine, pediatrics, and obstetrics and gynecology) while benefiting their application, but also gave the patient some experience shadowing a DO—something many DO schools require. This student, if asked on interviews and essay prompts, can speak more knowledgeably and convincingly about the differences and similarities between MDs and DOs while increasing the number of schools at which they are eligible to interview.

## 13.7 Summary

Shadowing is witnessing a "day in the life" of a doctor. It is a relatively efficient, easy, and cheap means of improving your application, and is also a great way for you to explore different aspects of the profession. Some schools require shadowing to even consider your application. There are multiple ways to obtain shadowing experience; these include contacting doctor's directly, or going through an official hospital channel. Every applicant should do at least some shadowing, but there is no good data on the right amount of shadowing time to experience. The best answer depends on assessing your own strengths and weaknesses as an applicant. In addition, your shadowing experience will be much more meaningful if you do some background reading and ask informed questions on what you see. You should also take note of the aspects of shadowing that you genuinely enjoy vs. despite. These insights will help you better understand *why* you want to become a physician (or why you might *not* want to become a physician!) and what aspects of medicine you may be drawn to.

# 14 Volunteering

*Phillip Wagner and Landon Cluts*

Medicine is an opportunity to serve people. Physicians impact so many lives, making volunteering an important aspect of any medical school application. However, it is not just enough to perform volunteering; you must also be able to articulate convincingly what that volunteering means about you as a candidate.

For application purposes, there are two types of volunteering: medical volunteering and nonmedical volunteering.

## 14.1 Non-Medical Volunteering

This is volunteering in a nonhospital or clinical setting. For many applicants, this will be less helpful than medical volunteering, which also counts toward clinical experience. Nonetheless, nonmedical volunteering can still be beneficial in terms of demonstrating that there is more to you than your interest to be involved in medicine—that you are not just an automaton designed for the purpose of getting into medical school. For example, let's suppose you had spent several hours every week volunteering at a women's shelter, or working for a sexual abuse hotline; these can be powerful, formative experiences that can shape your outlook and compassion as a future doctor, and may even affect what type of specialty you decide to pursue. For that reason, these experiences are allowed to be taken as seriously as you decide, and in some cases can even make up the most significant part of your application.

Examples of this type of volunteering include, but are not limited to:
- Volunteering in a soup kitchen.
- Helping out with a clothing drive.
- Volunteering at the animal shelter.
- Organizing an event for charity (marathons, auctions, drives, etc.).
- Tutoring/mentoring others without pay.
- Starting your own charity group or organizing your own event.
- Literally any type of volunteering that isn't explicitly medical!

If you are involved in nonmedical volunteering in a notable administrative, creative, or leadership capacity, this can help tremendously in displaying who you are and what you are capable of to an admissions team. Did you volunteer weekly in a soup kitchen for several years? That is certainly admirable and worthy of inclusion in your application. However, it can be even more impressive that you lobbied your college to fund a group that you founded that puts on weekly soup kitchens in your city. You had the idea, you used an interdisciplinary skill-set to bring it all together, and you have the social skill, leadership ability, and organizational prowess to keep this organization running smoothly. Many of these skills are universal, and it does not matter that they were displayed in a nonmedical setting. Not every experience needs to be this impressive, but we did want to illustrate just how illustrative this type of experience—one that is often overlooked—can be regarding your skills, initiative, and leadership ability.

## 14.2 Medical Volunteering

Medical volunteering is some type of volunteering that is done in a medical setting. The opportunities available for this type of experience are very accessible.

Examples of this type of volunteering include:
- Hospitals (most have volunteering departments).
- Nonprofit organizations (Red Cross, homeless shelters, free clinics, etc.).
- College (many schools or the clubs they sponsor carry out some type of medical outreach). If these fail, many schools have a prehealth advisor; ask them about what experiences have students really benefitted from in the past. Look around your area! More importantly, if you don't see something you want to be a part of, create something that fills that niche. It is more work, but chances are, if you want something, you can find a group of like-minded individuals who can share the load.

## 14.3 Which Type to Engage in?

Like other experiences, not all medical volunteering experiences are created equal; some are not only better for your application, but better for creating the type of person that will succeed in medical school and beyond. It may even influence what type of medicine you want to eventually practice. When selecting your experience, select for those types of experience that:

- **Allows you ample access to patients in a significant way:** Being a hospital greeter may be easy and low-stress, but volunteering to talk to terminally ill patients or play with children in the oncology ward is going to give you better insight into the patient experience and the hardships that accompany it (i.e., specific formative experiences that you can speak about in your applications and interviews). So, **be selective**, and do research/ask around for advice on what type to engage in.
- **Allows you ample access to health professionals:** Learning from patients is important, but if you can secure time working with medical professionals as well, it is only going to benefit you. You can watch physicians, nurses, and technicians talk to patients; you can see what works and what doesn't when communicating, relating, and treating. Sitting and talking with a patient in some inpatient section of the hospitals can give you insight into the nature of the multidisciplinary nature of modern medical care, a helpful experience when it comes time for interviewing, when you have to portray yourself as being in touch with the state and format of modern medical care. It is never too early to develop the interpersonal skills necessary for the practice of medicine by talking to patients and an insight that comes from watching the practice of healthcare happen around them.

## 14.4 Some Important Points

- Like any other experience recorded in your American Medical College Application Service (AMCAS), quality is more important than quantity. Just like a single major with a GPA of 4.0 is better than a triple major with a 2.6, having a nonmedical volunteering experience that shows the aforementioned desirable personal qualities over a significant period of time, aggregate amount of hours dedicated is more important than three short, simple, one-dimensional experiences.
- If the experience is significant enough, this can be a great source of a letter of recommendation.
- These experiences—again, if significant enough—can be excellent illustrative talking points during your interviews and personal statement/supplemental essays, and strong indicators of a factor very important to medical schools: evidence of interest in medicine.
- Pick experiences that allow you a quality longitudinal experience. Not all compelling moments are felt in an epiphany—like instant on your first day of volunteering. Many of them, in fact, are the cumulative buildup of many small experiences that change who you are, and how you think about medicine and patient care. To do that, you need to clock a good deal of hours over a significant period of time.
- If possible—show some creativity, initiative, leadership, and other medically transferable skills. This is more difficult with preset volunteering positions like the ones offered through preexisting hospital and community outreach organizations. However, once comfortable enough in the position—and you have stuck around long enough—you can talk to supervisors about changing the position in ways you think will benefit both patient care and volunteer experience, or creating entirely new positions that serve a novel function. Otherwise, much of these extra skills can be developed and portrayed by finding a medical problem that can reasonably be addressed by your limited time as a pre-med student, and finding a way to bring together resources and energy to make it a reality.

## 14.5 Do You Need to Do Volunteering to Get into Medical School?

The answer is—like most questions about what you need to do to get into medical school—specific to you and your situation. What have you done already, where do you want to go, and what do you want to do with your career? So, this is unfortunately a question we cannot definitively answer for you, but we should be able to give you the information you need to make this decision for yourself. Below are the points you should consider when making this decision.

- **The vast majority of matriculants volunteered:** Per the 2020 AAMC Matriculating (Medical) Student Questionnaire, 88.2 and 92.9% of MD matriculants participated in nonmedical and medical volunteering, respectively.[1] So how much volunteering makes you competitive? The University of Utah Medical School keeps data on their applicant pool, and has been able to give specific recommendations for what competitive applicants have done in regard to quantity and quality of experience for not just volunteering, but for research, GPA, and MCAT for their specific institution. For volunteering specifically, they recommend applicants complete 36 hours over 4 years, and that competitive applicants complete around 100 hours over that same time span. Just to put this in perspective: that is, minimally, 45 minutes of volunteering time, per month. To be competitive, that is just 2 hours a month. The theme: Quality volunteering, done over a long period of time, does not have to be time-consuming to be an integral component to your application, to make you a more competitive applicant. Nonetheless, for any applicant who wants to err on the side of caution: we recommend at least 300 hours of longitudinal volunteering experience.

- **Some schools not only emphasize volunteering when ranking applicants, but even require volunteering as a prerequisite for interview:** While it's hard to get medical schools to reveal any clear components of the rubric they apply when judging and grading applicants, certain schools are very forward about how much they value this in an applicant, going so far as to even require volunteering once you are a medical student there. State medical schools often place a premium on volunteering, so make sure to look out for that when applying locally.
- **Participating in volunteering is an easy way to gain a competitive edge:** Depending on where you are in your life, your education, or your stage of learning, making yourself a more competitive applicant can be challenging. Maybe you don't have a lot of research available at your school, maybe much of your free time is taken up trying to work your way through college (pay your way), or maybe going back to school to improve your GPA or taking an expensive class to improve your MCAT score just is not feasible. Maybe you are enrolled in a difficult undergraduate program where maintaining your high GPA takes most of your time. However, adding significant volunteering experience is often a very cheap, easy, efficient, and rewarding way to get you leadership experience, demonstrate an ability to help others, and make you a more competitive applicant in as little as a couple hours per week.
- **You should just do some volunteering anyway:** Medicine is a volunteering profession. The profession is loaded with paperwork, regulations, stress, and long hours that doesn't specifically or directly involve helping people. If you can't stand volunteering in any capacity or minimal amount, this may not be the most rewarding choice of a career for you.

## 14.6 So, Do You Really Need to Volunteer for the Application Process?

Basically yes. Again, for almost all applicants, it is a good idea and makes you more competitive, and it increases the number of schools that may consider accepting you (if they require it). Let us give you some examples about someone who should participate in volunteering, and someone who might not *strictly* "need" to (because just do some!).

*Applicant A:* A 21-year-old male is majoring in biology at a well-regarded state school. He has a GPA of 3.65. He has no volunteering experience, but is active in a couple of campus clubs, but is not involved in a leadership capacity. He has helped out on a research project, but has obtained no poster presentations, no abstracts, and no publications. His MCAT is a 510 (81st percentile). He spends his free time exercising or hanging out with his friends. His father was a doctor, and he wants to join the family profession. He has spent 200 hours shadowing in the field.

*Applicant B:* A 29-year-old computer science major who is getting a Master's in biomechanical engineering at a prestigious private university. She has participated in several research projects, presenting two posters, and is a first author on one of her publications. She only is active in the Improv club, but has been doing it for years, and is the president of that organization. Her GPA is 3.94, and her MCAT is 517 (95th percentile). She became interested in medicine while doing one of her research projects in partnership with doctors from the local university hospital, and has decided to pursue a career as a physician-scientist.

---

[1] https://www.aamc.org/media/50081/download

So which one needs to do some volunteering? Both should, but applicant A really needs to. Applicants can look very similar, especially when there are 50,000 of them nationally. His GPA is great—but only average when comparing it to the median applicant, and likely below average for those applicants who are accepted coming from his tier of institution and among those who are accepted in medical school. His MCAT is average as well, and around 70 to 80% of applicants have helped out with a research project. His shadowing and the fact that he is applying are the only real indicators of his interest in medicine, not necessarily the most convincing evidence of an applicant's interest and commitment. He hasn't gone out of his way to obtain an impressive amount of life experience or leadership experience, and as he is a traditional applicant (Undergrad straight to medical school); he doesn't have any work experience to lean on either. Applicant B, on the other hand, stands out for her above average GPA and MCAT, impressive research work. She only has one extracurricular activity of note, but she has done it for years, and is in a leadership role. Which do you think has an application that could benefit from volunteering experience? Who do you think appeals more to an admissions committee?

## 14.7 How to Record Your Volunteering

Here we will present examples of how you may present both medical and nonmedical volunteering in an AMCAS description or personal statement to help your writing process when it comes time to apply. Example A will describe the experience, while example B will show one possible way to write about that experience (in the context of the personal statement or secondary application).

*Example 1A:* I am a student applying to medical school and have volunteered in a Children's Hospital every week for 2 years. I have volunteered for approximately 150 hours and my job is to deliver art supplies and toys to the patients of the hospital and, if needed, help the nurses.

*Example 1B:* For the last 2 years, I have had the opportunity to serve at Children's Hospital of Philadelphia. I am responsible for bringing arts supplies and toys to the patients and to be available to help the nurses care for patients and help attend to the needs of families. Throughout my time at Children's Hospital, I got to form close relationships with some of the long-term patients and was able to closely observe the inner workings of a care team. Seeing a patient recover from a broken arm or a major infection or—sadly—see their seizures get worse, showed me the realities of medicine. I experienced the joys of a healing patient, and the tragedy of a struggling one and the care team that is with them every step of the way. I was able to develop my own interpersonal skills when interacting with patients and had to learn how to communicate with families from many backgrounds. I remember a specific family who spoke very little English, so we played almost a game of Pictionary to discover the type of toy the patient wanted me to retrieve for them. It was a simple moment, but we connected in that moment and it has driven me toward a career in medicine to make those connections with other families, but in the capacity of taking care of their health...

*Example 2A:* I worked as a counselor at a youth summer camp. Youth of all ages came throughout the weeks and teamwork among the staff was vital.

*Example 2B:* Last summer, I had the opportunity to be a counselor at the camp I grew up attending as a camper. It was not just a chance to be a mentor, but to also give back to a place that shaped who I am in an incredibly significant way. We were responsible for guiding our campers through a week of games, singing, swimming, and growth. The best memory I have of being a counselor is when one of my youngest campers who was afraid of the rope swing finally had the courage to swing with the encouragement of the friends he had made throughout the week. We had spent the whole week setting goals for ourselves and his was to use swing. His excitement after he ran and how proud he was let me know that I had done my job as a counselor. The rest of the staff and I cheered for him and I realized how important it is to care for and support everyone, especially children because it will help them grow. This experience helped me realize that value of being a physician because it is a career where you heal, mentor, and work together toward a common goal and you have the opportunity to change someone's life and guide people through some of their toughest moments...

There are of course many ways to write about your experience, and these are just a few examples. We encourage you to think deeply about what each volunteering opportunity means to you and make sure the committee sees what that opportunity has done for you and how it will make you a better physician.

Medicine is an incredibly challenging career but one with immense purpose. One of the greatest gifts a physician can give not just to the community but also to himself is to volunteer his time. This means that volunteering—especially in medicine—is not just what you do as a pre-med or medical student but a life-time commitment. And above all, you should pick an experience that genuinely moves you to sacrificing your own time among your other commitments.

## 14.8 Summary

Volunteering is essentially necessary for medical school admissions. For admissions purposes, it can be divided into medical and nonmedical volunteering. Both can bolster your application in different ways. Ideally, you will find medical and nonmedical volunteering opportunities that allow for longitudinal commitments over years that ultimately culminate in a leadership position, major project, fantastic letter of recommendation, or some combination thereof.

# 15 Research

*Jorna Sojati and Joel Thomas*

Research is an important driver of progress in modern medicine and is an increasingly important factor in matching into a competitive residency program, so it's no surprise that many medical schools are increasingly valuing applicants who have research experience.

Student research can present itself in all sorts of varieties, especially for those interested in medicine. It may include spending time in a basic research laboratory studying the mechanisms of biomedical processes (which is so often the image of research we have ingrained in our heads: the medical student pipetting away for hours on a lab bench), but it can also involve collecting and analyzing patient data from clinical studies, designing and implementing analyses based on existing research data from the comfort of your own home, or even pushing yourself out of your comfort zone and doing field work. Across several disciplines, from the health sciences to language studies and even business, the beneficial impact of conducting undergraduate research has been proven to enhance critical thinking skills,[1] improve GPA and other academic outcomes,[2] increase intrinsic motivation and independence,[1] and strengthen communication skills among others.[1,3,4,5,6,7,8] These are just a few of the reasons that medical schools consider involvement in research to substantially elevate a student's application, and many institutions have even altered their curricula to make research participation an essential component of medical education.

Here, we'll discuss how to determine if research is right for you (keeping in mind that research experience is not a required component in medical school applications, and may not be the right path for everyone), how to circumvent a lack of research experience on medical school applications, how to go about finding an ideal research experience, how to find the right mentor(s) as a researcher, and how to choose among different "flavors" that research can come in.

## 15.1 Research: Does It Spark Joy in You?

At this point, the competitiveness of medical schools should come as no surprise, nor should the toll that the demand of having a typical "well-rounded" application takes on a student. Your time becomes very valuable, and it is incredibly important in your pre-medical years to allocate it wisely: to recognize what facets of the pre-medical experience matter most to you and strengthen your passion for medicine, and to not waste time with activities that simply don't excite you as much. It is essential to recognize that while research does benefit your application, the idea of spending numerous hours mixing biological reagents or doing heavy, complex statistical work may not appeal to everyone. Luckily, there are some questions you can consider to make sure that pursuing research is the right track for you:

---

[1] Petrella JK, Jung AP. Undergraduate Research: Importance, Benefits, and Challenges. Int J Exerc Sci 2008;1(3):91–95. Available at: https://www.ncbi.nlm.nih.gov/pmc/articles/PMC4739295/. Accessed July 8, 2022.

[2] Sell AJ, Naginey A, Stanton CA. The Impact of Undergraduate Research on Academic Success. Available at: https://www.cur.org/download.aspx?id=3696. Accessed July 8, 2022.

[3] Melissa LA, et al. A social capital perspective on the mentoring of undergraduate life science researchers: an empirical study of undergraduate–postgraduate–faculty triads. *CBE Life Sci Educ* 2016; 15(2). PubMed Central, doi:10.1187/cbe.15–10–0208.

[4] Timothy WC, et al. Undergraduate research participation is associated with improved student outcomes at a Hispanic-serving institution. *J College Student Dev* 2017; 58(4): 583–600. PubMed Central, doi:10.1353/csd.2017.0044.

[5] David L. Undergraduate research experiences support science career decisions and active learning. *CBE Life Sci Educ* 2007; 6(4): 297–306. PubMed Central, doi:10.1187/cbe.07–06–0039.

[6] Medicine and health. *American Sociological Association*, http://www.asanet.org/topics/medicine-and-health. Accessed January 11, 2019.

[7] Deborah M-E, et al. What do medical students understand by research and research skills? Identifying research opportunities within undergraduate projects. *Med Teacher* 2010; 32(3): e152–60. Taylor and Francis + NEJM, doi:10.3109/01421591003657493.

[8] Susan RH, et al. Benefits of undergraduate research experiences. Science 2007; 316(5824): 548–549. science.sciencemag.org, doi:10.1126/science.1140384.

### 15.1.1 Does *Curiosity*, the Ability to Ask Novel Questions and Seek Answers to Them, Drive Your Motivation for Medicine?

The very premise of research is to quench the inquisitive nature that many of us have: to recognize a gap in knowledge and find ways to fill that gap.

### 15.1.2 Is There a Subject You Are Passionate about and Hope to Contribute to?

The ability to advance knowledge in a particular field of study is one of the primary appeals of research. Research, especially if conducted longer-term, allows one to become recognized in their area of study and establish greater connections with existing experts in that field and other like-minded peers.

### 15.1.3 Do You Have the *Time* to Commit to Research?

The significant time commitment that a research project requires is often vastly underestimated by students, and, if not addressed immediately, can become a point of contention between themselves and their research mentor. Before deciding to pursue research, ask yourself not only if there is room in your schedule for taking on research, but also how much time you can realistically devote to a research project. When meeting with a research mentor, keep this number in mind and be honest with them about your availability. Not all projects require the same amount of time, and, by making your expectations clear, research advisors will be much more likely to find a feasible project for you that best works with your schedule.

### 15.1.4 Are You Willing to Put in the Effort Toward Becoming a Student Researcher?

The mental exertion of undertaking a research project can be a factor just as important as time, passion, and curiosity. The research portion of your project often begins much earlier than when you first step foot in a lab or pick up your first clinical case file. It is first important to read and understand major papers in that field of study, find articles focused on the potential projects you might be working on or techniques you'll be using, and continuously update yourself with the work in that subject and related subjects so that your research questions remain relevant. This requires both a lot of additional reading as well as the ability to absorb the important existing information and filter out the less pertinent data, which can certainly take some getting used to. The patience required when conducting research can also be mentally draining, especially when your experiments do not go as planned (which is very often the case). It is called "re"-search specifically because of the amount of time spent repeating experiments to troubleshoot your errors, optimize your results, and reproduce your findings. To make your transition into an academic researcher smoother, make sure to account for this added time of literature review, troubleshooting, and repetition when assessing the level of commitment you can realistically give to your project. Another way to mitigate this exertion is to set small, incremental goals rather than larger ones. Chances are, you likely will not have found the answers to your research questions within a few months, but you may have picked up a new technique, designed an experimental procedure, or created a new cell line that is useful to your lab. Recognize these as small victories themselves—ones that push your project tremendously forward, and bring you one step closer to answering the bigger questions.

### 15.1.5 Ideally, You Should Pursue Research that Sparks Your Interest and Contributes to Your Narrative

For example, are you a musician? Perhaps you could look into research about diseases of the larynx/vocal cords. Or the pathology of ear disease? Sometimes connections don't need to be so obvious, so as long as you can incorporate the experience into your story or motivation. At the same time, we recognize that participating in a research project that genuinely excites you with a supportive mentor in a lab that is *also* highly productive in terms of publications and presentations is a golden goose. **The most important features to gain from your research experience is an appreciation and understanding of the scientific process that you can articulate during application time, as well as a strong relationship with a mentor who can vouch for you in a letter of recommendation.** A subject area that genuinely interests you will make this easier to achieve, however. In addition, publications and presentations can serve as icing on the cake but are absolutely *not* expected.

## 15.1.6  Are You Considering an MD/PhD Program (or Other Research Dual Degree, e.g., MD/MS)?

The one program for which extensive research experience is an absolute must is a dual-degree MD/PhD program. This is an ideal path for students who are interested in a career that involves tackling medical problems as both physicians and scientists, and want to devote their career to both patient care and medical research. This may not appeal to everyone, and there are many other ways to pursue research as a physician, but these are wonderful training programs for students committed to a career that integrates their scientific and clinical interests. Please see Chapter 25, Dual-Degree Programs: MD/PhD, MPH, MBA, JD, and Others for more information on this track.

## 15.2  Navigating Medical School Applications Without Research Experience

It may turn out that, from asking yourself the questions above and reflecting on your career goals, research does not seem to be a good fit for you. Luckily, medical school admissions committees have become significantly more holistic in their review process in recent years. In fact, according to the AAMC's 2020 Matriculating Student Questionnaire, only 58.7% of accepted applicants at MD schools had any laboratory research experience.[9] If you are a pre-medical student with little to no research experience, here are some considerations for strengthening your application in other ways.

### 15.2.1  Devote More Time to Your Other Pre-Medical Endeavors

It is pertinent to convince medical committees of your commitment to medicine, and to show that by not taking part in research you were able to deepen your commitment to other extracurricular endeavors. This can include things like taking on greater service hours and more volunteer opportunities, doing more clinical shadowing, becoming a tutor for pre-medical courses, or taking on a leadership role in a club or organization about which you are passionate.

### 15.2.2  Enter the Application Cycle with a Strong GPA and MCAT Score

The ability to do well academically, as referenced by your GPA and MCAT scores, is certainly important to admissions committees, and perhaps even more so for students who are lacking in a certain aspect of their application (i.e., no research experience, limited service, few extracurriculars). It helps to prove that, while you may not meet every expectation that a school has for pre-medical candidates, your academic competence and the ability to excel in medical school courses remains high.

### 15.2.3  Find the Right School for You, but also Recognize that not Having Research Generally Hurts Your Application

Keep in mind that different medical schools have different priorities when it comes to training their students, and it is crucial to find a school that best prepares you for the type of physician you'd like to be. For instance, there are some schools that consider research a top priority, and structure their medical curriculum to the training of their students as clinical scientists. On the other hand, there are medical

---

[9] Matriculating Student Questionnaire. Available at: https://www.aamc.org/media/50081/download. Accessed July 8, 2022.

institutions that may put greater emphasis on primary care, community medicine, or holistic medicine. You can learn about the academic priorities of different medical schools by going online and reading the mission statement of each school, the objectives of their curriculum, and even the types of elective classes they offer beyond the basic biomedical course blocks. Keeping in mind that applying to medical school is a long, exhausting, and expensive process, so be sure to find the schools that best prepare you for the type of career you envision. That said, if you don't have research experience on your application, you will be less likely to be admitted to research-heavy schools that may not be great fits for you.

At the same time, we want to again emphasize that ~60% of applicants are not admitted to *any school*. In addition, most medical school matriculants will have had some research experience, even though only a minority of physicians end up ultimately practicing in academics.[10] Therefore, it appears to be the case that medical schools value research experience in applicants while also recognizing that most matriculants will ultimately not participate in research as practicing physicians. As such, even if research does not genuinely spark joy in you, we recommend sticking through with a longitudinal research experience—if you can tolerate it and be competitive in other areas of your application—to make yourself more competitive for admission at *any* school and to gain valuable insight about the process of scientific discovery. Admissions Committees (ADCOMs) will understand if you communicate honestly to them that you explored many research avenues in college—and are potentially considering additional, alternate research opportunities in medical school—but are still not 100% committed to a research career.

### 15.2.4 Consider Postgraduate Research Opportunities

With the majority of accepted students matriculating being between the ages of 23 and 25, many applicants now decide to take time off after their undergraduate studies in order to mature their applications. If you are interested in exploring research, but did not have the chance to do so during your college years, there are now a number of research assistantships for postgraduate students. The Links guide at the end of this chapter has a few of these listed to get you started.

## 15.3 Finding Opportunities for Research

So you've made the decision to pursue research as a pre-medical student! The next step is to find a project that you're excited about, but it can seem like a daunting task (especially as an undergraduate) to find a suitable mentor and research environment. Listed here is a suggested strategy for finding research opportunities that might prove useful, which we call the *four R's of finding research*: Reflect, Review, Reach out, Realistic expectations.

### 15.3.1 Reflect

Think about the research areas that most appeal to you—this can be influenced by your academic major, the type of medicine you are considering, or any field of study that you'd like to learn more about. Use these interests as inherent "filters" when looking for research projects.

### 15.3.2 Review

Once you've done your homework and found a few laboratories or researchers that fit your areas of interest, the next step is to learn more about the laboratory and the type of projects in which they are involved. Review the literature listed on the laboratory's website or look up the publication list of the Principal Investigator (PI) using engines such as NCBI PubMed or Google Scholar. PIs are basically the bosses who run labs. Often they hold advanced degrees like a PhD or MD. Try to read through a few of their most recent papers, or at the very least skim the abstracts, to see if the work that they do excites you. This technique also proves very advantageous when applying for a research position. Being able to show that you've read about a laboratory's projects and taken a genuine interest in their work makes you a much more appealing candidate.

---

[10] The Long-term Retention and Attrition of U.S. Medical School Faculty. Available at: https://www.aamc.org/data-reports/analysis-brief/report/long-term-retention-and-attrition-us-medical-school-faculty. Accessed July 8, 2022.

## 15.3.3 Reach Out

Once you've found a lab, and PI, or a project that suits your general interests and has exciting projects available, the next step is to reach out to the PI (or his/her administrative assistant if that does not work). The most convenient way to send an inquiry is via email, since the email addresses of most PIs can be found on their institution or school's website. While this may seem rather difficult, the key to writing an effective research inquiry is to: introduce yourself, explain why this lab appeals to you (referencing knowledge of their papers and projects), express your desire to join the lab or work with the PI, and include your CV *with emphasis on relevant skills and experiences* (e.g., computer programming languages, statistical analysis, laboratory techniques, prior abstracts/publications).

Here's an example:

*"Hello,*
*(Introduce yourself) My name is Mary Smith, and I am a student at East Falls College who is interested in gaining research experience. (Explain your interests in the lab, citing specific projects) I am fascinated by the study of infectious diseases, and your laboratory's work on identifying key molecules involved in HIV pathogenesis greatly appealed to me. In particular, your recent project looking at proteins involved in HIV binding and entry really captured my attention. (Express your desire to join) I was hoping to have a chance to speak with you about potentially joining the laboratory and becoming a part of the research team. (List the best way to get in touch with you.) If you have any time in the coming weeks, I would really enjoy the chance to talk further with you about the lab and available research projects. I am happy to meet in person or continue this conversation by e-mail (msmith@efalls.edu) or phone number (XXX-555–5555) at your convenience. Thank you for your time and consideration."*

Also a few extra points of advice for once you've set up a meeting:
* *Before the meeting:* Make sure you know the background of the researcher, their lab, and a few of their publications. It's helpful to think of questions to ask about the experiments and implications of the results. What specifically was exciting or interesting about the research to you? In addition, if you have previous research experience, make sure to re-read your own papers and be able to explain what you did.
* *For the meeting:* Remember to dress nicely. Be respectful, cordial, and enthusiastic! Bring a copy of your curriculum vitae (CV). If you have previous research experience, it's helpful to bring organized binder of your past research and printouts of any posters on standard copy paper. Relax! You've got this!

If you are looking to do research on your college grounds or at a local research facility, it actually might be more beneficial to find research opportunities by using the connections you already have in place. This can include asking professors of yours for research recommendations, shadowing faculty members that you already know who conduct research, and, rather than blind emailing, stopping by during a professor's office hours and setting in-person meetings to specifically discuss their research. The advantage to this method (should it be an option for you) is a better opportunity to really see the lab and its investigators in action, converse more deeply with the PI to figure out whether this could be the right mentor for you (more on this later), and also the opportunity to meet and speak with graduate students, postdoctoral fellows, and other colleagues of this PI in order to get a better sense of their personality and their expectations for research students.

One last tip I'll leave is for those looking to reach out and find research positions in more distant locations (i.e., summer research programs, postgraduate research opportunities, internships, etc.), but that you might have some connection to (if your family or friends live there). Many students in this predicament end up utilizing the "local address strategy" to their advantage, in which they'll use an address local to that region (perhaps a family home or a friend who wouldn't mind you using their information) for more comprehensive consideration of their application and overall better chances of acceptance. It's no surprise that research facilities would prefer to hire someone who lives nearby, as these applicants have less problems traveling to work, less restrictions on their research time, and are more likely to stay on in that same research environment in a longer-term position.

Regardless of your method, there is really no bad way to reach out. Showing that you are motivated, curious, and willing to learn is really all that most PIs look for (and, arguably, all it really takes to become a great researcher).

### 15.3.4 Realistic Expectations

Once you find a mentor that is willing to take you on as a research student, it can become very easy to overcommit yourself to the laboratory and exaggerate your number of available lab hours in hopes of making a good impression. While this may seem harmless, it can lead to devastating outcomes long-term and actually harm the student–mentor relationship. As mentioned earlier in this chapter, it is important to be realistic with yourself and your mentor about the amount of time you can actually devote to being in the laboratory, especially as an undergraduate student doing research during a term. This affects the type of project you are assigned as well as how much progress on that project the PI expects.

While this may be a tough conversation to have, it is absolutely necessary for setting attainable research goals for both yourself and your mentor. So, in that first meeting, be honest about your time commitment, and that honesty will be rewarded in the long run. Likewise, do not feel sheepish about explicitly asking your mentor about prior students' outcomes (e.g., published abstracts and papers, presentations) in the lab. All things equal, you should aim to work with a mentor with a documented history of getting students' names on papers and presentations. Likewise, be tactful but explicit about your hopes to contribute significantly and ultimately present and publish. Again, we emphasize that while quality of mentorship and educational experience are more important than publications, papers and presentations in peer-reviewed journals can strengthen your application. Unfortunately, there is much variation by individual school and ADCOM members regarding the importance of publications. Collectively, publications appear to be of "lowest importance" for medical school admissions,[11] but we have personally run into ADCOM members that value them so much that we recommend including them in update letters to *all* schools that have wait-listed you (more in Chapter 36, Wait-List and Update Letters).

## 15.4 Mentorship

Mentorship is incredibly crucial for not only becoming an effective researcher, but also an ideal medical school applicant. It is important to find people, whether in your undergraduate institution, at a job, or perhaps in a research lab, that will not only speak on your behalf, but actually take the time to teach you new skills, deepen your perspectives, and motivate you to find and build on your passions. No one comes into college with an established "how-to" guide for becoming a great medical school applicant (even this book can't help you figure everything out!), and so it's important to use the wisdom and resources of those around you to your advantage.

### 15.4.1 The Principal Investigator (PI)

The PI of your lab has the potential to be the most influential mentor in your life, and his/her recommendation can do wonders for your medical school application. However, if you choose to stay in a research environment where the PI does not take an active mentorship role, the lack of a recommendation from them could potentially be damaging to your application. Different PIs have different personalities, which shapes their research environment and the expectations they have for their students. It is important to figure out which personality types are most conducive for your learning, and whether the researchers that you meet with have the traits that you're looking for. This highly popular cartoon done by Alexander Dent, a faculty member at Indiana University College of Medicine, showcases some of the very common PI personality types he encountered during his time at the NIH (▶ Fig. 15.1).

As this cartoon touches upon, there are upsides and downsides to the personalities of every PI. Likewise, from meeting with different PIs, you might find certain aspects of their personality that are very different from yours, which can create big problems in communication and make it difficult for you to recognize their expectations. In general, you should aim to foster an ongoing relationship with your PI. *If you rarely interact with your PI on the job, schedule regular meetings to touch base and discuss your ongoing progress and potential future directions.*

The PI–mentee fit is a necessary consideration for any research student, and, sadly, many students end up in a research environment where they encounter problems with the PI, other lab members, or

---

[11] https://www.aamc.org/download/462316/data/mcatguide.pdf. Publications ranked by committees as "of lowest importance" in 2022 application cycle.

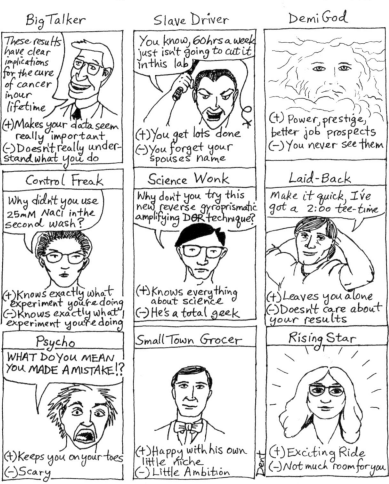

**Fig. 15.1** The nine types of principal investigators. Source: Dr. Alexander Dent.

the nature of the work in general. When this happens (and it commonly does), I urge you to take action and find a more suitable place for you. First, do a "self-inventory" and see whether these problems with your current lab situation can be remedied—this can include speaking to the PI and other lab members about your concerns, but also being honest with yourself and recognizing whether there's any changes you can personally make that would help you better adapt to this environment. If the problems are too large to fix, do not be afraid to set your sights elsewhere. Think of this past research experience as a learning opportunity—one that now allows you to better recognize the traits that don't work for you, so you can start the process of finding new research projects with a much better sense of your ideal lab environment.

## 15.4.2 Everyone Else

While it's important to have a PI that you get along with, there are some research environments (especially in larger labs) where you'll actually get very little interaction with the PI. In these cases, you might find yourself working under the guidance of a graduate student or postdoctoral fellow, and it's much more likely that they will instead take on the role of mentor for you. For this reason, it's also necessary to consider the personalities of not only the PI, but also the other members of your research team. When meeting with a potential PI about research opportunities, it might be helpful to also ask for the contact information of some of their graduate students and postdocs and reach out to them as well. This will not only give you a better sense of their lab environment, but these members of the research team (who are often younger and earlier in their training) tend to also be more honest about the pros and cons of that particular research lab.

### 15.4.3 You

Regardless of where and with whom you work, you should aim to be *proactive*. Ask your mentors if you can take on additional responsibilities if you believe you can do so. Speak up during lab meetings about potential avenues to take the research project; even if you don't feel 100% confident, mentors will recognize and appreciate your input if you demonstrate that you have done your research.

## 15.5 Types of Research and Publications

Finally, we will finish off this chapter by describing four of the major types of research that pre-medical students often engage in: basic, clinical, translational, and social research. We'll also touch a little bit upon the types of publications in these research fields and their value.

The kind of study you choose will notably shape your research experience, and so I urge you to think carefully as you read these descriptions about the project types that work best for you.

### 15.5.1 Basic Research

This involves what we traditionally consider to be "bench research"—the use of biological, chemical, or physical techniques to study molecular and cellular properties, mechanisms, and functions in a laboratory setting. Most basic research projects that appeal to medical students are ones that examine the characteristics of pathological (disease) states. This can be anything from identifying tumor markers for specific cancers to studying cellular processes that underlie inflammatory responses. This type of research is usually one of the most accessible for students (numerous university faculty often run basic research laboratories), and can leave students with a huge sense of gratification. The ability to improve medicine by better understanding the mechanisms of disease is something that most students never thought they'd be able to do as undergraduates, especially from behind a lab bench. Another factor to consider is that basic research requires a significant amount of time spent in the laboratory, whereas other research types may be more conducive for doing off-site work. But if you're looking to greatly expand your scientific skill set and learn a number of new experimental techniques and procedures, basic research is certainly the right environment to do so.

### 15.5.2 Clinical Research

Clinical research is dedicated to the study of different medical interventions in actual human participants. This can include a number of different research designs, such as observational studies that track subjects with exposure to certain interventions or factors of interest, experimental studies that involve conducting clinical trials with patients in a controlled environment, or meta-analyses of existing studies done with human subjects. What makes clinical research so appealing is the opportunity to work with patients and, depending on the project, even play a direct role in their care. If you are someone who doesn't see the appeal of basic research but is interested in studying new methods of patient care and treatment, this may be an ideal research experience. Clinical research is often not as accessible as basic research for undergraduates, due to most studies being conducted in a hospital setting and requiring a number of clearances. However, clinical research has the unique advantage of allowing a short time from project inception to publication. Many "chart review" projects simply entail sifting through an electronic health record and identifying whether particular clinical variables are associated with outcomes of interest based on a hypothesis surrounding a plausible mechanism. For example, one might ask whether the use of statin medications impacts long-term survival in patients diagnosed with degenerative muscle diseases because patients taking statins for high cholesterol tend to experience side effects associated with muscle damage. Such chart reviews often require no funding (and therefore no grant applications) or even full approval from an ethical board. *They can even be done entirely remotely, i.e., "from your couch,"* as long as you have remote access to the electronic health record from your computer. As a result, such projects are frequently undertaken by medical students to maximize their quantity of "abstracts, publications, and presentations" when applying to medical school. Other types of "easy" (i.e., short time from conception to publication) include case studies (writing up an interesting clinical case and including discussion of the clinical reasoning) and review articles (summarizing the current state of literature on an interesting question). Essentially, anything that requires analyzing preexisting data (e.g., patient records, literature reviews) will take substantially less time to publish compared to anything that requires producing and polishing *new* data (e.g., laboratory experiments, randomized controlled trials).

It should be noted - however - that some of this "easy research" may not be clinically meaningful, reproducible, or even true. This is **not** because researchers are intentionally committing fraud en masse. Instead, it's largely due to incentives in academic medicine that reward quantity of research (i.e., sheer number of presentations and published articles or abstracts) over quality of research (e.g., hypothesis-driven work on clinically meaningful questions with reproducible findings and careful quality control to maximize the odds of generating accurate results - basically the stuff requires a lot of time and funding to generate publications). Of course, you can absolutely be a rockstar clinical researcher who delivers on both quality and quantity, but we want to make you aware of this active issue in academia so that you hopefully don't contribute to the problem.[12] That said, we strongly emphasize exploring clinical research for the applicant who has no strong preferences regarding type of research, wants early experience with the most commonly done type of research in medical school, and hopes to maximize their documented productivity (i.e., publications, abstracts, and presentations) for medical school applications.

### 15.5.3 Translational Research

What if both clinical and basic research projects appeal to you? What if your goal is to both understand the etiology of a disease and to use this knowledge in developing new treatment approaches? Luckily, there is an area of research that allows you to do both—to manage patient care from the "bench to the bedside." This is the very premise of translational research laboratories, who conduct basic research using relevant cell lines or animal models, apply these findings to the design of new therapies, and ultimately test these promising therapies with clinical trials in human subjects. Similar to clinical research, working in a translational research environment is also less accessible, as these studies are also often conducted in a hospital setting, and requires long-term commitment due to longitudinal patient follow-up, as well as advanced clearance. However, working in this type of environment does have the benefit of exposing you to both basic and clinical research techniques, and is perhaps the most representative of a true physician-scientist career path. In addition, because of its multidisciplinary nature, choosing a translational research experience allows for networking and collaboration with numerous doctors and medical scientists. If translational work appeals to you as not just a research experience, but potentially a career track, see Chapter 25, Dual-Degree Programs: MD/PhD, MPH, MBA, JD, and Others for more information on physician-scientist programs.

### 15.5.4 Social Research

This research type involves the use of scientific techniques to better understand and describe society. In the context of medicine, this can include studies that examine the efficacy of healthcare systems in varying local and global communities, uncover the prevalence of illness among different populations, and better uncover socioeconomic barriers to healthcare treatment. Social research is incredibly multifaceted: just a few areas of study that fall under the category of social research are epidemiology, community health, population medicine, healthcare policy, medical ethics, psychology, economics, and human behavior. In addition, it is an ideal field of research for those who are more inclined to examine healthcare from a social perspective rather than a biomedical one. It is important to note that different social research projects can require vastly different levels of time commitment: for instance,

---

[12] Ioannidis JPA. Why Most Clinical Research Is Not Useful. PLoS Med. 2016;13(6):e1002049. Available at: https://www.ncbi.nlm.nih.gov/pmc/articles/PMC4915619/. Accessed July 8, 2022.

studies that rely on existing data banks of social surveys or already-published statistics may require less time and can be done off-site, while community-centered projects are more time-intensive and may require weeks of observation or interviewing at a site. Finally, in recent years, the psychosocial considerations of medicine have proven to be much more imperative than we previously thought, and there is increasing demand for physicians that can recognize and tackle the sociological problems that our healthcare system currently faces.

While these are four major branches of research that currently exist, it is important to realize that your options are not limited to the ones mentioned above. I hope that, by now, you are convinced of research being much more than just students mixing chemicals on a lab bench. It can come in so many unique flavors, but what matters most is finding a project that teaches you how to ask and answer scientific questions, exposes you to new skills, and (perhaps the most crucial element) gives you something to be excited about.

We'll conclude this chapter by including links to a few great research programs run by fantastic organizations (think of this as a thank-you for making it to the end). Now get out there and make some discoveries!

## 15.6 Summary

Research is not necessary for medical school admissions, but a slight majority of MD matriculants participate in research. Research comes in many different forms (e.g., basic experimental, clinical, social, theoretical), and we encourage you to explore the different options available to find something you're intellectually curious about. Participating in the production of knowledge can give you a deeper understanding of the scientific process, which may give you additional insights into the practice of medicine and potentially even veer you toward the MD/PhD route!

Student research is also a great way to foster strong mentorship relationships, which can ultimately lead to fantastic letters of recommendation. That said, your choice of mentor will likely be the single most important factor affecting your research experience. Ideally, you will stay with a single mentor for many years to build a strong professional relationship. As with any relationship, there may be bumps in the road and moments of tension; we encourage you to keep an open-mind during these moments to see your commitment through to the end. At the same time - as with any relationship - sometimes there is genuine incompatibility that you could not have reasonably predicted in advance. If you genuinely feel that you and your mentor have exhausted all reasonable options to produce a healthy professional relationship, then you should not be afraid to respectfully part ways to seek a new mentor.

### 15.6.1 Short-term Research Opportunities

- Summer Undergraduate Research Program Listing from the American Association of Medical Colleges: https://students-residents.aamc.org/choosing-medical-career/article/summer-undergraduate-research-programs/
- National Institutes of Health's Summer Internship Program: https://www.training.nih.gov/trainees/summer_interns
- National Association of Advisors for the Health Professions (NAAHP) Listing of Summer Opportunities for Pre-Health Students: https://www.naahp.org/public-resources/student-resources/student-announcements/student-opportunities
- National Cancer Institute Summer Research Internship: https://ccr.cancer.gov/training/summer-internships

### 15.6.2 Longer-term Research Opportunities

- National Institutes of Health's Postbaccalaureate Intramural Research Training Award (NIH IRTA) *1–2 year commitment*: https://www.training.nih.gov/programs/postbac_irta
- National Institutes of Health's Postbaccalaureate Research Education Program (NIH PREP) *1–2 year commitment*: https://www.nigms.nih.gov/training/PREP/Pages/default.aspx
- Fellowship Listings by the Center for Disease Control and Prevention (CDC) *Includes both short-term and long-term experiences*: https://www.cdc.gov/fellowships/index.html

### 15.6.3 International Research Opportunities

- Fulbright U.S. Student Program Open Study/Research Award—Many locations *Traditionally a 1-year commitment*: https://us.fulbrightonline.org/about/types-of-awards/study-research
- DAAD-RISE (Research Internships in Science and Engineering) Summer Program, Germany: https://www.daad.de/rise/en/rise-germany/
- Pasteur Foundation Summer Undergraduate Internship Program—France: http://www.pasteurfoundation.org/scientific-careers/summer-internship
- ThinkSwiss Research Scholarship Program—Switzerland: https://thinkswiss.org/research-scholarship/
- EURO (European Undergraduate Research Opportunities) Scholars Program—Many locations: https://euroscholars.eu/

# 16 Gap Years, Employment, Graduate Degrees, and Post-Baccalaureate Fellowships

*Phillip Wagner and Joel Thomas*

The median age of matriculation to MD schools from 2018 to 2020 was 23[1]; the mean age of matriculation to DO schools in 2020 was 23.[2] Many, if not most, of these matriculants likely did not plan to take time between college graduation and medical school matriculation when they began their pre-medical journey. The practice of taking gap year(s) has become increasingly common among those applying to medical school, and it does not hurt your chances of acceptance. Those that go straight from undergrad to medical school are called traditional applicants, and those that take time off are deemed non-traditional applicants, and distinction is becoming less valid as the number of non-traditional applicants and traditional applicants is now roughly equal.

There are many valid reasons to take time off between graduating college and starting medical school, and many of these things can actually enhance your application and make you more competitive. While many people are non-traditional applicants by accident (had a previous career and decided to switch to medicine, for instance), there are other reasons that people choose to pursue a more non-traditional route, either for leisure sake (maybe you want a break between undergrad and medical school, and you aren't in a rush to become a physician) or for strengthening perceived weaknesses in your application.

## 16.1 If You Just Want to Take a Breather…

Not wanting to go to medical school right away is completely reasonable, and ultimately a personal decision. After all, the process of building a competitive medical school application is exhausting, and it is perfectly acceptable to take some time to recharge and explore other interests before rushing headfirst into the rigors of a medical career. If you *are* putting distance between ending undergrad and applying to medical school, make sure that you are doing something with your time that—at least on paper—is professionally enriching. You can do things specifically targeted to make your application stronger (as described below), especially if you have some glaring weaknesses, but otherwise you can focus on what interests you. Every year, people with strong applications decide they want to slow down a bit and do other things, and it does not hurt their chances. Do research, volunteer, join the peace corps, play a professional sport, take care of a sick loved one, spend a few years teaching at a charter school, whatever you want. *Just don't do nothing the entire time (a few months off is fine).*

For those of you that will be taking a break in order to fix or strengthen your application, the rest of this chapter is for you. If you are in the above group, however, feel free to take ideas for how to spend your time off, even if your application doesn't need the help.

## 16.2 If You Need to Strengthen Your Application…

A quick word on weaknesses: some are absolute, and some are relative. If you are an applicant who has great grades, scores, letters, and superb basic science research whose application has pointed in the direction of medical researcher, yet is lacking anything resembling a clinical experience, and you have just decided you would rather not be a doctor than do one more minute of medical research—you might have a weakness now that you didn't have before. You were initially considering MD/PhD combined programs only, but now you want to focus on a career centered only on clinical medicine. While you are still no doubt a strong applicant and still may have more than your share of medical schools eagerly offering you admission, some schools may question rightfully, "How do you know you only want to do clinical medicine? What evidence do we have other than your word? Have you had any experience in a clinical setting?" Your application has a weakness now, albeit a relative one, that you didn't have before.

---

[1] Matriculating Student Questionnaire. Available at: https://www.aamc.org/media/50081/download. Accessed July 8, 2022.
[2] 2020 AACOMAS Profile Applicant and Matriculant Report. Available at: https://www.aacom.org/docs/default-source/data-and-trends/2020-aacomas-applicant-matriculant-profile-summary-report.pdf?sfvrsn=d870497_20. Accessed July 8, 2022.

If you were the kind of person that wanted time off too, a focus on gaining clinical experiences would not only fix this relative weakness, but also actually help you in deciding if clinical medicine is actually something you want to do (remember, you haven't had any significant experience in this before). Gaining some experience, if you do not like it, might actually tell you that medical school is not for you and will save you a great deal of time and effort.

As mentioned above, there are infinite impressive ways to spend your gap year(s). What follows is a discussion of some of the more traditional ways to spend your time to improve your application. Remember, not only can these fix weaknesses, but can also just strengthen an already well-rounded application to make it more targeted.

## 16.2.1 More School

- Self-guided coursework at a university.
  - Nothing's stopping you from enrolling in a local university as a non-degree-seeking student and taking required coursework piecemeal. For the applicant who simply needs to make up missing coursework, this is likely the most affordable option. Keep in mind, however, that financial aid will likely be limited and that you probably have to cover expenses out-of-pocket.
- A certificate program.
  - Not a traditional or popular way that applicants enhance their application; this is much more popular in fields other than medicine, and are generally used by working professionals to do some quick targeted graduate learning. However, a quick perusal of the graduate certificate landscape does return several options for aspiring medical professionals that don't need the boost of a post-bacc or Master's program. Northeastern University in Boston, for instance, offers grad certificates (four courses each) in health management, human-centered informatics, quality assurance in biomedical product regulation, biopharmaceutical regulations, among others. These obviously are not for everyone, but for the right applicant, they could be the targeted final boost. They aren't cheap, but will cost less than getting a second Bachelor's. If you work for an institute of higher learning, some of these courses are often free.
- A second Bachelor's degree.
  - *Don't do this.* Medical schools accept applicants with Bachelor's in philosophy, sociology, economics, and other unrelated studies every year. This is time-consuming, expensive, and unnecessary. All you need is a 4-year degree, and the prerequisite pre-med courses, the latter of which can be achieved with much less money and effort than attaining another Bachelor's in many other ways.
- A Master's degree.
  - A good option if you don't have any glaring weaknesses and you want to focus on something a little more specific and extensive than a post-bacc will allow. Typical choices are Master's of public health, which has obvious benefits for someone interested in becoming a doctor and is interested in the prevention aspect of healthcare. However, these programs are notorious for being less rigorous than undergrad in terms of grading. Therefore, a 4.0 in these programs will not fix your poor grades or help you study for the MCAT. Likewise, poor grades in these programs will often sink your application as well, as they are nowhere near as difficult as medical school. Other popular options are MBAs, but again: do not expect the grades to save your application for similar reasons. That said, these programs can greatly strengthen your narrative with in-depth extracurricular opportunities, demonstration of an advanced academic interest, and additional research output.
- A post-baccalaureate program (post-bacc).
  - This type of program traditionally involves 1 year of intense pre-medical education (biology, chemistry, organic chemistry, physics, genetics, and some related courses), and is targeted for those trying to get into a professional school in the health sciences. This is the tried and true option for a wide range of non-traditional applicants to get them ready for medical school. Post-baccs are intense, expensive, and time-consuming. They are perfect for people whose chief flaws in their application are (1) poor grades, (2) completion of a non-STEM Bachelor's without the prerequisite pre-medical course work, or (3) long time spent out of school, spent working in another career. They have the added benefit of being excellent MCAT prep if you have not taken the test or would like a higher grade and plan on retaking it. Keep in mind, you can take your missing pre-medical courses without admission or adherence to a specific pre-medical post-bacc program, as this option is often cheaper and more

flexible. These strict programs have some added benefits, however, ranging from minor to significant, the most notable of which are targeted advising, committee letters, and *linkage to certain medical schools* that ranges from increasing your admissions chances to *guaranteed admission* contingent on fulfilling certain requirements within the program. There are a wide range of options to pick from, and an updated list is curated constantly by the AAMC.[3] Be aware, however, that financial aid for these programs varies greatly: some will offer scholarships and grants, whereas others don't even qualify for federal loans. In addition, be extremely skeptical of any program that does not explicitly mention their success rates in getting students into medical school. Do your due diligence!

- A Special Master's Program (SMP).
  - A high risk, high cost, high reward option. An SMP is a 1- to 2-year Master's program specifically targeted to getting the applicant into medical (and occasionally dental) school. Much like an intense post-bacc program with several extra things (the specifics vary by program) but with one weighty addition: it's a try-out. You take the first year of a program's medical school curriculum alongside medical students at the same time, and are evaluated the same way, and are even graded against their students. If you do well, most SMP boast a very high success rate of their participants gaining acceptance to medical schools (MD), even approaching ½-²/₃ rds of the class. However, the risk is tremendously high as well. If you do poorly, it's likely a death sentence to your medical school hopes, at least as it pertains to MD schools. If a program boasts a 50% success rate, it also means the other half of people spent 1 to 2 years of their lives, often more than $50,000 dollars without the benefit of financial aid (scholarships for aid for these programs is incredibly rare) without much to show for it.

- A PhD Degree.
  - This never should be used to enhance your ability to get into medical school, and consequently almost no one does this. It does however demonstrate a level of research prowess, dedication, and focus that medical schools find attractive, and those with PhDs looking to become doctors do *very* well when applying for medical school (assuming other admission criteria are met).

## 16.2.2 Employment

Almost any job, as discussed above, is fine during your gap years. Popular jobs people use to add to their application by adding to their Clinical Experiences are EMT/paramedic, medical assistant, medical scribe, and research coordinator/assistant (also in research). Sometimes people do whatever work they want, but use that to support themselves while they continue to engage in unpaid clinical volunteering and research opportunities that improve their application success. Ideally, an applicant with a particular deficiency (e.g., research, clinical experience) will secure employment that addresses that deficiency, however. Of course, you shouldn't feel forced to engage in one of these above options if you want to pursue other options and your application is already strong.

## 16.2.3 Research

- You can choose to engage in formal paid research or unpaid research. These are great boosts for your medical school resume, as many higher end medical schools look for applicants with research experience and interest.
  - Paid research positions are incredibly helpful as you can somewhat support yourself on your research salary (depending on the city). This gives you prolonged, significant exposure to a research mentor (and possibly an excellent letter of recommendation), attractive research experience (either fixing a weakness in your application or just making it stronger), a chance at publications (which will often benefit you your entire medical career), and a chance at actually getting a better understanding of the research world with all its good and bad qualities. It may make you more interested (or less) in research, and change what you want to do with your career—this happens all the time. The downside of these experiences: most research mentors know this is a popular medical school preapplication target, and will require you to sign a 2-year contract of employment as it's hard for them to keep training assistants that immediately leave for medical school or who miss 20 days immediately while

---

[3] Postbaccalaureate Premedical Programs. Available at: https://mec.aamc.org/postbac/#/index. Accessed July 8, 2022.

traveling for interviews. That said, 1-year contracts are still fairly common, and we encourage applicants to be upfront about asking for them if they desire them.[4]

- Unpaid opportunities can be incredibly beneficial as well, but come with the obvious downside of you needing to support yourself another way. Unpaid opportunities can unlock all the same benefits as paid research, but also has the added benefit of more options. Some researchers have funds to pay you, but others do not. Thus, if you are willing to research for free, your lab may let you work on projects that you couldn't if you were only willing to accept paid work. It also allows you to have much more flexibility with your gap years or with focusing on other parts of your application. It's not an uncommon tactic for students in their gap year to work on research projects piecemeal, (e.g., 0 to 10 hours a week the whole year), or in intense bursts (an entire summer, full time) and do other things accordingly.
- Research programs: Things to consider if you are interested in well-known research opportunities include: Rhodes, Fulbright, and Marshall's Scholars' programs as well as others. A well-curated list with associated descriptions is available here.[5] These programs are well-known, and offer a combination of research and associated experiences that is often very impressive, enriching, and beneficial to a medical school admission attempt but also for a career as a physician researcher.

## 16.2.4 Miscellaneous

As described above, there are a ton of worthwhile ways to spend your time between undergraduate and medical school. The options described above are just popular suggestions. Other popular ways that don't necessarily fit into the category above include nonprofit work (Peace Corps, Teach for America, AmeriCorps) which are often nonmedical but offer valuable experience with other cultures, underserved populations, and a livable wage.

Of course, our suggestions are not exhaustive, and we encourage you to be creative and explore as many options as possible to make the most out of your best gap year(s)!

## 16.3 Summary

Gap years before medical school are becoming increasingly common. There are many different reasons to consider gap years, including strengthening your application, taking a break before going down the gauntlet of medical training, or just broadening your personal and professional horizons with unique opportunities. Whatever you do, make sure you have *something* to show for your time and are able to tie it to your narrative toward medicine as a whole.

---

[4] We particularly recommend the NIH IRTA post-bacc paid research program (https://www.training.nih.gov/programs/postbac_irta). The author of this chapter did a 1-year paid research year and found it an incredibly rewarding opportunity that was commented on very favorably by multiple top 20 medical schools.

[5] Office of External Fellowships and Scholarships. Available at: https://www.rollins.edu/external-competitive-scholarship/major-scholarships/. Accessed July 8, 2022.

# 17 Crushing the MCAT

*Landon Cluts and Joel Thomas*

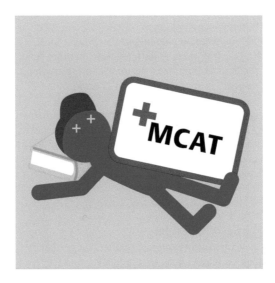

The Medical College Admission Test (MCAT). The big kahuna of your undergraduate career. This is the test you have heard about for years, and now it is time to fight. So, how do you prepare yourself mentally, emotionally, and physically for this beast of a test? There are many resources, strategies, and timeframes that people use, but the most important advice in this chapter is that you should use *whatever* strategy works best for *you* that allows you to get the best possible score you can on your first—and ideally only—attempt. We will discuss a few of the big-name resources and their pros and cons, as well as a few general strategies that tend to be successful for most test-takers. The rest depends on you and your unique circumstances leading up to the test (e.g., how comfortable you are with the pre-req material, how much time you have to prepare, and what type of learning works best for you). You have made it this far in college, and if you are reading this chapter to learn about the MCAT, you probably already have developed studying and test-taking strategies that you will simply need to refine for this test.

## 17.1 The Test

- The MCAT has undergone significant changes since it was first introduced as a tool for normalizing academic aptitude among medical school applicants, with the most major overhaul being MCAT 2015 that added a section on psychology, sociology, and behavior. In addition, MCAT 2015 shifted its focus to chemistry and physics topics in the context of living systems, de-emphasizing abstract concepts such as pulleys, lenses, and atomic phenomena in isolation. Success on the MCAT is predictive of success on the United States Medical Licensing Exam (USMLE) and Admissions Cmmittees (ADCOMs) collectively rate MCAT scores as "highest importance" for determining which applicants receive interviews.[1] In addition, higher MCAT score correlates with a higher chance of admission, even when controlling for grade point average (GPA) (▶ Fig. 17.1).[1]
- The average MCAT score for all matriculants to MD schools from 2020 to 2021 was 511.5 (83.5th percentile). For DO matriculants, the average score was a 504 (58th percentile). Note that this differs for under-represented minority (URM) applicants (for additional context, read more in Chapter 21, Before You Begin: Application Strength Analysis). "Black or African American" matriculants to MD programs

---

[1] Using MCAT® Data in 2023 Medical Student Selection. Available at: https://www.aamc.org/media/18901/download. Accessed July 8, 2022.

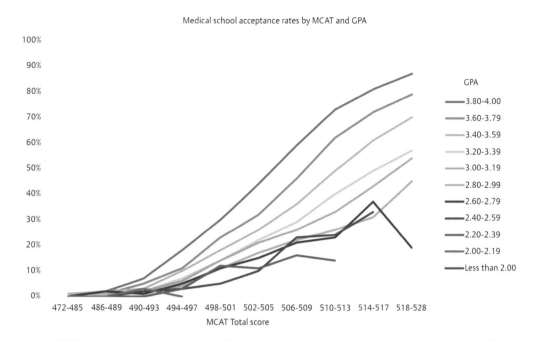

**Fig. 17.1** Percentage and number of 2018, 2019, and 2020 applicants accepted into at least one medical school, by Medical College Admission Test (MCAT) total score and undergraduate grade point average (GPA) ranges.

had an average MCAT of 505.7 (67th percentile), Hispanic/Latino/Spanish applicants 506.6 (70th percentile), Asian 513.8 (89th percentile), White 512.2 (85th percentile), American Indian/Alaska Native 503.8 (60th percentile), and Native Hawaiian/Pacific Islander 507.3 (70th percentile).

- As of 2020, the MCAT consists of 230 questions over 7 hours and 30 minutes (~6 hours of actual test-taking time at 90 minutes per section) split into four sections (Biological and Biochemical Foundations of Living Systems; Chemical and Physical Foundations of Biological Systems; Psychological, Social, and Biological Foundations of Behavior; and Critical Analysis and Reasoning Skills).
- There is a mix of stand-alone questions and reading passages with multiple associated questions including topics in psychology, sociology, biology, biochemistry, chemistry, organic chemistry, physics, and general prose critical reading.
  - The questions assess your ability to extrapolate general principles you learned in your prerequisite courses and apply in the setting of novel information and scenarios. For example, a passage in the physics section may describe an experiment using lenses in meticulous detail, and the associated questions may ask you to infer what happens if various parameters are changed (e.g., different type of lens, different image distance, etc.).
  - You will have a periodic table available during "Biological and Biochemical Foundations of Living Systems" and "Chemical and Physical Foundations of Biological Systems."
  - On the Critical Analysis and Reasoning Skills (CARS) section you may be asked to analyze and scrutinize a wide range of passages, ranging from clearly written literary analysis about Hamlet to incredibly obtuse passages about postmodern philosophy.[2]
- You get a 10-minute break between after the first and third section and a 30-minute break after the second section so that you can eat the healthy, good-for-your-brain lunch that you packed.
- If you do not prepare, this test will be grueling, and you will leave stressed and desperate for your score. If you prepare and practice, you will have a pretty good idea of how you did, and you will be able to take a well-deserved nap when you get back home.

---

[2] The author was a philosophy major, and even he struggled tremendously with these passages.

## 17.2  The Logistics

- You will be provided a locker to keep your lunch and other personal items. One of these items *should not be your phone* because you *cannot* look at it during your breaks, if you do there will be severe consequences.
  - It is best to just leave your phone in your car.
- Whenever you enter or exit the exam room you must be signed in and out and they will search any pockets you have and will look at things like glasses.
- Wear clothes with as little pockets as possible to save time during this process and leave any unnecessary accessories at home for the day.
- The night before your exam be sure you have any documents you need, especially your license.
- You will be provided paper and pencil to take notes during the exam so you do not have to bring many extra items. You will have a tutorial section at the beginning of the exam. Use this time to write down all of the rote memorization material (e.g., physics equations, amino acid structures) that you struggle to memorize so you don't have to struggle to keep them in your mind.

## 17.3  Student Perspective: Exam Day

**Landon Cluts:** I arrived at the test site, which was on the fourth floor of a multistory building. I arrived very early, and it turned out I was the second person to get in. I picked up a large laminated sheet with numbers. The numbers turned out to be the order they called you in to get situated in the test room. There were several other people who soon arrived after me. No one was really talking to each other, and no one was really studying any material. People seemed understandably nervous. When it was time, the proctor called us over to her desk by number. We gave her out basic info, and she took fingerprint scans and pictures of our faces with the computer. We were given a locker key if we wished to store our bags and food. The lockers were quite small. The proctor made me turn my pockets inside-out to check for anything illegal. Then another employee led me inside the test room, which was just a closed room with many computers separated by dividers. The computers were PC's with fairly large flat LCD screens. I sat down at the assigned computer and immediately began. I also used earplugs, which I brought with me. The earplugs were approved beforehand by the employee sitting outside. After the first section was done, I got up and went back outside the test room. The employee took my fingerprints and made me sign a sheet. Then I raced to the bathroom and back since the timer was going. I ate half of a banana that I had in my locker, which may or may not have been a good idea. I signed back in and passed the pocket check and fingerprint scan again. I had only a few seconds before the next section began again. Then I went on with the rest of the exam, which followed the same pattern. After the exam was done, I did a final sign-out, fingerprint scan, and returned the key. I was in a daze but glad the MCAT was over. Little did I know, that a month's wait to find out the score was going to be torture...

## 17.4  The Results

- In the test's current form, you will receive a score between 472 and 528 (56-point range) that is fit to a bell curve, with confidence intervals reported for each section score.
- Each of the four sections is scored out of 132 points.
- Your score will take about a month to get to you, so do yourself a favor and do not think about the test again until the day that scores are released. Just relax and do not speculate.
- A 500 is approximately the mean, 510 is approximately the 80th percentile, and 514 is approximately the 90th percentile.
- Your interpretation of your score is up to you. We recommend discussing your score with an academic advisor and to also set up a score goal.
- Each school has a different mean MCAT score so you will have to consult a resource such as the Medical School Admissions Requirement Database (MSAR) to determine which schools you are competitive at.

- A high MCAT score is absolutely NOT a guarantee that you will be accepted to medical school or even get an interview. It is just one of many parts of your application that will contribute to a Committee's final decision.

## 17.5  The Classes to Take Before You Take the MCAT

- There is a reason the prerequisite classes for medical school are what they are, so it is a good idea to try and get these classes done or mostly done before the MCAT because they are the content pool that will show up there.
- Other helpful but *optional* classes include human anatomy and physiology, cell biology, molecular genetics, neuroscience, and philosophy.
- Do well in these classes and that will not only set you up well for the MCAT, but medical school applications and medical school itself.
- Be familiar with all the content on the official topics list,[3] but also be aware that this list is likely not exhaustive.

## 17.6  So What's the Best Way to Prepare?

Again, there's no one-size-fits-all approach. Do whatever it takes to ensure that you get the highest possible score on full-length practice exams taken in a realistic test-day setting several days before you take the actual test. At the end of the day, the common denominators for success are the number of practice problems/passages done, hours spent in deep focus review material, mitigating test-day anxiety, maintaining wellness throughout the intensive study process, and doing practice passages under test-day conditions. If you are *not* in range of your target score, then **delay your test date, no matter how much money it costs.** That said, here are some of our best tips used by people who were accepted to medical school.

## 17.7  Timeframe

- Once you have an idea of when your exam test will be, you will need to decide when you will start preparing for the exam.
- If you are sure medicine is what you want to do for the rest of your life when you come to college, then you may be able to start studying from day 1. What this really means is that you do well in your pre-med classes—with an emphasis on *deeply understanding the material on a conceptual basis* versus simply memorizing and doing well on tests—and get an MCAT resource to focus on the material that will be tested in tandem with studying the lower-yield material.
  - We recommend signing up for an "MCAT Question of the Day" email subscription from the first day of college.
- Usually, however, people start studying no more than two semesters (1 year) before the exam and in most cases, people take about a semester to prepare and some even take the month or two between the school year ending and their test. On average, students that perform well on the exam spend between 200-300 hours total over several months studying for the exam.[4]
  - For an up-to-date resource on how students prepare for the exam, check out the most recent MCAT post-MCAT-questionnaire released by the Association of American Medical Colleges (AAMC).
- No matter the length of time you want to study for the MCAT, it is important to do it systematically.
  - Make a calendar from the first day you start studying to your test day laying out clear timeframes and what you will be studying each day.
  - Google image search "MCAT study schedules" and look at some of the examples there to help form your calendar.
  - *Before you start any intensive studying, go through the official content list and highlight the topics you don't know well to pay extra attention to them as you go through your study plan.*

---

[3]  Taking the MCAT® Exam. Available at: https://www.aamc.org/students/download/377882/data/mcat2015-content.pdf. Accessed July 8, 2022.
[4]  https://www.princetonreview.com/med-school-advice/mcat-study-guide/mcat-study-timeline

- Organization and time management are key in preparing for the MCAT, studying randomly is a good way to fall behind and not retain as much information.
- Exercise often, sleep 6 to 8 hours a night, take appropriate time off (e.g., at least 1–2 days a week and *whenever you feel burnt out or as if you are not retaining material*), eat healthily (avoid simple sugars, alcohol). Again, it's a marathon, not a sprint, and you'll want to "sharpen the saw" to the best of your ability.
  - Consider practicing stress reduction techniques (e.g., deep breathing exercises, meditation) early in your study period so that you can best use them to mitigate exam stress during your practice and real exams.

**Student Perspective: Study Schedule**

Landon Cluts: I began studying on January 2nd and planned to take the exam on May 19th. I woke up at 6 a.m. every morning and studied until 10 a.m. and then from 10 p.m. to midnight. I went through the Kaplan books twice. The first time I went through, I made flashcards of the bold topics. The second time I went through, I answered the review questions throughout the book and took more detailed notes on the more difficult topics I didn't quite understand. Additionally, I watched Khan Academy videos to help visualize those topics. I also took 10 practice tests from Kaplan, AAMC, and Princeton Review, along with 2 diagnostics (1/3 length tests) from Kaplan. Three of those exams were in the three weeks leading up to the exam.

## 17.8  Resources

- There are numerous exam study resources out there including Kaplan, Princeton Review, Examkrackers, the AAMC, the Berkeley Review, classes and free resources such as Khan Academy that can be used to supplement some of those hard topics.
- This list is not exhaustive but these are—by far—the most used resources for budding physicians taking the MCAT.
- Whichever books or methods you use, you should do it systematically and should go over the material more than once. *Likewise, all students should read through the AAMC Official MCAT Guide at least once.*
- We strongly recommend looking through this extremely exhaustive list of resources and study schedules on reddit.com/r/MCAT:
  - https://www.reddit.com/r/Mcat/wiki/contentreview, the Student Doctor Network (SDN) MCAT Study Plan Thread: https://forums.studentdoctor.net/threads/mcat-study-plans-study-strategies-and-ask-me-anything-ama-threads.1262572/, and the 509 + MCAT Study Habits thread on SDN: https://forums.studentdoctor.net/threads/509-mcat-study-habits.1143569/
  - Of note, the 3-month (100 Day) MCAT Study Schedule on SDN is very popular: https://www.studentdoctor.net/3-month-mcat-study-schedule/

## 17.9  Kaplan versus The Princeton Review

- These are both the most well-known and truly excellent MCAT review resources.
- Their books are a comprehensive review of all the science you need to know for the big test.
- The main difference between the two is that Princeton Review has significantly more difficult practice exams and they probably should not be the first practice test you take.
- You should, however, end up taking practice tests from both resources which will be discussed later in this chapter.
- Find someone who has these books and see which one appeals most to you.

## 17.10  Classes

- Some people find taking a class is the best for them because it provides a regimen for you and has regular diagnostics along with resources to ask questions.
- These classes tend to be quite expensive and are like adding another class to your school schedule.

- Think back to how you prepared for the SAT. Did you use a class? If so, was it useful for you? If not, do you wish you did in retrospect?
- Before you sign up for a class, be sure you ask people who have taken them to ensure it is the best for you.
- If you do decide to take a class, be sure you stay committed and keep up with it or else, you will be wasting money and points on your test.
- Both Kaplan and Princeton Review have classes and may have sites near your school, and you will inevitably get emails or pamphlets describing their services. Be wary that there are *many* scam programs that are expensive and unhelpful; make sure to do your research on a program if it's not well established.

## 17.11  Other Options

- A more recent development in the exam study world is a spaced repetition program called Anki.
  - It is a flashcard system used to memorize huge amounts of information over long periods of time (i.e., months to years).
  - You will have to search the Internet for MCAT review decks or make your own cards.
  - Once you start an Anki regimen it is best to keep up with it *daily* while you are walking around, on a bus, or before you go to bed.
  - This is also a valuable resource in medical school so you can practice now.
  - Refer to reddit.com/r/MCAT for additional info on Anki.
- Wikipremed.com is also a great resource for understanding enough about a topic to be adequately prepared for the MCAT.
- Khan Academy has a wealth of videos for many topics but the ones that are important for you are all of their videos from the sciences you have taken and will help you learn some of those difficult topics (like Physics) and can be used in conjunction with most resources and even during your classes before you start your MCAT preparations. In addition, the AAMC has partnered with Khan Academy to provide 1,100 free videos and 3,000 practice questions.[5]

## 17.12  Practice Exams

- These are some of the most important tools in your MCAT preparation tool kit because they will introduce you to the questions and passages you will see, and they will help you with your time management during the real thing so you will not run out and be forced to randomly guess on the last few questions.
- Kaplan, the AAMC, and Princeton Review all offer tests and you usually get a few free depending on what book set you get and when you sign up for the test the AAMC gives you one.
- It is worth buying extra practice tests from each of these entities so that you end up taking 8 to 12 practice exams before your test date.
- It is a good idea to take a diagnostic test (usually ⅓ length) through AAMC or Kaplan to see where you are starting from and to practice using the system before the full-length test comes into play.
- When taking your practice exams, it is important to take them in the most sterile environment you can to closely match what you will experience on test day.
  - This means only take the breaks when you would on test day, no phone, and a silent room.
- After each exam it is important to go through each question, even if you got it right.
  - You want to take detailed notes on questions you got wrong and why you got them wrong and make sure you got the ones right for the right reason.
  - Likewise, even if you got the question right, go over the answer choices to understand why each wrong answer is wrong. Typically, the wrong answer choices relate to topics that are tested in other questions.
  - Consider keeping a notebook record of which problems in particular were really hard or caused you to make a mistake. After all your review is done, you should come back to these problems and make sure you can do them cold.

---

[5] Test prep MCAT. Available at: https://www.khanacademy.org/test-prep/mcat. Accessed July 8, 2022.

- Finally, you will be given the approximate score you would have gotten if this was the real deal.
  - This is mainly useful to see your improvement over time.
  - Do not get stressed if your first practice exam score or diagnostic test is lower than you want your actual score to be, this is a marathon and your score will grow as you practice.
- It is important to remember that Kaplan, AAMC, and Princeton Review have different practice exam difficulties.
  - Princeton Review > > Kaplan > Real MCAT > AAMC in terms of difficulty.
  - It is important (usually) to not take the Princeton Review practice first.
    - Imagine if the first time you went to the gym and you tried to bench 400 pounds.
    - If you worked your way up to that heavy weight over time (with Kaplan and AAMC) you will get much more out of your workout and will eventually get something out of benching 400 pounds.
- In general, you should just switch between all of them and not take exams from the same company back-to-back.
- Keep a notebook or excel sheet of your scores to see your progression and also spend the time to create a document of the questions you missed or were particularly difficult so that you are forced to go through them thoroughly and have easy access to them.

## 17.13  Practice Questions

- Many of the companies that have been mentioned throughout this chapter also have question banks available.
  - These are useful to increase the number of questions and answers you see, but remember you are not doing them under time restraint.
- UWorld offers a huge MCAT question bank that may be a good option to massively increase your practice question reps.
- A good strategy for these is to get them much earlier than when you truly start studying so that you can start getting used to the question style you will see (this is like doing small free weights in the gym).
- Take one early practice test to see what you're up against.
  - If you take the test and do so well on it that it encourages you. Congrats. On the other hand, if the test makes you feel completely demoralized, then that's probably a pretty normal outcome. Don't let a low score kill your confidence. At least now you will take the MCAT seriously. Just know that the MCAT is a big mountain and from working hard enough for a long time, anyone can climb it.

## 17.14  Critical Analysis and Reasoning

- The Critical Analysis and Reasoning section (CARS) of the MCAT is quite different from the others.
- You will be presented nine 500- to 600-word reading passages and five to seven questions that go along with each.
- You will essentially have 10 minutes for each passage-question set, so time is often most tight on this section.
- The reading passages may be something wholly outside of science, meaning that you will have to truly understand what you are reading because you are unlikely to know about the topic beforehand. *All of the information required to answer the questions is contained solely in the passage. Do NOT extrapolate on outside information to answer the questions.*
- The best way to practice for this section is to:
  - Practice CARS and review them on practice exams.
    - Get a timer. Do two passages a day. Time yourself, and aim for 5 minutes or lower per passage.
    - Don't get too cocky in this section because the practice tests are usually easier than the actual exam for this section, in our opinion.
    - Experiment with reading strategy in this section to see what works for you, if you have time. If you are within a month of taking the exam, avoid changing up strategy too much.
  - Read articles, difficult books across a variety of genres, and short stories and think about them critically (best done in the years leading up to the exam—hopefully you were a lifelong reader!).
  - Think about what the author is trying to say, if they are biased, where their logic falls flat, etc.
    - Approach each passage with the questions, "Why is the author writing this?" and "How is he trying to convince me/frame the argument?" Specifically, pay close attention to words like "despite,"

"therefore," "nonetheless," etc., that shape logical connections between the premises of the argument and the ultimate conclusion.[6]

  ○ Read every single word of the passage. Do *not* skim, as you will likely miss important subtleties and make assumptions that will lead you to pick distracting incorrect answer choices.
  ○ Take a *short* mental break after you finish reading and answering the questions for each passage before you move onto the next passage, as you will need to—again—muster intense focus.

- There is not a set of knowledge you must know for this section; it is purely based on your ability to read quickly and gather as much insight as possible from what you read.
- This is probably where time will be least on your side and is notorious for being the lowest section on many MCATs so take a little extra time to practice this section to not fall victim to CARS. Since there are nine passages with 90 minutes for the section, plan to spend no more than 10 minutes per passage (assuming you will not use time left over to recheck earlier passages).
- Try to force yourself to be interested in or engage with the author's passage. Realistically, many of them will be extremely dry and academic, and you will be more likely to make careless mistakes if you half-heartedly skim through the passage without any interest in the material whatsoever.

## 17.15  Other Sections in General

- The content you will need to know for the MCAT will be in the resources that we discussed earlier in this section.
  - Know your organic chemistry, cell biology, etc.
  - Know how to interpret various charts and how to synthesize conclusions from them.
- These sections will have discrete questions (stand-alone questions) and questions that will be from a passage or set of data and may be part of a series of several questions.
- The best way to practice for these sections is to know the material like the back of your hand and do practice question after practice question *after practice question*. It's acceptable to do them under more "forgiving" conditions earlier in your study period, but move onto doing them under test day conditions (e.g., 10 passages in a row with 95 min).

## 17.16  Biochemical Foundations

- Know your organic chemistry basic reactions cold. Know *some* of the more uncommon amine reactions as well since it ties well with biochemistry.
- Lately there is more emphasis on genetics so it doesn't hurt to know the basic molecular techniques such as electrophoresis, chromatography, and Western blotting.
- Know your physiology, including heart depolarization, muscle depolarization, kidney, blood acid/base.

## 17.17  Chemical and Physical Foundations of Biological Systems

- Know the basic physics equations cold. Know the math shortcuts. You will not have time to look up any equations, even if they give the simple ones to you. You have to have enough time to examine and understand the *complicated* equations they throw at you. Remember that you don't have to understand the equation completely, but just the *relationships*.
- Remember to check units in the answer early. Sometimes you can pick the answer by just picking the one with the right units. *Guestimate guestimate guestimate*.
- Our best advice—*for this section especially*—is to do practice problem after practice problem.

## 17.18  Test-Taking Strategies

- Do yourself a huge favor and only take the MCAT when your goal score is the average of your practice test scores.

---

[6] In an argument, a premise is a statement that substantiates a conclusion. An argument may have multiple premises, and the premises themselves may be implied (i.e., not explicitly written out). A conclusion may also be a premise for another conclusion.

- If you are not reaching that score, you may need to re-evaluate your studying.
  - Talk to an advisor about what may be going on.
- Each one of you knows how to take a test. You have spent time honing your ability to work through a chemistry and physics exam and in doing so you have unknowingly been practicing for the MCAT.
- The MCAT is about answering as many questions correctly as possible and is not only a small fraction of an individual class; it is 100% of your final grade and each question is weighed the same.
- As you go through the exam it is important to not get hung up on one question; this is a powerful time waster and you will lose out on easy to get answers.
  - If you find yourself struggling on a question for even about 20 seconds, mark it and move on to easier questions so that you do not run out of time and miss them.
  - At the end of each section you will be able to go back to those tougher questions and get them, but you will not be able to if you waste time stewing over them and at this point you have missed even the easiest of questions.
- When you are learning physics and chemistry you will learn a lot of math, for the MCAT a lot of times you can use logic to eliminate many wrong answers before you must do calculations and may not need to do any at all. Be sure you seek out mathematical shortcuts to make those long formulas easier on the exam.
  - Many of the companies that have been mentioned will describe how to do this.
- When you are taking the test, it is important to eliminate answers which are definitely wrong which will allow you to increase your chances of being correct on a guess if it comes down to it.
  - This brings up a critical point that *no question should be left unanswered*. A guess has more of a chance of being correct than a question that goes unanswered.
- Do not do intensive studying the day before your test. Continue the healthy habits you have been doing regularly throughout your study period, and do something relaxing for most of the day. The night before, you can consider a brief review of straight-memorization topics (e.g., physics equations), but avoid doing entire passages.

## 17.19 Retake or Not to Retake?

- General scenarios in which you're highly encouraged to retake your MCATs are:
  - You scored significantly lower than your target schools' average MCAT.
  - You scored much lower than the average score of your practice tests.
  - There were some extenuating difficult or stressful events occurring when you were studying or taking the MCAT.
  - Your scores are considered expired by schools, due to the date you have taken them.
    - MCAT scores do *expire* after 3 years.
- That said, retaking the MCAT *may* be a strategic decision for most applicants. Consider the data from the AAMC on MCAT retakers from 2016 to 2018 (▶ Fig. 17.2).[7]
- Across a wide range of scores, the median change on retaking the MCAT was an increase in two to three points. All other factors remaining constant, it appears that this has a fairly substantial increase in acceptance rate, considering the following data of acceptance rates across MCAT scores (▶ Table 17.1).
- Very few students who retook the MCAT did worse. On one interpretation, the risk/costs of retaking the MCAT are fairly low (statistically speaking, at least), and the potential benefits seem to outweigh these risks. On the other hand, the admissions data alone does *not* allow you to straightforwardly conclude that—all things equal—an increase in MCAT score of two to three points will make a substantial difference in *your* likelihood of acceptance. For one thing, schools will generally be able to see all of your MCAT scores, and different schools may evaluate multiple scores in different ways (e.g., average of all scores vs. weighted score with greater emphasis on a more recent attempt).[8] As such, while it may be the case that—on average—there's a 10% difference in acceptance rates between "Total MCAT score of 498–501" versus "Total MCAT score of 502–505," it's not clear that an ADCOM will see *your* scores

---

[7] MCAT Examination Repeat Policies and Data. Available at: https://www.aamc.org/media/36216/download. Accessed July 8, 2022.

[8] MCAT Examination Repeat Policies and Data. Available at: https://www.aamc.org/media/36216/download. Accessed July 8, 2022.

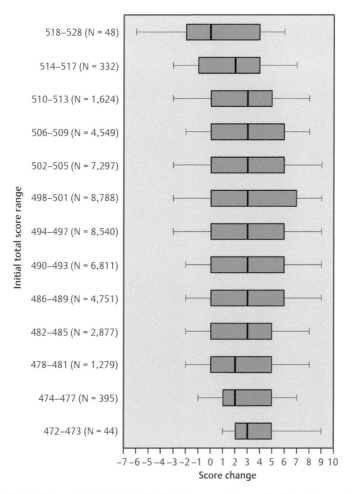

**Fig. 17.2** Changes in Medical College Admission Test (MCAT) total scores between the first and second attempts for MCAT examinees from 2016 to 2018 who retested.
**Note:** These box-and-whisker plots show changes in MCAT total scores from the first to the second attempt for examinees ($N = 47,335$) who took this version of the MCAT exam for the first time during this 3-year period and then tested a second time in this same window.

of—say—a 500 and 503 as significantly different. The takeaway here is that you're likely to get a two- to three-point increase on retaking the MCAT, but there's no good data on how ADCOMs would interpret an increase of this magnitude. The best we can confidently say is that it's unlikely to hurt you, and it *may* help you, albeit to an unknown extent.

- Note that you cannot take the MCAT over three times in a single testing year, four times in a 2-year period, or seven times altogether. Failure to show up for an examination and voiding an examination both count toward these limits. Students can appeal for special permission to exceed the limits, however.

## 17.20 Final Thoughts

I like to imagine the MCAT like a punching bag—a target that never moves. With enough practice you realize that it is a one-trick pony and not a moving target. There's a lot of material out there that can help you get a good score so all you have to do is supply the will power. At the same time, there are simply too

**Table 17.1** MCAT and GPA grid for applicants and acceptees to US MD-Granting Medical Schools, 2019–2020 through 2021–2022 (aggregated)

| Acceptance rate for applicants | | Total MCAT scores | | | | | | | | | | All applicants |
|---|---|---|---|---|---|---|---|---|---|---|---|---|
| | | Less than 486 | 486–489 | 490–493 | 494–497 | 498–501 | 502–505 | 506–509 | 510–513 | 514–517 | Greater than 517 | |
| **Total GPA** | | | | | | | | | | | | |
| Greater than 3.79 | Acceptees | 2 | 7 | 44 | 297 | 1,002 | 2,466 | 5,092 | 7,630 | 7,790 | 8,819 | 33,149 |
| | Applicants | 169 | 327 | 793 | 1,741 | 3,541 | 6,127 | 9,251 | 11,044 | 10,046 | 10,473 | 53,512 |
| | Acceptance rate % | 1.2 | 2.1 | 5.5 | 17.1 | 28.3 | 40.2 | 55.0 | 69.1 | 77.5 | 84.2 | 61.9 |
| 3.60–3.79 | Acceptees | 5 | 5 | 60 | 299 | 938 | 1,917 | 3,433 | 4,924 | 3,984 | 2,573 | 18,138 |
| | Applicants | 460 | 650 | 1,334 | 2,605 | 4,414 | 6,437 | 8,228 | 8,426 | 5,784 | 3,463 | 41,801 |
| | Acceptance rate % | 1.1 | 0.8 | 4.5 | 11.5 | 21.3 | 29.8 | 41.7 | 58.4 | 68.9 | 74.3 | 43.4 |
| 3.40–3.59 | Acceptees | 9 | 10 | 39 | 260 | 701 | 1,244 | 1,963 | 2,386 | 1,647 | 872 | 9,131 |
| | Applicants | 689 | 855 | 1,574 | 2,702 | 3,989 | 5,084 | 5,842 | 5,026 | 2,875 | 1,357 | 29,993 |
| | Acceptance rate % | 1.3 | 1.2 | 2.5 | 9.6 | 17.6 | 24.5 | 33.6 | 47.5 | 57.3 | 64.3 | 30.4 |
| 3.20–3.39 | Acceptees | 3 | 9 | 31 | 150 | 411 | 700 | 882 | 957 | 628 | 280 | 4,051 |
| | Applicants | 823 | 898 | 1,468 | 2,057 | 2,790 | 3,154 | 2,993 | 2,418 | 1,259 | 509 | 18,369 |
| | Acceptance rate % | 0.4 | 1.0 | 2.1 | 7.3 | 14.7 | 22.2 | 29.5 | 39.6 | 49.9 | 55.0 | 22.1 |

*(Continued)*

**Table 17.1** (*Continued*) MCAT and GPA grid for applicants and acceptees to US MD-Granting Medical Schools, 2019–2020 through 2021–2022 (aggregated)

| Acceptance rate for applicants | | Total MCAT scores | | | | | | | | | | All applicants |
|---|---|---|---|---|---|---|---|---|---|---|---|---|
| | | Less than 486 | 486–489 | 490–493 | 494–497 | 498–501 | 502–505 | 506–509 | 510–513 | 514–517 | Greater than 517 | |
| 3.00–3.19 | Acceptees | 3 | 4 | 16 | 95 | 248 | 348 | 405 | 352 | 203 | 121 | 1,795 |
| | Applicants | 903 | 743 | 985 | 1,416 | 1,623 | 1,684 | 1,542 | 1,095 | 479 | 230 | 10,700 |
| | Acceptance rate % | 0.3 | 0.5 | 1.6 | 6.7 | 15.3 | 20.7 | 26.3 | 32.1 | 42.4 | 52.6 | 16.8 |
| 2.80–2.99 | Acceptees | 3 | 5 | 9 | 25 | 86 | 137 | 137 | 106 | 56 | 35 | 599 |
| | Applicants | 686 | 528 | 607 | 679 | 765 | 777 | 601 | 367 | 173 | 75 | 5,258 |
| | Acceptance rate % | 0.4 | 0.9 | 1.5 | 3.7 | 11.2 | 17.6 | 22.8 | 28.9 | 32.4 | 46.7 | 11.4 |
| 2.60–2.79 | Acceptees | 0 | 4 | 3 | 14 | 38 | 45 | 49 | 35 | 18 | 7 | 213 |
| | Applicants | 523 | 325 | 350 | 346 | 383 | 273 | 210 | 146 | 59 | 25 | 2,640 |
| | Acceptance rate % | 0.0 | 1.2 | 0.9 | 4.0 | 9.9 | 16.5 | 23.3 | 24.0 | 30.5 | 28.0 | 8.1 |
| 2.40–2.59 | Acceptees | 0 | 0 | 2 | 5 | 6 | 7 | 19 | 7 | 4 | 3 | 53 |
| | Applicants | 383 | 171 | 169 | 152 | 127 | 102 | 77 | 38 | 17 | 10 | 1,246 |
| | Acceptance rate % | 0.0 | 0.0 | 1.2 | 3.3 | 4.7 | 6.9 | 24.7 | 18.4 | 23.5 | 30.0 | 4.3 |
| 2.20–2.39 | Acceptees | 0 | 0 | 0 | 3 | 5 | 3 | 8 | 3 | - | - | 24 |
| | Applicants | 229 | 76 | 75 | 65 | 48 | 36 | 33 | 18 | - | - | 584 |
| | Acceptance rate % | 0.0 | 0.0 | 0.0 | 4.6 | 10.4 | 8.3 | 24.2 | 16.7 | - | - | 4.1 |

*(Continued)*

**Table 17.1** (*Continued*) MCAT and GPA grid for applicants and acceptees to US MD-Granting Medical Schools, 2019–2020 through 2021–2022 (aggregated)

| Acceptance rate for applicants | | Total MCAT scores | | | | | | | | | | All applicants |
|---|---|---|---|---|---|---|---|---|---|---|---|---|
| | | Less than 486 | 486–489 | 490–493 | 494–497 | 498–501 | 502–505 | 506–509 | 510–513 | 514–517 | Greater than 517 | |
| 2.00–2.19 | Acceptees | 0 | 0 | 0 | 0 | 0 | 0 | - | - | - | - | 4 |
| | Applicants | 109 | 36 | 37 | 10 | 11 | 13 | - | - | - | - | 235 |
| | Acceptance rate % | 0.0 | 0.0 | 0.0 | 0.0 | 0.0 | 0.0 | - | - | - | - | 1.7 |
| Less than 2.00 | Acceptees | 0 | 1 | 0 | - | - | - | - | - | - | - | 1 |
| | Applicants | 50 | 13 | 10 | - | - | - | - | - | - | - | 90 |
| | Acceptance rate % | 0.0 | 7.7 | 0.0 | - | - | - | - | - | - | - | 1.1 |
| All applicants | Acceptees | 25 | 45 | 204 | 1,148 | 3,435 | 6,867 | 11,988 | 16,402 | 14,334 | 12,710 | 67,158 |
| | Applicants | 5,024 | 4,622 | 7,402 | 11,780 | 17,692 | 23,690 | 28,791 | 28,582 | 20,701 | 16,144 | 164,428 |
| | Acceptance rate % | 0.5 | 1.0 | 2.8 | 9.7 | 19.4 | 29.0 | 41.6 | 57.4 | 69.2 | 78.7 | 40.8 |

Abbreviations: GPA, grade point average; MCAT, Medical College Admission Test; SD, standard deviation; Undergraduate Grade Point Average (UGPA).

**Notes:** 1. The frequencies are combined totals of 3 y.

2. The means and SDs of MCAT scores are calculated based on data from applicants who applied with MCAT scores (each year, approximately 2% of individuals apply without MCAT scores). Specifically, 60,334 applicants and 21,942 matriculants in 2021 were included in the calculations; only the most recent MCAT score is used for individuals who took the exam more than once. The means and SDs of UGPA are calculated based on applicants with available GPA data. Specifically, 62,140 applicants and 22,483 matriculants in 2021 were included in the calculations.

3. Dashed cells indicate the MCAT/UGPA range combinations with fewer than 10 applicants; blank cells indicate MCAT/UGPA range combinations with zero applicants.

4. Each academic year includes applicants and matriculants that applied to enter medical school in the fall of the given year. For example, academic year 2021–2022 represents the applicants and matriculants that applied to enter medical school during the 2021 application cycle.

many resources out there for any individual to make full use of, and you will ultimately run into diminishing returns with your studying. Eventually, you will just need to trust your gut and face the beast with full fury. Keep all of the above in mind and you will be on your way to destroy the MCAT. Good luck!

## 17.21 Summary

You need to do well on the MCAT to get into medical school. Preparation starts with your pre-req courses, as obtaining a deep conceptual understanding of the sciences will make the months of preparation before the exam significantly easier. Once you get to the months leading up to the test, you will find that there are many different study strategies; stick to whichever works best for you and allows you to do as many practice problems as possible under test-day conditions. Familiarize yourself with the logistics of test-day; have a detailed plan of action for how you will spend the day taking the test. Take care of yourself during the months of intensive study before the exam. Lastly, the decision to retake the exam should be very carefully considered; most test-takers who retook the MCAT did not score four or more points on a retake, and the percentage of those who did score four or more points on a retake gets lower as their initial MCAT score gets higher.

# 18 Self-Care and Wellness

*Joel Thomas and Eva Roy*

Personal wellness is critically important to success in medicine and *life in general.* If you are not physically and mentally well, you will suffer across virtually every aspect of your life, including not only your pre-medical career, but also your ability to physically navigate the world, handle complex relationships, and to provide for those who depend on you. Wellness also suffers from being a "hot topic" that gets superficial, band-aid solutions from administration (e.g., "meditate more!") because they are under pressure to demonstrate that *something* is being done. In addition, many people assume that they are doing well if they are not suffering from severe, obvious symptoms (e.g., frank depression, physical injuries). The reality is that wellness exists on a spectrum ranging from "suicidal" to "nirvana." In this chapter, we will discuss why you should *actively* focus on your wellness. We will also explore the modern science of wellness while being highly critical of "feel-good" popular solutions that ultimately fail to deliver their promises for long-term wellness.

It's easy to get bogged down by the amount of work there is always to do. As a pre-medical student, you will always find yourself balancing classes, extracurriculars, jobs, and relationships. Amid this chaos, taking care of yourself may become last on the list of things to prioritize. It's natural to think that all of those tasks take precedence because the short-term perceived benefits of—say—staying up late to cram for a test may be immediate, whereas the long-term effects of chronic stress and sleep deprivation are insidious and delayed. If you do not take care of yourself now, your health will slowly deteriorate and consequently affect your performance in *all* aspects of your life. To make matters worse, just as the harms of neglecting wellness develop slowly over time, recovering your wellness once you're in a dark place will also take sustained commitment to (re)establishing healthy habits. On the other hand, being proactive about wellness is reinforcing. You will notice that you generally feel better and perform closer to your maximum potential across all dimensions. Your life won't be perfect, however. You will still experience defeats and sadness—this is simply a normal part of being human. You will, however, be much more resilient in the face of hardship. Ideally, you will become *antifragile*[1] and actively thrive against adversity.

Keep in mind that this chapter gives recommendations for *optimizing* wellness, i.e., the ideals you should *strive* for. Realistically, we do not expect you to do everything recommended. If anything, this chapter can help you identify and implement strategies to fix low-hanging fruit in your lifelong journey to wellness (e.g., getting started with exercise, fixing poor sleep hygiene, etc.).

## 18.1 Why Care Now?

Unfortunately, the balancing act only gets harder as you progress in your career. Therefore, we emphasize that college is a critical time to lay down the foundation of good wellness habits. The journey to becoming a physician is an endurance test rather than a sprint. You have to do well today, but make sure you are healthy and mentally ready to do well tomorrow, next month, next year, and next decade. We encourage you to periodically check in with yourself physically and mentally (e.g., through regular journaling), to carefully consider the material in this chapter, and to experiment with different strategies for optimizing wellness if you feel that you have room to improve.

## 18.2 So How Do I Get Started and Keep the Ball Rolling?

*"We are what we repeatedly do. Excellence, then, is not an act, but a habit."*

— Will Durant

Wellness is a state-of-being—a continually maintained goal that arises from repeated *habits.* Thus, in order to optimize wellness, you will need to consistently prioritize certain habits, even (or especially) when it may seem easier in the short term to pick the option that leads to worse well-being in the

---

[1] A Definition of Antifragile and its Implications. Available at: https://fs.blog/2014/04/antifragile-a-definition/. Accessed July 8, 2022.

long term. As such, most readers will need to achieve *long-term habit/behavior change*, which is arguably one of the hardest things for anyone to do (ask any primary care physician!).

Fortunately, the science of behavior change has made tremendous strides. Borrowing from James Clear's *Atomic Habits,*[2] you will need to change your environmental conditions, (i.e., the system), *to minimize the level of resistance* required to do whatever leads to optimal wellness. For example, if you find that the activation energy required to get out of your apartment during the winter and walk to the campus gym is too high for a regular exercise routine, you may change the environment by investing in a pull-up bar for your apartment and adjustable dumbbells. We also urge you to conceptualize wellness as a core part of your *identity* and not simply things that you try to do consistently. As discussed in *Atomic Habits:*

*Imagine two people resisting a cigarette. When offered a smoke, the first person says, "No thanks. I'm trying to quit." It sounds like a reasonable response, but this person still believes they are a smoker who is trying to be something else. They are hoping their behavior will change while carrying around the same beliefs.*

*The second person declines by saying, "No thanks. I'm not a smoker." It's a small difference, but this statement signals a shift in identity. Smoking was part of their former life, not their current one. They no longer identify as someone who smokes.*

Likewise, you turn down the donut at breakfast not because you are *trying to lose weight* but because *you* don't eat sweets.

In the following sections, we will give you information and recommendations for optimizing wellness, but it is ultimately up to you to identify ways to automate these choices so that they feel as natural to you as reflexively checking your phone when you hear it ring. We encourage you to *track* how often you do these habits (e.g., with a habit tracking app) so that you can identify what's working and what isn't to adjust accordingly. Don't get too discouraged in the beginning; habits are psychological associations (i.e., "cue-response" patterns) that arise from conditioning, and the strength of the association—and underlying neural circuitry—will grow stronger over time as you continue to reinforce it.

## 18.3 Physical Components of Wellness

### 18.3.1 High-Quality Sleep

We want you to rake through your brain and burn *every* association you have with "being a successful future physician" and "compromising sleep." Yes, there will be rare occasions (e.g., long call shifts as a resident) when you will be sleep deprived, but your goal for *every single day* should be to get 7 to 9 hours of high-quality sleep. We emphasize quality in addition to quantity because it is now known that environmental conditions, (e.g., noise pollution and light in the room), can lead to nonrefreshing sleep by disrupting the percentage of deep refreshing sleep, as well as by increasing circulating stress hormones.[3] In the short term, this can lead to greater daytime fatigue and irritability. In the long term, this can predispose to a variety of chronic illnesses associated with a chronic stress response (e.g., diabetes, hypertension, and certain cancers). In addition, the growing literature on *even slightly reduced* quality and quantity of sleep on working memory,[4] long-term memory consolidation,[5] mood,[6]

---

[2] This is one of the most influential books the author has *ever* read and helped him *tremendously* in reframing his approach to quitting bad habits and taking up good habits *for good. We urge everyone to read this book at least once.* And this is coming from someone who *hates* self-help books and finds them incredibly unscientific and clichéd. This book does an impressive job in compiling the most up-to-date science on behavior change in an actionable way.

[3] How Noise Can Affect Your Sleep Satisfaction. Available at: https://www.sleepfoundation.org/bedroom-environment/how-does-noise-affect-sleep. Accessed July 8, 2022.

[4] Xie W, Berry A, Lustig C, Deldin P, Zhang W. Poor Sleep Quality and Compromised Visual Working Memory Capacity. J Int Neuropsychol Soc 2019;25(6):583–594. Available at: https://www.ncbi.nlm.nih.gov/pmc/articles/PMC6620134/. Accessed July 8, 2022.

[5] Rasch B, Born J. About Sleep's Role in Memory. Physiol Rev 2013;93(2):681–766. Available at: https://www.ncbi.nlm.nih.gov/pmc/articles/PMC3768102/. Accessed July 8, 2022.

[6] Triantafillou S, Saeb S, Lattie EG, Mohr DC, Kording KP. Relationship Between Sleep Quality and Mood: Ecological Momentary Assessment Study. JMIR Ment Health 2019;6(3):e12613. Available at: https://www.ncbi.nlm.nih.gov/pmc/articles/PMC6456824/. Accessed July 8, 2022.

metabolic health,[7] and overall well-being[8] make it abundantly clear that it's non-negotiable. Make sure you get 7 to 9 hours of high-quality sleep every night[9] with the following habits:

- Fall asleep at roughly the same time every night and wake up at roughly the same time every morning. *Even on weekends and vacations. Even when your schedule changes dramatically for rotations.*[10]
- Keep the bedroom dark, quiet, and slightly cool (~68 °F). Use your bed only for sleeping.
- Avoid eating a large meal within 2 hours of sleep. Minimize alcohol intake (clear association with reducing quality of sleep) and nicotine.
- Minimize caffeine intake in the afternoon.
- *Prioritize high-quality sleep.* Don't compromise on sleep to study more or to talk to friends. There *will* be free time available sometime in the day, especially if you stick to a schedule and are more efficient in getting your work done because you had enough high-quality sleep!
- Avoid overstimulation before bed. This includes strenuous exercise, as well as mental stimulation (e.g., checking emails and social media) and natural light—specifically *blue light*. Blue light is poorly filtered by the eyes and will get to the retina, blocking melatonin production and ultimately keeping you up at night.[11] Various apps (e.g., iPhone settings, F.lux[12] for computers) will gradually lower blue light as you get closer to bedtime, but you can also consider buying glasses that filter out blue light for nighttime work, as preliminary data seems to suggest that they may help some people achieve better sleep (although this area of research is still very much up-in-the-air).[13]
- Consider taking over-the-counter melatonin for sleep. The evidence appears to be mixed as to what dose and timing relative to sleep works best.[14]
- If you are lying in bed for over 30 minutes and unable to fall asleep, get up *out of bed and into another room*, do something *mildly* mentally engaging but boring (e.g., reading the user manual for your computer), and then try to fall asleep again.
- Consider meditating before bed (more in the meditation section).
- To optimize sleep quality, try earplugs, blackout curtains, and a sleep mask to minimize subclinical disruptive stimuli.
- Consider **power naps** in the day if you're forced to operate on suboptimal sleep (e.g., adjusting to night shift). We recommend this excellent article by MedSchoolInsiders: "How to Nap and NOT Wake Up Groggy."[15]

## 18.3.2 Exercise

It's incredibly easy to become sedentary when you have to study and write papers for hours at a time. As such, you will need to prioritize some exercise, *ideally every day*. Most universities have a gym that you have access to and may even have discounted workout classes. In addition, some universities may even offer exercise classes for credit which is a great way to get moving and an easy A for your GPA (great strategy for boosting your semester credit load without overwhelming yourself). If you're new to exercising, start slow and increase the intensity and frequency over time. Every Olympic athlete started horribly out

---

[7] Robertson MD, Russell-Jones D, Umpleby AM, Dijk DJ. Effects of three weeks of mild sleep restriction implemented in the home environment on multiple metabolic and endocrine markers in healthy young men. Clinical Science 2013;62(2):204–211 Available at: https://www.metabolismjournal.com/article/S0026-0495(12)00279-X/fulltext. Accessed July 8, 2022.

[8] Sleep Health. Available at: https://www.healthypeople.gov/2020/topics-objectives/topic/sleep-health. Accessed July 8, 2022.

[9] The exact number will vary from person to person. Some people will be just as refreshed on 7 hours vs. 9 for others.

[10] Obvious exception being night shift or any other schedule that would require you to be awake when you would otherwise be sleeping.

[11] Tosini G, Ferguson I, Tsubota K. Effects of blue light on the circadian system and eye physiology. Mol Vis 2016;22:61–72. Available at: https://www.ncbi.nlm.nih.gov/pmc/articles/PMC4734149/. Accessed July 8, 2022.

[12] f.lux. Available at: https://justgetflux.com/. Accessed July 8, 2022.

[13] Shechter A, Kim EW, St-Onge MP, Westwood AJ. Blocking nocturnal blue light for insomnia: A randomized controlled trial. J Psychiatr Res 2018;96:196–202. Available at: https://pubmed.ncbi.nlm.nih.gov/29101797/. Accessed July 8, 2022.

[14] UpToDate®. Available at: https://www.uptodate.com/contents/physiology-and-available-preparations-of-melatonin#H722735623. Accessed July 8, 2022.

[15] How to Nap and NOT Wake Up Groggy. Available at: https://medschoolinsiders.com/video/how-to-nap-productively-tips/. Accessed July 8, 2022.

of shape at some point. Reshape your *identity* and think of yourself as someone who is in shape and thrives off of peak physical performance. Altogether, we recommend both aerobic (e.g., running, cycling, swimming, rowing) and anaerobic (e.g., weight lifting) exercise.

## Aerobic Exercise

Current medical recommendations for adults are 150 minutes of moderate-intensity per week (i.e., maintaining a target heart rate of 50–70% of one's maximum heart rate) or 75 minutes of high-intensity aerobic exercise per week (i.e., maintaining a target heart rate of 70–85% of one's maximum heart rate[16]).[17] The benefits of regular aerobic exercise are dramatic, ranging from *direct* improvements in memory and learning[18] (including improved cognition after a single exercise session with persistent effects after regular exercise,[19] as well as increased grey matter[20] and neuron growth[21]), immediate gratification through endorphin release,[22] and long-term mood improvements through antidepressant and mood-stabilizing effects.[23]

- For anyone new to aerobic exercise, we recommend speaking with a doctor or trainer first to safely and gradually increase your participation. Once you are safe to participate, ask them for ways to gradually increase your weekly physical activity to meet 150 minutes of moderate or 75 minutes of vigorous exercise weekly.
- Couchto5k[24] is a fantastic program that does exactly what the name suggests: it gradually builds up running intensity so that even the previously sedentary can run a 5k without stopping. The author of this chapter used it and was very impressed!
- Other options to explore include trialing ClassPass[25] (which lets you try out different classes), walking to class as much as possible (walking more steps per day appears to be associated with lower all-cause mortality with a dose-dependent effect[26]), and participating in intramural sports.

## Anaerobic Exercise

Current medical recommendations are **at least 2 days per week of muscle strengthening exercise.** Adding muscle mass increases one's basal metabolic rate, which keeps it easier to maintain a lower body fat

---

[16] Maximum heart rate = (220 – age in years). A 25-year-old should aim for a target heart rate between 98 and 137 bpm for moderate aerobic activity and between 137 and 166 bpm for vigorous aerobic activity.

[17] What Exactly Is "Moderate-Intensity" Aerobic Exercise? Available at: https://www.pennmedicine.org/updates/blogs/metabolic-and-bariatric-surgery-blog/2012/january/what-exactly-is-moderate-intensity-aerobic-exercise. Accessed July 8, 2022.

[18] Physical activity, brain, and cognition. Available at: https://www.semanticscholar.org/paper/Physical-activity%2C-brain%2C-and-cognition-Erickson-Hillman/309e97018cb1927f12d3e851f0ae296b98d049a8. Accessed July 8, 2022.

[19] The Effects of Acute Exercise on Mood, Cognition, Neurophysiology, and Neurochemical Pathways: A Review. Available at: https://content.iospress.com/articles/brain-plasticity/bpl160040. Accessed July 8, 2022.

[20] Batouli SAH, Saba V. At least eighty percent of brain grey matter is modifiable by physical activity: A review study. Behav Brain Res 2017;332:204–217. Available at: https://pubmed.ncbi.nlm.nih.gov/28600001/. Accessed July 8, 2022.

[21] Servick K. How does exercise keep your brain young? Available at: https://www.sciencemag.org/news/2018/09/how-does-exercise-keep-your-brain-young. Accessed July 8, 2022.

[22] Boecker H, Sprenger T, Spilker ME, Henriksen G, Koppenhoefer M, Wagner KJ, Valet M, Berthele A, Tolle TR. The runner's high: opioidergic mechanisms in the human brain. Cereb Cortex 2008;18(11):2523–31. Available at: https://pubmed.ncbi.nlm.nih.gov/18296435/. Accessed July 8, 2022.

[23] Schuch FB, Vancampfort D, Rosenbaum S, Richards J, Ward PB, Stubbs B. Exercise improves physical and psychological quality of life in people with depression: A meta-analysis including the evaluation of control group response. Psychiatry Res. 2016;241:47–54. doi:10.1016/j.psychres.2016.04.054.

[24] Kamb S. Should You Do Couch to 5K? Don't Make These 5 Mistakes. Available at: https://www.nerdfitness.com/blog/couch-to-5k-crucial-things-to-know-before-you-start-training/. Accessed July 8, 2022.

[25] classpass. Available at: https://classpass.com/. Accessed July 8, 2022.

[26] Saint-Maurice PF, Troiano RP, Bassett Jr DR, et al. Association of Daily Step Count and Step Intensity With Mortality Among US Adults. JAMA 2020;323(12):1151–1160. Available at: https://jamanetwork.com/journals/jama/fullarticle/2763292. Accessed July 8, 2022.

percentage.[27] Adding strength training to aerobic exercise also yields better improvements to cognition than aerobic exercise alone.[28]

- As with aerobic exercise, consult with a doctor or trainer if you are new to weight lifting.
- Popular starting routines include "Starting Strength" (the author also used this to great success) and "Strong Lifts."

### 18.3.3 Healthy Diet

It's incredibly common to fall into unhealthy diet patterns in college. You likely ate whatever your parents made up till this point, and now you have free reign to eat whatever you want. Moreover, you're dealing with new stressors, and the late-night options (as well as what you end up scarfing down on your nights out) aren't exactly the most wholesome. While it's perfectly acceptable to splurge here and there, we recommend following a healthy, sustainable diet that allows you to maintain a healthy BMI (i.e., not becoming overweight or obese[29]). There are many options for a healthy diet (e.g., keto, low-carb, vegetarian/vegan, Mediterranean, intermittent fasting), but we generally recommend minimizing processed foods and sugar-sweetened beverages, as well as eating reasonable portion sizes (you can still become obese from eating unprocessed foods—nut butters and oils are very calorie dense!). We strongly recommend adhering to a healthy diet to maintain a healthy body weight because mood appears to be best at normal to slightly overweight BMI[30] and processed food intake appears to be associated with depression (though it's unclear what the direction of the association is).[31] On a more discouraging note, there is very real bias against overweight and obese applicants in the medical profession;[32] while this alone shouldn't be the compelling reason for anyone to attempt weight loss, it *is* a fact to be aware of.

- If you're short for time, consider meal-prepping, or many meals at once and storing them in to-go containers. Reddit.com/r/MealPrepSunday has many suggestions! You can even do this with your roommates.
- Consider a delivery service (e.g., Hello Fresh) or Whole Foods Delivery, which is free with Amazon Prime (which is also discounted for students).
- Speak with your doctor if you're overweight or obese and unsure of how to lose weight and keep it off.
  - *Weight loss is almost entirely diet;*[33] you can spend hours burning calories by running, only to gain them all back in a few seconds by eating Oreos (and you'll probably be hungrier since you burnt so many calories).
  - Reddit.com/r/loseit is an *excellent* community for understanding how to lose weight and to keep it off. Check out the links and material on the sidebar.
  - Many individuals also report success with Noom,[34] an app-based service that heavily integrates behavioral psychology for weight loss.

---

[27] Byrne HK, Wilmore JH. The Effects of a 20-Week Exercise Training Program on Resting Metabolic Rate in Previously Sedentary, Moderately Obese Women. Available at: https://journals.humankinetics.com/view/journals/ijsnem/11/1/article-p15.xml; https://academic.oup.com/ajcn/article/60/2/167/4732054?login=true. Accessed July 8, 2022.

[28] Cohen R, et al. Neuroimaging Approaches to the Study of Cognitive Aging. N.p.: Frontiers Media SA; 2020:119.

[29] Calculate Your Body Mass Index. Available at: https://www.nhlbi.nih.gov/health/educational/lose_wt/BMI/bmicalc.htm. BMI has less utility for athletes with significant muscle mass. It's more important to maintain a healthy body fat percentage, i.e. 8–19% in men and 21–33% in women. Accessed July 8, 2022.

[30] de Wit LM, van Straten A, van Herten M, Penninx BWJH, Cuijpers P. Depression and body mass index, a u-shaped association. BMC Public Health 2009;9:14. Available at: https://www.ncbi.nlm.nih.gov/pmc/articles/PMC2631467/. Accessed July 8, 2022.

[31] Lachance L. Food, Mood, and Brain Health: Implications for the Modern Clinician. Mo Med 2015;112(2):111–115. Available at: https://www.ncbi.nlm.nih.gov/pmc/articles/PMC6170050/. Accessed July 8, 2022.

[32] Maxfield CM, Thorpe MP, Desser TS, et al. Bias in Radiology Resident Selection: Do We Discriminate Against the Obese and Unattractive? Acad Med 2019;94(11):1774–1780. Available at: https://pubmed.ncbi.nlm.nih.gov/31149924/. Accessed July 8, 2022.

[33] Exercise alone does not help in losing weight. Available at: https://www.sciencedaily.com/releases/2015/08/150817142140.htm. Accessed July 8, 2022.

[34] NOOM. Available at: https://www.noom.com/. Accessed July 8, 2022.

## 18.3.4 Avoiding Unhealthy Substance Use

We're not your parents. We're not going to give you an insipid lecture about how "drugs are bad." You have probably heard about the risks. Realistically, if you're at the point of considering self-medicating with drugs and alcohol, then you are dealing with enough to conclude that the immediate, short-term gratification of using substances is worth whatever abstract, hypothetical risks may occur many years down the line. In addition, you might think that the risks probably don't apply to *you* as an individual. After all, you're a highly intelligent, hard-working future doctor who doesn't have the other risk factors seen in the typical "alcoholic on the street."

- Check yourself before you wreck yourself. Reach out to friends and family if you find yourself even at the precipice of an unhealthy pattern of substance use. Identify people in your life with whom you can have reasonable, nonstigmatizing conversations about the topic.
- It's important to recognize that the scientific and clinical understanding of substance use has evolved from black-and-white conceptions of "addict" versus "normal" to a spectrum of risk and impairment.[35] You may not be at the point of frank impairment in your life, but most individuals who begin using substances insidiously increase their level of use until some catastrophic event occurs in their life. You don't need to hit rock bottom to change your behavior.
- If you're physically dependent on a substance (i.e., experiencing significant withdrawal symptoms on cessation), then we *strongly recommend* speaking with a medical professional about safe detoxification. At the same time, we recognize that not everyone who uses a substance will need to engage with professionals for cessation. Someone who uses marijuana once at a party and resolves to never do it again, for example, does not necessarily need to disclose this to a physician, especially considering the draconian implications this may have for medical licensing (e.g., having a documented diagnosis of "cannabis use disorder" that may require disclose for licensure in certain states, even though the documented diagnosis does not actually capture the individual's pattern of use[36]).

## 18.4 Mental Components of Wellness

While the interventions we just discussed will undoubtedly improve mental health, it is also crucial to discuss mental health directly. It is perfectly normal to experience the full spectrum of human emotion, which can include pure elation, crushing defeat, painful embarrassment, glowing pride, gnawing envy, crippling anxiety, and even transient alexithymia. Chances are high that everyone around you has felt these emotions at some point or another. At the same time, when you're experiencing a negative emotion, it's very easy to conclude that you're the only one who has ever felt that way and that no one else could ever truly understand. In addition, as a pre-med, it is very easy to compare yourself to others and to feel like you're not doing enough. As such, you should be proactive about safeguarding your mental health.

We have done extensive reviews of the current psychological literature—while being mindful of the fact that many findings in psychology and functional neuroimaging are plagued with reproducibility crises[37]—to compile robust, actionable recommendations for optimizing your mental health as a pre-med. That said, we are *not* clinical psychologists. Trust but *verify* our recommendations. Always seek professional guidance if in doubt about anything we present.

---

[35] Laurence E. The "Addiction Spectrum" Challenges You to Think About Substance Abuse Differently. Available at: https://www.wellandgood.com/what-is-addiction/. Accessed July 8, 2022.

[36] Physician-Friendly States for Mental Health: A Review of Medical Boards. Available at: https://www.idealmedicalcare.org/physician-friendly-states-for-mental-health-a-review-of-medical-boards/. Accessed July 8, 2022.

[37] This is what happened when psychologists tried to replicate 100 previously published findings. Available at: https://digest.bps.org.uk/2015/08/27/this-is-what-happened-when-psychologists-tried-to-replicate-100-previously-published-findings/. Accessed July 8, 2022; Poldrack RA, Baker CI, Durnez J. Scanning the horizon: towards transparent and reproducible neuroimaging research. Nat Rev Neurosci 2017;18(2):115–126. Available at: https://pubmed.ncbi.nlm.nih.gov/28053326/. Accessed July 8, 2022.

**Positive psychology** is the relatively new branch of psychology that rigorously studies flourishing, well-being, and happiness.[38] A meta-analysis of 49 studies in 2009 showed that specific interventions that improved well-being and lowered depression included *writing gratitude letters, learning and applying optimistic thinking, replaying positive life events*, and *social interaction*.[39] Well-being is also related to *having engaging work, religion or spirituality, leisure*, and *subjective health*.[40] Other contributing factors include a sense of self-acceptance, autonomy, and purpose in life.[41] In line with these findings, we offer the following recommendations:

- **Practicing gratitude:** Gratitude is the feeling of being thankful or appreciative for something. It's a ubiquitous feature of human psychology. *Practicing* gratitude, however, involves taking the time to deliberately think about things that you are grateful for and to *write them out* to consciously reorient your mind. A growing body of research suggests that consciously and regularly *practicing gratitude* (e.g., writing gratitude letters directed at specific people,[42] gratitude journal apps) improves subjective well-being over time.[43]

- **Learning and applying optimistic thinking:** We tend to think of ourselves as optimists, pessimists, realists, etc. Emerging evidence, however, suggests that forcing yourself to become an optimistic, (i.e., cognitive reframing)[44] of negative events by considering them in a positive light, leads to improved overall well-being.
  - **Replaying positive life events:** Similar to practicing gratitude and cognitive reframing, vividly imagining prior positive life events appears to be an intervention that improves well-being. We recommend doing this when you feel "meh" about life, as it's probably easier to reorient your state of mind then (vs. forcing yourself to replay positive life events when something immediately distressing is happening).

- **Social connectedness:** When you are busy with school, it's easy to push off opportunities to connect with friends and family. After all, your friends and family will always be there next week, whereas the chemistry quiz is tomorrow! Over time, you might inadvertently find yourself becoming more and more reclusive in the hopes of maximizing your productivity. *The reality is that deteriorating social connections will lower your overall well-being, which will impact your performance across all aspects of life.* We recommend creating scheduled times—at least once a week—to give focused, interrupted attention to close friends and family.

- **Having engaging work:** We reiterate a constant theme we have been pushing throughout the book: *whenever possible, do things that you genuinely enjoy.* This is easiest with extracurriculars but also applies to choosing majors. That is, all other things roughly equal (e.g., research opportunities, ease of obtaining a high GPA, etc.), you should give significant weight to genuine interest when choosing a major. Every long-term pursuit has less-glamorous drudgery, however. You can minimize needless suffering by recognizing and accepting this fact (i.e., setting realistic expectations), as well as by choosing pursuits with the most personally engaging drudgery.

- **Religion or spirituality:** If you are religious, we recommend regular participation in your faith (e.g., going to services weekly). If you are not religious (and even if you are!), we—*again*—recommend engaging in *mindfulness meditation* daily. We have been paying homage to this practice throughout the book so far—we will now give it our full attention.

---

[38] Concepts that held the center stage in philosophy and literature for thousands of years but did not receive the same level of *scientific* scrutiny as mental illnesses, or "negative psychology."

[39] Sin NL, Lyubomirsky S. Enhancing Well-Being and Alleviating Depressive Symptoms With Positive Psychology Interventions: A Practice-Friendly Meta-Analysis. Available at: https://onlinelibrary.wiley.com/doi/pdf/10.1002/jclp.20593. Accessed July 8, 2022.

[40] *Positive Psychology in a Nutshell.*

[41] Ryan RM, Deci EL. On happiness and human potentials: a review of research on hedonic and eudaimonic well-being. Annu Rev Psychol. 2001;52:141–166. doi:10.1146/annurev.psych.52.1.141.

[42] No need to actually send them to people, but bonus points if you do!

[43] Is Gratitude Good for Your Health? Available at: https://healthmatters.nyp.org/is-gratitude-good-for-your-health/. Accessed July 8, 2022.

[44] Scott E. How to Reframe Situations So They Create Less Stress. Available at: https://www.verywellmind.com/cognitive-reframing-for-stress-management-3144872. Accessed July 8, 2022.

## 18.4.1 What Is Mindfulness Meditation?

*Meditation* is an incredibly difficult term to define, and it has been used to mean different things in different contexts. Broadly speaking, it refers to a variety of practices in which one orients the mind and conscious awareness to achieve a state of internal emotional stability and calmness. *Mindfulness meditation* is a specific form of meditation in which one pays close, intense, and *nonjudgmental* attention to his subjective, conscious experience in the here-and-now. That is, one nonjudgmentally becomes aware of everything that is happening in the present moment, including whatever random thoughts may pop into his stream of consciousness, the waxing and waning of background noise, the shifting pressure sensations of proprioceptive input, and even the subtle differences in hues in one's visual field when the eyes are closed.

Mindfulness meditation is *not* trying to think about nothing. It is *not* about trying to reduce stress (although it has this effect with regular practice). It is *not* about trying to focus on the breath. It is simply a nonjudgmental attempt to widely focus attention on the here-and-now. Focusing on the breath, however, is often used as an introduction to mindfulness meditation. The practitioner will sit cross-legged with his back straight and hands on his knees. He will attempt to pay very close attention to the entire experience of breathing: the movement of the diaphragm, the changes in pressure on the legs and buttocks, the feel of air moving in and out of the lungs, the space in between inhalation and exhalation. Inevitably, his mind will begin to wander. *It is in **recognizing** this and reorienting his attention to the breath that he engages in mindfulness meditation*. In doing this over and over again, he becomes vividly aware that his thoughts can be as spontaneous as the noise in his apartment and that he does not necessarily need to identify with or agree with whatever pops into his mind.

Meditation had been researched for decades, but much of the early research was plagued by bias and methodological errors. Newer research, however, shows that practicing mindfulness has significant positive effects on a variety of cognitive domains—even after very limited practice in untrained practitioners. Beginning meditation appears to improve stress management,[45] response to chronic pain,[46] concentration,[47] working memory,[44] and emotional awareness and reactivity.[48] Regular mindfulness practice has the benefit of allowing the practitioner to arrive at a state of baseline calmness and well-being that isn't so dependent on externalities (e.g., doing well on exams) or easily displaced by negative emotion. *As a result, the author of this chapter—who taught mindfulness meditation to medical students—believes that it's one of the most cost-effective health interventions that virtually **everyone**[49] should practice.*

Unfortunately, it can be very frustrating to pick up and *maintain* a meditation practice. It took the author of this chapter about a year before he became consistent with daily meditation. Even now, he will fall out of doing it for up to a month or two at a time (mainly during busier rotations—he tends to practice immediately after waking, and getting sleep becomes much more tempting on rotations with early starts). We recommend using meditation apps, such as "Waking Up," "Headspace," and "Ten Percent Happier," to begin with short meditation sessions that allow you to gradually build up to longer sessions that you can continue daily.

---

45 Spijkerman MPJ, Pots WTM, Bohlmeijer ET. Effectiveness of online mindfulness-based interventions in improving mental health: A review and meta-analysis of randomised controlled trials. Clinical Psychology Review 2016;45:102–114. Available at: https://www.sciencedirect.com/science/article/pii/S0272735815300623?via%3Dihub. Accessed July 8, 2022.

46 Brown CA, Jones AKP. Psychobiological correlates of improved mental health in patients with musculoskeletal pain after a mindfulness-based pain management program. Clin J Pain 2013;29(3):233–44. Available at: https://pubmed.ncbi.nlm.nih.gov/22874090/. Accessed July 8, 2022.

47 Chiesa A, Calati R, Serretti A. Does mindfulness training improve cognitive abilities? A systematic review of neuropsychological findings. Clinical Psychology Review 2011;31(3):449–464. Available at: https://www.sciencedirect.com/science/article/abs/pii/S027273581000173X. Accessed July 8, 2022.

48 How Does Mindfulness Meditation Work? Proposing Mechanisms of Action From a Conceptual and Neural Perspective. Available at: https://www.semanticscholar.org/paper/How-Does-Mindfulness-Meditation-Work-Proposing-of-a-H%C3%B6lzel-Lazar/9cc501b90381f125b1ea8747cf661cedf9dd144a. Accessed July 8, 2022.

49 As with any intervention, there are qualifications. There is some concern that mindfulness should only be undertaken with medical supervision by those with increased predisposition for unstable psychotic disorders: https://www.heretohelp.bc.ca/visions/mindfulness-vol12/is-mindfulness-useful-or-dangerous-for-individuals-with-psychosis, https://www.frontiersin.org/articles/10.3389/fpsyt.2020.00600/full

- **Leisure:** You need healthy outlets for treating yourself, e.g., video games, bubble baths, creative pursuits, reading "lowbrow" literature. If these outlets also *happen* to improve your medical school application, then that's great. That said, it's probably better for your well-being to have genuine, free sources of leisure—things that you don't feel pressured to optimize or refine on a competitive level. The author—for example—genuinely loved playing guitar as a form of self-expression, playing up to 10 hours a day at one point. At some point, however, he fell into the trap of feeling the need to become the best guitarist impossible. Practice sessions became much more structured and—honestly—felt more like a chore. Something that used to be a free, healthy outlet slowly became a source of stress. The author is still working on rediscovering his original "safe" hobby and recommends that readers take care to keep their competitive natures away from their free sources of leisure!
- **Subjective health:** Curiously, the positive psychology research suggests that one's *subjective perceptions* about their health are better predictors of well-being than *objective health* (e.g., control of chronic diseases, BMI). Of course, the two are likely related to an extent, but we recommend making *personal hygiene* non-negotiable to optimize your personal (and hopefully objective!) health. Give yourself enough time in the day to shower, brush your teeth and floss, clean your living space, do laundry, dress nicely. On a practical level, abundant research on the halo effect demonstrates that simply looking and presenting yourself better will lead to being evaluated more positively across multiple dimensions.[50] On a personal level, being well-groomed and dressing well tends to improve our confidence, and some argue that it can lead to improved mood.[51]

Beyond recapitulating the positive psychology findings, we also recommend the following:
- **Personal organization:** *Use technology to make your life easier.* Be proactive about putting all deadlines into your Google Calendar at the beginning of the academic term. Aggressively schedule your time as per Chapter 9, Timing, Class Structure, and Personal Schedules.
  - Don't get overwhelmed by large, seemingly insurmountable obstacles. Break them down into individual, constituent goals and focus on achieving each small goal. Your achievement will build momentum and propel you to carry on.
  - Have concrete goals for the day, week, month, semester, year, etc., and reassess along the way. Go over your plans for the next day before you go to bed—even if just for a few minutes.
- **Financial health:** Feeling financially secure is a key component to overall well-being.[52]
  - Have a budget and stick to it. We recommend the Mint app for understanding where your money goes.
  - Know where you have emergency funds available (e.g., savings, loans, parents) to be secured against whatever unexpected punches life throws at you.
- **Optimize your environment:** Altogether, these interventions themselves are no substitute for optimizing your environment, (i.e., the *causes* of your stress). Are you still engaged in toxic relationships? Are you pursuing extracurriculars you are not genuinely passionate about? Are you gradually beginning to realize that medicine is *not* what you want to do with your life but you still feel pressured to pursue it to appease others? If so, then take concrete steps to fix these conditions *in addition* to practicing the wellness guidelines we recommend.

## 18.4.2 When Should I Talk to a Professional?

As physicians, we are committed to eliminating mental health stigma. In our ideal world, everyone would feel comfortable opening up about their depression or anxiety, just as they are about their diabetes and

---

[50] Lorenzo GL, Biesanz JC, Human LJ. What is beautiful is good and more accurately understood. Physical attractiveness and accuracy in first impressions of personality. Psychol Sci 2010;21(12):1777–1782. Available at: https://pubmed.ncbi.nlm.nih.gov/21051521/. Accessed July 8, 2022.

[51] Clothes and Your Mood: How Your Outfits Can Make You Feel Better. Available at: https://medium.com/@serendipity12th111/clothes-and-your-mood-how-your-outfits-can-make-you-feel-better-eda2e9a8058c. Accessed July 8, 2022.

[52] A surprising connection: Financial wellness and your overall health. Available at: https://www.purdue.edu/hr/CHL/healthyboiler/news/newsletter/2020-01/finances-health.php. Accessed July 8, 2022.

hypertension. In addition, no one would hesitate to get professional evaluation of distressing symptoms (e.g., intermittent feelings of hopelessness, burnout, loneliness, drinking alcohol more often, etc.) *before* they lead to significant dysfunction. **At the same time, we recognize that there are very real concerns to seeking mental healthcare as a future physician.** The reality is that many states still ask highly invasive questions about your history of treatment for *anything* related to mental health, ostensibly for the sake of "public safety."[53]

For example, Alabama asks if you have "…received any therapy or treatment for… mental health issues?"

Alaska asks, "'Have you ever been diagnosed with, treated for, or do you currently have', followed by a list of 14 mental health conditions including depression, seasonal affective disorder," and "any condition requiring chronic medical or behavioral treatment."[54]

Being forced to answer "yes" to these questions can lead to severe consequences, ranging from significant delays to renewing your medical license yearly to forced participation in Physician Health Programs—some of which may mandate non-evidence-based practices[55] (e.g., participation in drug rehabilitation programs without any history of drug abuse) *at one's own expense.*[56] Fortunately, the trend appears to be that most state licensing boards are updating their mental health questions to avoid being overly draconian. We hope that it is because they recognize that such questions likely lead to professionals' delaying seeking treatment at *earlier, more treatable* states of mental illness. Instead, they are forced to wait until the consequences for not seeking treatment (i.e., intolerable dysfunction) outweigh the potential risks of seeking treatment, (i.e., expensive and punitive recourse from professional agencies).

We bring up these ugly facts to make you aware that mental health stigma *still exists in medicine* and that there *are still risks to seeking professional counsel.* The good news is that most states' licensing boards ask more reasonable questions along the lines of, "In the last 5 years, have you had…" or "Do you currently have a mental health condition that *impairs your ability to practice medicine*?" This is much more consistent with reasonable standards for other medical conditions. After all, while a physician with well-controlled epilepsy should be able to practice medicine, it is reasonable to restrict licensure to a physician with uncontrolled seizures.

So, what is the takeaway here? We regrettably recommend getting as much information as possible about avenues for mental healthcare available to you, as well as getting as much collateral information about your level of dysfunction before seeking professional counsel. Are the records accessible to your residency program (i.e., within the same healthcare system?). Do the counselors have a potential conflict of interest? (i.e., does a counselor also work for the Physician Health Program?). Have you exhausted all other individual behavioral strategies (e.g., diet, exercise, avoiding substances, seeking meaningful social contact through friends and family, meditation, personal hygiene) before seeking mental healthcare? How *bad* is your level of dysfunction? Are you acutely suicidal or homicidal? Are you seeing or hearing things that your friends and family don't see or hear? Are people in your life *seriously* worried about you and think you need immediate professional help?

All things considered: you probably stand to gain much more than you could lose from seeking mental healthcare—especially if you intend to practice in a more progressive state. As with all symptoms and illnesses, we recommend erring on the side of caution and getting evaluation before things get out of control. That said, if you are considering obtaining medical licensure in a state with more draconian, invasive questioning, then the cost/benefit calculus to seeking mental healthcare for mild symptoms may be radically different—especially if you are able to overcome your symptoms with more conservative treatment (e.g., personal care, social support, etc.). Yes, it's an unfortunate situation. We—as physicians—often have

---

53  State licensing boards *do* run a risk of licensing a physician with a history of depression—who could become acutely depressed while working with patients—compared to one without depression. Just like they run a risk of licensing a physician with diabetes—who could have symptomatic hyperglycemia with patients—compared to one without.

54  Physician-Friendly States for Mental Health: A Review of Medical Boards. Available at: https://www.idealmedicalcare.org/physician-friendly-states-for-mental-health-a-review-of-medical-boards/. Accessed July 8, 2022.

55  Lenzer J. Physician health programs under fire. BMJ. 2016;353:i3568. Published 2016 Jun 30. doi:10.1136/bmj.i3568.

56  Boyd JW. Doctors Pay Up or Else Don't Work. Available at: https://www.psychologytoday.com/us/blog/almost-addicted/201912/doctors-pay-or-else-dont-work. Accessed July 8, 2022, Boyd JW. Why Physicians Who Need Psychiatric Care Go to Kansas. Available at: https://www.psychologytoday.com/us/blog/almost-addicted/201904/why-physicians-who-need-psychiatric-care-go-kansas. Accessed July 8, 2022.

the loudest voices about ending mental health stigma. At the same time, we actively perpetuate it by disincentivizing our practitioners from seeking early care.

### 18.4.3 What Is Burnout, and Why Should I Care about It Now?

Burnout is a word you will become all too familiar with as you progress on your journey through medicine—both because it's an ever-present danger and because it's something of a buzzword that the administration will often attempt to treat with quick "solutions." It is the feeling of being overworked or too tired to continue on, but you have no choice to continue. It is characterized by overwhelming feelings of apathy/emotional exhaustion, depersonalization, and the feeling that you're not accomplishing anything of worth. The long hours of studying and pressure to do well can be tolling. In addition, applying to medical school can be stressful. Unfortunately, medical school and residency continue to be stressful on the mind and body. This is where individual wellness techniques can come in and help reduce that feeling of burnout.

At the same time, it *must be stated that burnout is often a systems-based issue, (i.e., the natural consequences of a dysfunctional work environment).* Even the most mentally well-adjusted person will experience burnout in a sufficiently toxic work environment. As such, you should actively seek to avoid such environments (e.g., needlessly competitive, cut-throat institutions and workplace cultures) whenever possible. Unfortunately, malignant programs will not overly advertise these facts about themselves. Therefore, you will need to learn how to read between the lines when choosing among different medical schools, residency programs, extracurricular organizations, jobs, etc., because burnout is frighteningly common among physicians, ranging from 40 to 60% depending on the specialty![57] Moreover, even though new medical students begin with similar or *better* mental health than their age-matched controls,[58] physicians ultimately end up with a suicide rate greater than *twice* that of the general population—the highest of *any profession*![59]

These are critical habits to form **now**, as your good habits will become more automatic as you reinforce them over time. Unfortunately, you only get busier as you advance in your career. We know a lot of this information may be things you already know or practice, but we wanted to emphasize just how important wellness is in whatever path you choose, and *especially* in medicine. Read this chapter over several times; taking care of your physical and mental health is equally important if not more important than everything else we have discussed so far.

### 18.5 Summary

Maintaining personal wellness can be incredibly difficult in medicine because of multiple significant systemic issues (e.g., long hours, sleep deprivation, relatively poor pay, increasing scope of practice from midlevel providers, etc.). In addition, many discussions about wellness are superficial and inadvertently shift blame onto trainees vs. the system itself and how it contributes to burnout. Nonetheless, you will still need to put in active efforts toward maintaining personal wellness through high-quality sleep, diet, exercise, and avoidance of unhealthy substance use. Positive psychology interventions may also be worth considering. You should also be mindful that there may be consequences to seeking mental healthcare. Reassuringly, the stigma appears to be decreasing with time.

---

[57] https://www.ama-assn.org/practice-management/physician-health/report-reveals-severity-burnout-specialty.

[58] Staying Sane: Addressing the Growing Concern of Mental Health in Medical Students. Available at: https://www.amsa.org/2015/09/08/staying-sane-addressing-the-growing-concern-of-mental-health-in-medical-students/. Accessed July 8, 2022.

[59] Anderson P. Doctors' Suicide Rate Highest of Any Profession Privacy & Trust Info. Available at: https://www.emedicinehealth.com/script/main/art.asp?articlekey=212270. Accessed July 8, 2022.

# 19 Finding Mentors

*Christian Morrill*

## 19.1 What Are Mentors and Why Should I Care about Them?

In the business world, the chief executive officer (CEO) is the highest-ranking executive in the company and is routinely tasked with making decisions that affect the future of the company. Rarely, if ever, do CEOs make decisions without insight, direction, and approval from their board of directors. A board of directors consists of successful individuals across multiple disciplines and backgrounds whose collective wisdom and counsel serve to grow the company while avoiding potential pitfalls. Like a successful business, you as a pre-med will be tasked with making decisions that will significantly impact your career development, professional aspirations, and personal growth. Your ability to make the best possible choices, however, is largely contingent on experiences you have yet to acquire. This is why you need your very own "board of directors"— mentors!

At their core, mentors should be invested in your personal success and willing to invest time and resources in your development. They should be people with whom you share a similar passion or interest and are willing to advise you on how they were able to find success and how to follow in their footsteps. Your mentor may be a physician you shadowed and with whom you really connected. Another mentor may be a college professor who offers you a research project in a field about which you are passionate. Community leaders who share your passion for advocacy and are willing to help you better understand local health policy can also be instrumental mentors if you have interests in public health.

Mentors are profoundly important to your development in college. As mentioned earlier, the 2014 Gallup-Purdue Index found that a mentor who encouraged your goals and dreams was found to more than double the odds of being engaged at work beyond graduation for college students.[1]

## 19.2 What Attributes Should I Look for in Mentors?

Mentors are important and can do lots to guide you not only successfully through your pre-med years but also throughout your career. What exactly should you be looking for in a mentor? We've listed some of the most important attributes to look for.

### 19.2.1 Desirable Success

A stellar mentor is successful in achieving one or more of *your* personal or professional goals. Perhaps that is running a successful medical practice or research laboratory, balancing a family and a medical career, holding a competitive appointment at a major hospital, or being recognized as a leader in their field. Whatever the goal, you want to learn from someone who has demonstrated they can be successful in the things you are interested in. In addition, you ideally want to find a mentor who has a strong track record of successful mentees that he or she has mentored throughout the years.

### 19.2.2 Nurturer

No amount of success can make up for not being able to invest time and energy into your growth. For many reasons, you may not want the "most" successful person as a mentor if he/she cannot give you meaningful time and invest in you personally. A mentor should nurture you by giving you responsibilities, opportunities, and feedback. It might be entrusting you with a difficult research project or pushing you to present a project at a national meeting.

---

[1] Great Jobs Great Lives: The 2014 Gallup Purdue Index Report. Available at: https://www.gallup.com/file/services/176768/The_2014_Gallup-Purdue_Index_Report.pdf. Accessed July 8, 2022.

### 19.2.3 Network of Resources

A good mentor readily acknowledges they are not the best resource for all your interests and will readily connect you with *other* individuals within their own network better suited to help you. These mentors don't know everything, but they know people that do. A good mentor facilitates your success by helping you to meet the *right* people and get into the right places (internships, interviews, jobs, etc.).

### 19.2.4 Strategic Coach

Coaching is an important aspect of mentoring. Your mentor should help you see the big picture and help you understand your specific timeline. A good coach will add insightful perspective on your strengths and weaknesses. Together you can build a plan that accentuates your strengths and builds on your weaknesses.

### 19.2.5 Cheerleader

Mentors are not your parents, but ideally they will cheer for you like parents would. This type of mentor should bolster your confidence and be there to pick you up when you're down. Having once been in your shoes, they understand the road is long and that it takes sustained effort to be successful. This mentor helps you to keep going when times are tough.

### 19.2.6 Honest Critiques

A good mentor should keep you accountable to your goals and tell it to you straight. They won't hold back from honestly sharing their concerns for you when you're making questionable choices. They will offer you both pros and cons of your choices. Although it can be hard to hear, these mentors will honestly give you their assessment of your competitiveness for programs. Whether it's a borderline GPA, applying to the wrong schools, or needing to take a year off to strengthen your application; good mentors are not afraid to have difficult discussions about where you stand.

## 19.3 Five Mentors to Start With

Not all mentors are created equal and very rarely will you find all the best attributes within a single mentor. Like all of us, mentors have their strong points and their weak points. As you fill your "board of directors," identify what each individual mentor' strengths are and aim to find mentors that complement each other. You may want to start with these five mentors alone, but these are just suggestions.

### 19.3.1 The Physician

It is highly recommended to find a physician as a mentor. This is the mentor who has made it to where you want to be someday. Keep in mind that on your board of directors, the physician may not play as active a role as others due to his/her schedule. At the same time, something as simple as having someone to shadow, give you advice, and provide feedback on your progress is invaluable. Having a physician that can vouch for your candidacy for medical school is a major strength when you apply for medical school. If you want to go to an allopathic school, find an MD (if osteopathic is your future, find a DO—as many DO schools require this).

### 19.3.2 The Upperclassman

When it comes to applying to medical school, these are the individuals that often give the best advice on the day-to-day struggles and hurdles. Find either someone who successfully made it into medical school or a first- or second-year medical student who will let you pick their brain. Ideally, this is a current student or alumnus from your undergraduate institution who can speak specifically to how he/she prepared for medical school with a similar background. Upperclassmen are invaluable resources when it comes to learning about different schools to apply to, essay preparation, and interviewing at different programs. They also went through the process recently, and have a more complete and up-to-date knowledge of how to help you.

### 19.3.3  The Researcher

Whether research is in your future or not, your ability to understand and critically analyze research will be utilized often as a physician in any specialty. Finding a research mentor early in your undergraduate career will allow the most time and opportunity for you to develop these critical skills as a pre-med (assuming you choose to pursue research as a pre-med). Letters of recommendation from research mentors are greatly valued by medical school admission committees. You can further develop the mentor relationship by taking a course with this professor and regularly meeting with them in office hours to ask intelligent questions (i.e., *not* questions you already know the answer to).

### 19.3.4  The Role Model

More than just career success or research papers, you want to identify someone whom you sincerely respect and hope to emulate. Perhaps this is someone who has the life–work balance you want, practices medicine in the community you hope to settle down in, or has the doctor–patient relationship that made you want to go into medicine. These individuals can be your best cheerleaders and help you maintain your individuality throughout your medical career.

### 19.3.5  The Classmate

You and your classmates have great potential for mentoring each other. Find one of your classmates whose strengths are different from you and whom you'd benefit from interacting with. Pre-med is hard but having peer-mentors in your corner can do a lot to build camaraderie and strengthen each other.

## 19.4  The Key to a Successful Mentor Relationship

It's no secret! You get out what you put into relationships. Mentoring relationships are no different. For an effective mentoring relationship, you need something to bring to the table. For 98% of pre-meds that something is (1) time, (2) enthusiasm, or (3) a good work ethic (hopefully all three). At this time of your life, you probably won't have many—if any—marketable skills, insight, or education that will "impress" your mentor and entice them to mentor you. However, *you have time*, something that becomes more and more precious the deeper you get into your career. Your mentors likely have limited time for pursuing their own interests or projects not directly related to their day to day. As a mentee, you can take the lead on doing the groundwork to develop your mentor's projects and interests. It's a win-win relationship! Second, *you have enthusiasm*, and enthusiasm is contagious. It's just as easy to get stuck in the drudgery of day-to-day life as a pre-med student as it is as a physician. Working with enthusiastic pre-med students often reminds mentors of when they were in your position and their reasons for pursuing their career! Lastly, as a pre-med student you have a *good work ethic*. This conveys to your mentor that you are the real deal. It is unfair, and unreasonable to presume your mentor will work any harder than you do. In my experience, mentors will match the level of effort you put in. Want a great mentor? Be a fastidious enthusiastic hard-working mentee.

## 19.5  My Mentor Relationship Isn't Working!

If your mentor doesn't seem to be working out or the relationship isn't going where you hoped, then there are several things you should do. First, re-evaluate your effort level and whether there is more you should be doing. Are you keeping your promises with your mentor and doing what you said you would? If there is no problem with your level of effort, then it may be a problem of communication. Miscommunications are common in any relationship, and can be avoided proactively by asking your mentor how best to communicate with them (email, text, phone calls, bi-weekly meetings, etc.). If you haven't determined the best mode of communication with your mentor, don't stress but determine communication expectations as soon as possible.

There are many reasons individuals grow out of, pause, or end a mentorship relationship. Except for cases of abuse, assault, and fraudulent behavior, it is important to give your mentor the benefit of the doubt for a time and ensure you're not making a decision overly based on your current emotional status. Sleep on it. Outside of how you're feeling in the moment, try to identify why specifically you think you should end/pause your mentoring relationship. It could be that your circumstances changed and you are no longer able to meet with them regularly or you discovered an unknown passion in an unrelated field that is demanding your time and attention. When navigating this topic with your mentor it is important to remove emotion from the substance of the conversation and focus on the facts of your situation. Although intimidating, honest conversations about poor fit or "moving on" will most commonly leave your mentors happy for you and supportive of your choices. Often, mentors will help introduce you to individuals more pertinent to your interests and situation.

## 19.6 Letter of Recommendation and Your Mentor

When choosing a mentor, it's important to think about the roles a mentor will fulfill for you. One of these roles will likely be writing a letter of recommendation on your behalf. Mentors are ideally suited to write such letters because they should have a longitudinal professional relationship with you (best if the relationship is >1 year). Your mentor should be able to speak to your passion and goals, and he/she should be able to give concrete examples of your personal qualities (integrity, fortitude, patience, etc.). Your mentor should be a professional authority (physician, scientist, community leader, professor, etc.) whose judgment of you carries some weight.

## 19.7 Summary

Strong mentorship is one of the most important contributors to success after college. The ideal mentor provides motivation, access to resources and a professional network, honest critiques of your performance, and—come application time—a fantastic letter of recommendation.

# Section III

## Applying to Medical School

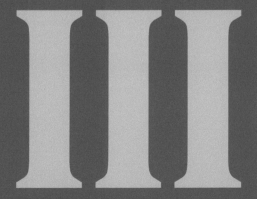

# 20 The Big Picture

*Joel Thomas*

It's finally time. You've poured countless hours into making yourself a competitive medical school applicant. You've probably re-evaluated your choices multiple times: is this *really* what you want out of life? Blood, sweat, and tears were undoubtedly shed, but you're now ready to take the bull by the horns and submit your medical school application.

Hold up one second. Recognize that simply applying to medical school is a *long, expensive, and stressful* process that requires coordinating multiple moving parts and strict attention to detail and deadlines. Many applicants unwittingly make themselves less competitive by not fully understanding the application process. You will not be one of those applicants. The upcoming chapters contain a *lot* of information, and much of it may have changed by the time you're reading this and applying to medical school. *Thus, our foremost recommendation is to cross-check this information with official sources (e.g., per The American Medical College Application Service (AAMCAS). The American Association of Osteopathic Medicine Application Service (AAOMCAS) Texas Medical and Dental Schools Application Service (TMDSAS) websites) online forums and blogs[1] (with a grain of salt), and your school's advisors.*

## 20.1 All Right, I Get It—This Might be Painful. So How Do I Apply to Medical School?

1. Learn how applicants from your school have historically applied and gotten into medical school.
   - Does your school have a pre-med advising office? If so, what are their specific policies for medical school applicants? *You will want to coordinate with your pre-med office throughout the process.*
2. Start the process of continual self-reflection and social media whitewashing (see Chapter 21, Before You Begin: Application Strength Analysis and Chapter 22, Before You Begin: Application Cycle Prophylaxis).
3. Decide *which* schools you are applying to (see Chapter 24, DO, MD, and International Schools, Chapter 25, Dual-Degree Programs: MD/PhD, MPH, MBA, JD, and Others, Chapter 26, Medical School Rankings, and Chapter 27, Making Your List: What Schools Do I Apply To?) because different schools use different application materials.
   - You will use tools such as *MSAR* or *ChooseDO* to determine your list of schools.
   - In 2020 to 2021, the average MD applicant applied to 18 schools,[2] and the average DO applicant applied to 9 schools.[3]
4. Broadly speaking, there is a standardized *primary application* that's sent to many schools (see Chapter 28, Primary Application: AMCAS, AACOMAS, and TMDSAS). These include the AMCAS for US MD schools, the AACOMAS for DO schools, and the TMDSAS for MD and DO schools in the state of Texas.
   - You will list which schools you are applying to on your primary application. All of these schools will receive the same primary application.
   - A completed primary application contains many components such as letters of recommendation, MCAT scores, personal statement, description of extracurriculars (with miniessays), and official transcript, among others. See Chapters 26 to 30 for discussions of specific primary application components.
5. Once an individual school receives your primary application, it will usually send a *secondary application* (see Chapter 33, Secondary Application) with questions and writing prompts that may be specific to that school.
   - These typically do not change over time. Thus, we recommend finding the prompts online and prewriting them.

---

[1] We generally recommend studentdoctor.net and reddit.com/r/premed (particularly the Wiki and FAQ).

[2] Table A–1: U.S. MD-Granting Medical School Applications and Matriculants by School, State of Legal Residence, and Sex, 2021–2022. Available at: https://www.aamc.org/system/files/2021-10/2021_FACTS_Table_A-1.pdf. Accessed July 8, 2022.

[3] aacom®. Available at: https://www.aacom.org/docs/default-source/data-and-trends/2020-aacomas-applicant-matriculant-profile-summary-report.pdf?sfvrsn=d870497_20. Accessed July 8, 2022.

6. Once a school has your completed primary and secondary applications, it may send you an invitation to interview (see Chapter 34, Interviews and Chapter 35, Interview Trail Travel and Attire).
   - After the interview, you may be accepted, wait-listed, or rejected (see Chapter 36, Wait-List and Update Letters; Chapter 37, Financial Aid; and Chapter 38, Acceptance and Decisions: What Really Matters when Choosing the One School).
7. As of 2019, you will need to narrow down your acceptances to three schools and ultimately commit to attend a single school (see Chapter 38, Acceptance and Decisions: What Really Matters when Choosing the One School).

This is a long process that takes about a year: you begin applying in spring the year before your matriculation in fall. For example, if you want to begin medical school in the fall after you graduate (e.g., Fall 2020), then you will begin your application in spring of your *junior year* (Spring 2019—applications open in *May*). As such, you should pick courses in your senior year that would allow absences for interviews, which are mostly held between September and February. If you are currently working, you will need to discuss time off for interviews with your employer. You will also need to think about finances, as you may need to pay for airfare, rental cars, +/− housing for the interviews, as well as the applications themselves.[4]

You will also begin many parts of the application (e.g., personal statement, secondary essays, contacting letter writers) before the application even opens in May to give yourself more time for revisions and feedback, as well as to account for unexpected circumstances (e.g., letter writer is suddenly MIA).[5]

## 20.2 Two Years Before Intended Matriculation

**Fall**—Contact your pre-medical office and let them know you will be applying to medical school next year (e.g., Spring 2019 for admission in Fall 2020). Keep an eye out for mandatory meetings and workshops your school may hold for medical school applicants.

## 20.3 One Year Before Intended Matriculation

1. **January–March:** Contact your letter writers, and ask them if they can write you a "strong positive letter of recommendation for medical school." Typically, you will need at least two science professors and one non-science professor. Alternatively, your school may use a *committee letter* (see Chapter 23, Letters of Recommendation).
   - You want to contact your letter writers 6 to 12 weeks before the application opens in May to give them enough time. Professors are busy people, and popular letter writers likely have multiple students to write for!
   - Your letter writers may also mysteriously become MIA. A large buffer time gives you the opportunity to try other forms of communication (e.g., contacting the department secretary) or contacting another letter writer.
2. **January–March:** Brainstorm and write a working draft of your personal statement. Get as much feedback as possible from different sets of eyes (e.g., English professors, pre-med advisor, family, close friends).
3. **March–early July:** Take Altus Suite if a school you're applying to requires it.
4. **~2 weeks before May**: Request an official copy of your transcript sent to your address. This will allow you to manually enter your transcript into your primary application exactly as written on your official transcript to minimize the chances of having verification of your primary application delayed.
5. **Beginning of May (~May 1):** Complete your primary application; this can take hours to days of effort depending on how prepared you are, and assuming you've finished your polished personal statement already. Also, request that your official transcript is sent to the primary application office for verification.

---

[4] Note: international schools (particularly Caribbean schools) operate on a completely different timeline and application process. While some of these schools accept AMCAS or AACOMAS, others may have their own application. Many of these schools have rolling admissions throughout the year with new batches of students beginning in winter, spring, and fall.

[5] There may be slight differences in timing depending on AMCAS, AACOMAS, and TMDSAS—refer to the specific application instructions online.

6. **~May 24:** This is the last day you can take your MCAT without delaying your application (you will get your score back at the end of June, and applications aren't sent to schools until end of June).

7. **End of May (~May 31):** *Submit your primary application as soon as you are able to (ideally the moment the application is open for submission).*
   - Schools evaluate applications on a rolling basis (and may take 4–6 wk to verify!). You are putting yourself at a disadvantage by not submitting your application as early as possible.

8. **June (and potentially earlier):** Prewrite your secondary application essays.

9. **End of June:** Applications are sent to MD schools (vs. mid-June for DO schools). Almost immediately, you will receive secondary applications from schools.

10. **August 1:** Deadline for *early decision* application for MD schools (see below).

11. **September–February of the year you matriculate:** Interview at medical schools.

12. **October 15:** First day to receive acceptance from US MD schools (including Texas).
    - DO schools will typically send out admission decisions several weeks after interviewing.

## 20.4  Intended Matriculation Year

13. **January–March:** Assess how your application cycle is going. If you genuinely feel that you will not gain admission this cycle, reach out to your pre-med office.
    - We also recommend *tactfully* reaching out to schools that have rejected you for honest feedback on your application. Most schools will likely ignore you, but you may get useful, actionable advice that you can use to strengthen your application for next cycle.
    - Additional advice is covered in Chapter 40, Plan B and Reapplication.

14. **February 19–April 30:** Applicants with multiple acceptances can select "Plan to Enroll" on AMCAS. This is nonbinding, but it allows schools to view the number of applicants who have selected this option to manage their wait-lists.

15. **April 15–April 30:** Applicants should narrow down their acceptance offers to three schools.

16. **April 30 to matriculation:** Pick "commit to enroll" at the school you will matriculate at. Withdraw applications to the other schools that have accepted you and *communicate* these decisions to the individual schools.

17. **October:** Primary application closes.

## 20.5  Early Decision Application

This is an option for US MD schools that allows you to initially apply to one and only one school, from which you will hear your admission status no later than **October 1** the year before matriculation. If accepted, you *must* attend this school. You cannot apply to any other medical schools unless you receive a rejection from this school. *We generally do not recommend this strategy unless you are a highly competitive applicant with personal, unique ties to that school, and the school has strongly suggested to you that you would be accepted.* More information in Chapter 27, Making Your List: What Schools Do I Apply To?

## 20.6  How Much Will This Cost?

- **MCAT:** $320 (also consider test preparation, which ranges from ~$100 for self-study to > $2500 for premium courses).
- **Altus Suite-CASPer:** $10 for the test, $10 *each* for every school you send your score to.
- **Letter of recommendation expenses:** $0 to $70 (some pre-med committees have administrative fees).
- **MSAR:** $28.
- **Primary application:**
  - **AMCAS:** $170 for the initial application (which includes one medical school) + $40 *each* for every additional school.
  - **AACOMAS:** $195 for the initial application (which includes one medical school) + $45 *each* for every additional school.
  - **TMDSAS:** $185 flat fee.

- **Secondary application:** $100 to $200 *per school.*
- **Interview attire (suit, shoes, dry cleaning)**: $300 to $500.
- **Travel**: Varies widely depending on whether you will be flying. A round-trip flight may be around $400 per school +/− taxi/uber/rental car. Budget $500 to $4000!

In total, expect to spend $3,000 to $10,000 (Or more)! Studentdoctor.net (SDN) offers a useful calculator for budgeting application expenses: https://schools.studentdoctor.net/cost_calculator/

However, the AAMC offers the *Fee Assistance Program*[6] for applicants earning up to 300% of the federal poverty level. This program allows applicants to apply to up to 20 schools (primary application) for free. It also provides official MCAT preparation resources, a reduced registration fee for the MCAT ($130), and complimentary MSAR access.

## 20.7  How Can I Keep Track of the Admissions Cycle for My Individual Schools?

The SDN forums have specific threads for each school during each application cycle (e.g., "2021–2022 MD Medical School-Specific Discussions" will have a thread for the 2021–2022 Application Cycle for Drexel University; "Osteopathic School Specific Discussions" will do the same for DO schools).

These are *not* official threads created by the schools themselves. Moreover, recognize that it's a self-selected group of applicants that chooses to actively participate in these threads. Do *not* assume that you are at the bottom of the applicant pile because every other poster on the threads has a near-perfect GPA and MCAT score; the applicants with lower scores are less likely to publicly admit as such.

However, these threads often have current medical students willing to share intimate details about their school. Remember that the application process is highly artificial in a sense: schools and applicants put on their best appearances (you don't normally meet people in a suit, for example), and it's actually quite difficult to get honest information about schools' weaknesses. This is where these forums shine, as anonymous students are more likely to be forthcoming about their dissatisfaction with their schools.

## 20.8  Student Perspective on Student Doctor Network School-Specific Threads

The threads are also a great source of information on real-time application updates. For example, my medical school released its admissions decision several days earlier than they stated on their website and on my interview day, and I was able to find out that I was accepted by following the forum thread!

## 20.9  What Are Update/Intent Letters, and When Do I Send Them?

As consuming as the cycle is, life still goes on after you've submitted your application. Ideally, you'll make new friends, cherish novel experiences, and maybe even publish a paper in your fall semester. If you accomplish something that would greatly strengthen your application and isn't on your originally submitted application (e.g., new leadership role, research publication, dramatic improvement in GPA—*not* demonstration of the same high GPA you already have), then we recommend strategically contacting your schools of interest with an *update letter*.

You'll have to use your best judgment to determine which schools and when to send your letter. Suggested examples include:

- It's November. You didn't receive an interview from your dream school, but other applicants on the SDN forums did.

---

[6] Fee Assistance Program (FAP). Available at: https://students-residents.aamc.org/applying-medical-school/applying-medical-school-process/fee-assistance-program/. Accessed July 8, 2022.

- You've interviewed at the school and are waiting on a final decision.
- You're on the wait-list—*this is arguably the most useful time.* However, a *letter of intent* may be better for your #1 school (but probably isn't—keep reading).

The update letter is different from the *letter of intent.* Basically, this is an update letter on steroids. In this letter, you explicitly tell your dream school that they are your #1 choice and that you will choose to matriculate if accepted. This is useful information to schools because accepting students is somewhat of a risk to schools. Many applicants will have multiple acceptances, and therefore not all accepted applicants to a school will matriculate at that school (because an applicant can only matriculate to a single school). As a result, schools typically accept more students than their intended class size. In doing so, they take the risk of overadmitting students, which leads to logistical and financial problems for the school—training medical students is expensive![7]

That being said, we advise caution with letters of intent. For one thing, it's bad form to renege on a letter of intent, and it's possible that a medical school may hold this against you down the line (e.g., barring you from residency positions). From an ethical perspective, it's also just dishonest.

There is no data above the anecdotal level that letters of intent affect the admissions process, and the real effect is debated. While no one believes these letters hurt your chances, it's more than likely that the vast majority of them don't affect admissions decisions at all. For those letters that do affect these decisions, they probably never turn a blatant "no" into a "yes." At best, they likely secure interviews for a few candidates that wouldn't be offered to them, and maybe (but probably not) move you up in the wait-list. Given the lack of downside of sending one of these letters—if sent honestly and thoughtfully to the one school you really would pick—it should be something you consider.

Something to keep in mind when you are considering pledging matriculation to a specific school: Financial aid packages are only offered to students after acceptances, often weeks to months later, and you may discover that your dream school costs three times as much to attend as another school that gave you a surprisingly good financial aid package. That pledge to go to a slightly higher ranked school may now come with a hefty price tag.[8]

## 20.10 Additional Resources

We always recommend knowing the official recommendations. The AAMC has a wealth of information available to applicants on their "Tools for Medical School Applicants" page. You also should read through *The Official Guide to Medical School Admissions: How to Prepare for and Apply to Medical School.* It's sold by the AAMC for $20, but your pre-med advising office might have a free copy.

## 20.11 Summary

The application timeline in ▶ Fig. 20.1 will provide you with a relative timeline of the process and components. Unofficial student forums can be a helpful guiding resource throughout the process as long as the content is taken with a grain of salt, and in the context of your specific situation. You can deviate from the standard application process by electing to apply to one school early and only via an early decision program, but for the vast majority of applicants the benefits of these programs do not outweigh the risks. Update letters are sent to schools to let them know about big changes (read: improvements) on your resume since you have submitted your application. A select few applicants may benefit from letters of intent, provided they write them openly and honestly, agnostic of possible future financial aid offers from schools.

---

[7] At the same time, it's questionable how much of an impact, if any, these letters actually have. Unsavory applicants have been known to renege on their letters of intent; schools would probably be wise to take these letters with a grain of healthy doubt.

[8] This is a more significant barrier for low income applicants where need-based aid can vary drastically between schools (between $0 and$ 40,000 per year, for instance). Applicants from wealthy families (many applicants) will likely not receive enough financial aid variation to affect a letter of intent.

## Application Time Line

### Fall

Advise pre-med office of your plan to apply to med school

Attend all school hosted meetings for med school applicants

### January—March

At least 6–12 weeks before application process opens in May request letters of recommendation

Working draft of personal statement

### March–July

Take CASPer if required by med school application

### May - June

2 weeks before May - request official transcript

May 1 - Complete primary application

Before May 24 - take MCAT

May 31 - Submit application

June - Prewrite secondary application essays

End of June - Applications are sent to schools

### August

August 1 — Deadline for early decision applications to MD schools

### September — February

Interview at medical schools

### October

10/1—Last date for early applicants to receive admissions decision

10/15—First day to receive acceptance from US med schools

### January—March

Assess your application cycle

Plan B or reapplication?

### Feb 19–April 30

If multiple applications = Plan to enroll on AMCAS

### April

April 15—April 30 Narrow down acceptance offers to 3 schools

April 30—Matriculation Commit to school Withdraw application to other schools

### October

Primary application closes

**Fig. 20.1** Application timeline.

# 21 Before You Begin: Application Strength Analysis

*Joel Thomas*

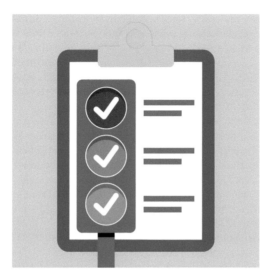

## 21.1 Check Your Readiness to Apply to Medical School

If you're still reading, then you're probably still serious about actually applying to medical school. Remember that even though only 40% of MD applicants gain acceptance *anywhere*, part of this is due to not fully understanding the application details and deadlines. Some applicants unknowingly apply to medical school when they're not reasonably competitive *anywhere*. As such, we'll take the time now to assess your pre-medical profile and to decide whether you should:

- Move forward with your application now.
- Take some time off to strengthen your application.
- Reconsider medical school altogether (rare).

Again, if your school has a pre-med office, you should absolutely work *with them* to brainstorm among these options.

Let's start with the basic requirements. Will you be done with the required academic prerequisites before *matriculating* to medical school?[1] The requirements vary a bit from school to school, but (as of 2020) the basic requirements are a year of college biology with lab, a year of inorganic/general chemistry with lab, a semester of organic chemistry with lab, a semester of biochemistry, a year of physics with lab, +/− genetics depending on the school, ~24 credits of humanities and social/behavioral sciences, and 4–8 credits of mathematics (calculus and/or statistics).

Note that different schools vary in whether they accept AP/IB, community college, extension/evening, foreign, and online courses. For example, if you have AP Biology credit for a semester of college biology, Johns Hopkins School of Medicine requests that you take 4 credits of upper-level biology.[2]

---

[1] It's a common misconception that you need all your pre-reqs completed before *applying* to medical school.

[2] Prerequisites, Requirements and Policies. Available at: https://www.hopkinsmedicine.org/som/education-programs/md-program/application-process/prerequisites-requirements-and-policies.html. Accessed July 8, 2022.

In addition, because the courses only need to be taken before matriculation, you can use your senior year (while applying) to take any requirements you may have missed. For example, you may want to take 4 more credits of mathematics if you only have 4 credits but a school you're interested in requires 8. That said, it's a *de facto* requirement that you complete your biology, (organic) chemistry, and physics requirements before taking the Medical College Admission Test (MCAT) to score well.

Next, what are your academic stats? Although medical schools evaluate applicants "holistically" (i.e., considering their life experiences and personal characteristics), they also expect minimum grade point average (GPA) and MCAT standards to be confident that you will pass the seemingly endless barrage of exams throughout your medical career. In addition, a typical medical school receives thousands of applications for ~130 spots. As a result, many use automatic academic cutoffs to screen the large number of applications they receive. *Thus, your academic metrics are the single most important variables in gaining acceptance to medical school.*

As discussed in Chapter 2, What Medical Schools Look For, the mean GPA ± standard deviation (SD) for matriculants in 2021 for US MD programs was 3.74 ± 0.25, and mean GPA ± SD using only science courses (i.e., "science GPA") was 3.67 ± 0.31. In addition, the average MCAT ± SD in 2021 for matriculants to MD programs was 511.9 ± 6.6, or the 84th percentile. For DO schools, the average GPA in 2018 was 3.54 ± 0.27, and the average MCAT was 504.3 ± 4.7 (58th percentile).[3] See also Table 17.1.

These numbers have also been increasing over time. Thus, if your GPA or your MCAT is below 1 standard deviation of the recent accepted average (e.g., GPA <3.49 for MD and <3.27 for DO schools or MCAT <505 for MD and <500 for DO in 2018[4]) we recommend:

- Post-bacc work to strengthen your GPA +/- applying to an SMP (see Chapter 16, Gap Years, Employment, Graduate Degrees, and Post-Baccalaureate Fellowships).
  - If your overall GPA is **<3.0**, we *strongly recommend* post-bacc work (<10% of applicants with this GPA were accepted anywhere).
  - If your GPA is in the **3.0–3.3** range, we also generally recommend post-bacc work unless you have *exceptional* circumstances (e.g., multiple published first-author papers in high-impact journals, a PhD, started a nonprofit, underrepresented minority [URM] status).
  - You will absolutely need to have at least the average MCAT—ideally higher than average and on your first take—if you go down this route. Schools are already taking an academic gamble on your GPA, and most will not take a two-hit risk.
- Retaking the MCAT after rehauling your study strategy (see Chapter 17, Crushing the MCAT) if your MCAT is low.
- Moving forward with the application cycle with realistic expectations (i.e., significantly strengthening your application *during* the application cycle with plans to potentially apply again next year).
  - We only recommend this strategy if your application is otherwise excellent in other areas (e.g., research, volunteering, URM status, legacy status, extremely high MCAT or GPA if the other stat is low).

---

[3] DO Programs: A Comprehensive Guide to Osteopathic Medical Schools. Available at: https://ingeniusprep.com/blog/osteopathic-medical-schools/. Accessed July 8, 2022.

[4] Assuming similar standard deviations.

## 21.2 Are You an Underrepresented Minority (URM) Applicant?

The AAMC defines under-represented minority (URM) applicants as, "those racial and ethnic populations that are underrepresented in the medical profession relative to their numbers in the general population." Their definition is fluid, as they shifted in 2003 from identifying specific ethnic groups to, "a continually evolving underlying reality. The definition accommodates including and removing underrepresented groups on the basis of changing demographics of society and the profession."

Prior to 2003, the definition explicitly included the following racial/ethnic groups:
- Black/African American.
- Native American (American Indian, Alaskan Native, or Native Hawaiian).
- Mexican American.
- Mainland Puerto Rican.

If you belong to one of these racial/ethnic groups, you almost certainly qualify for URM status. What this means is that—*all other things equal*—your odds of getting accepted by a medical school increase dramatically.

For example, the average GPA and MCAT for accepted Black applicants in 2019–2020 were 3.33 and 497.6, compared to a 3.64 and 504.7 for White applicants.

This is a controversial practice,[5] but it's one you should be aware of given its significant impact on admissions. It's also probably useful to understand why schools do this.

First, many URM students are believed to have encountered more obstacles in their pre-medical journey, (e.g., less exposure to role models with whom they can strongly identify), fewer financial resources for test prep.[6] Thus, it could be argued that the disadvantaged applicant with a 3.33 could have gotten a 3.64 if they had access to the same resources as a more advantaged applicant.

In addition, a body of literature supports the advantages of a diverse physician population. Black and Hispanic patients, for example, tend to report greater satisfaction with physicians of the same racial/ethnic backgrounds.[7]

An obvious criticism is that this process further disadvantages students who encountered hardships but do not fit URM description, e.g., low-income Asian Americans.[8] Moreover, it has been argued that these policies are disproportionately utilized by URM students from privileged backgrounds.[9]

We do not take any specific stance for or against URM recruitment, as the underlying sociopolitical and structural issues are beyond the scope of this book. However, we want you to be aware of its effects on admissions, and we encourage you to do your own research on the topic, as an understanding of social forces is critically important to being a compassionate physician (and human being).

If your GPA and MCAT are competitive, then congratulations! The next question is whether your extracurriculars are robust enough to be competitive. While there are no officially published data on extracurriculars as there are for GPA and MCAT, we recommend the following as rough guidelines *at minimum* for a competitive MD applicant[10]:
- At least 200 to 300 hours of clinical experience.

5  Blake V. Affirmative Action and Medical School Admissions. Available at: https://journalofethics.ama-assn.org/article/affirmative-action-and-medical-school-admissions/2012-12. Accessed July 8, 2022.
6  Lakhan SE. Diversification of U.S. medical schools via affirmative action implementation. BMC Med Educ 2003;3:6. Available at: https://www.ncbi.nlm.nih.gov/pmc/articles/PMC212493/. Accessed July 8, 2022.
7  Saha S, Komaromy M, Koepsell TD, Bindman AB. Patient-physician racial concordance and the perceived quality and use of health care. Arch Intern Med 1999;159(9):997-1004. Available at: https://www.ncbi.nlm.nih.gov/pubmed/10326942. Accessed July 8, 2022.
8  Hsu H. The Rise and Fall of Affirmative Action. Available at: https://www.newyorker.com/magazine/2018/10/15/the-rise-and-fall-of-affirmative-action. Accessed July 8, 2022.
9  Insight: How affirmative action helps rich people. Available at: https://www.sfchronicle.com/opinion/article/Insight-How-affirmative-action-helps-rich-people-13689137.php. Accessed July 8, 2022.
10 Adopted from the University of Utah recommendations: https://medicine.utah.edu/students/programs/md/admissions/

- At least 200 to 300 hours of volunteering.
  - 200 to 300 hours of volunteering in a clinical setting, (e.g., hospital volunteering), will take care of both the clinical experience and volunteering "requirements." However, we also recommend some additional nonclinical volunteering (e.g., soup kitchen, animal shelter, or whatever else interests you) as the cherry on top of your application.
- At least 100 hours of shadowing.
  - This should be done across multiple specialties, at least one of which is primary care: outpatient general internal medicine, family medicine, or outpatient general pediatrics.
- At least 200 to 300 hours of research if you're applying to any research-focused MD schools.
  - That being said, virtually any medical school will appreciate research experience.

Ideally, you'll have cultivated these experiences over several years to demonstrate longitudinal interest and commitment. For example, years of research in the same lab with multiple projects will likely be more useful than a focused summer experience immediately before applying to medical school. You should also be prepared to discuss how these experiences were meaningful to you and how they shaped your interest in medicine.

While these extracurricular "requirements" are *de facto* necessary for acceptance, they are not sufficient. Admissions committees will evaluate you for other characteristics such as passion, leadership potential, experience with diverse communities, and communication skills. Consider the "Core Competencies for Entering Medical Students" for assessing your strengths.[11] Passion, for example, is demonstrated through significant involvement in *any* extracurricular; if you're an award-winning juggler who can speak off the cuff about the nuances between two- and three-ball juggling, you better believe that medical schools will be excited to hear about your story.

Lastly, you'll have confidence in your letters of recommendation. Ideally, you'll have multiple authors with whom you've worked intimately over several years. We recommend asking your letter writers for a "strong, positive letter of recommendation for medical school," ideally in person (with email as a second choice). We also recommend giving your letter writer the "Guidelines for Writing a Letter of Evaluation for a Medical School Applicant."[12] Keep in mind that schools have minimum requirements for letters (e.g., two science professors and one non-science professor at minimum). If you suspect that one of your required letters may be lukewarm at best, we recommend asking an additional writer (e.g., employer, extracurricular faculty member) for an outstanding letter to strengthen your application.

Let's return to our decision tree from the beginning of this chapter. If you have all these pieces of the puzzle at minimum, then we'll move on with our application! If not, then it is our recommendation that, in general, you should not move ahead with your application. Feel free to check in with your pre-medical advisor for a second opinion. Applying to medical school is incredibly time-consuming, expensive, and stressful, and you start a lower chance of admission if you failed the first time and must try again as a reapplicant. Only apply to medical school once.

That said, we have already discussed when it would be appropriate to take time off to make up for a low GPA and/or MCAT. If your extracurriculars do not meet the minimum standards, then too we recommend taking time to make up for these deficits. Fortunately, extracurriculars are much easier to salvage than a low GPA or MCAT.

As far as reconsidering medical school altogether, we only recommend this for *extreme* cases. For example, significant academic dishonesty (e.g., cases of cheating), significant criminal history, or inability to meet the technical standards required by medical schools[13] should prompt serious introspection about whether medical school is your best choice.

Nonetheless, even these cases should be assessed on an individual basis. For example, while Stanford's Technical Standards include, "MOTOR FUNCTION: Candidates must possess the capacity to perform physical examinations and diagnostic maneuvers. They must be able to respond to emergency situations in a

---

[11] https://students-residents.aamc.org/applying-medical-school/article/core-competencies
[12] Guidelines for Writing a Letter of Evaluation for a Medical School Applicant. Available at: https://www.aamc.org/system/files?file=2019-09/lettersguidelinesbrochure.pdf. Accessed July 8, 2022.
[13] https://med.stanford.edu/md/mdhandbook/section-2-general-standards/section-2-3-school-of-medicine-technical-non-academic-standards.html

timely manner and provide general and emergency care," medical schools have made significant accommodations for extraordinary circumstances in the past (e.g., quadriplegic student[14]). Moreover, even felony criminal histories may theoretically be overcome with *years* of good behavior demonstrating a fundamental change in character. At this point, however, we urge you to consider how badly you want to commit to medicine versus the many other careers available. It's ultimately a decision that only you can make for yourself, but we implore you to take a birds-eye view of your pre-medical journey in the context of your life as a whole to avoid missing the forest for the trees.

## 21.3 Medical School Admissions Consultants

Medical school admissions consultants are expert advisors—typically former Admissions Committee (ADCOM) members at highly ranked medical schools—who work closely with you throughout the application process to maximize your chances of getting into medical school. They're basically like personal trainers for getting into medical school. They're often extremely expensive (frequently several thousand dollars), but the well-regarded ones are extraordinarily helpful resources for crafting the best possible application that an applicant can present. In addition, admissions consultants will work with you every step of the application process, reacting in real time to various setbacks and bumps in the road on the admission trail. If you have the money available, then the peace of mind of knowing that you exhausted every possible resource to get into the highest ranked medical school you could get into (or leverage the best scholarship you could get) may be worth it. This is especially the case if you have major weaknesses or specific deficits in your application that you're having trouble overcoming (e.g., disciplinary action, poor writing ability).

The vast majority of matriculants to medical school—including top medical schools—did not use admissions consultants. At the same time, it may be the case that they could have had better results if they did. How *much* better? It's hard to say, and it's ultimately a personal decision as to whether you feel the benefits are worth the costs (including the potential cost of losing an entire year's worth of attending salary because you didn't get into medical school).

If you *do* choose an admissions consult, we urge you to pick one with:
1. Experience on an ADCOM (preferably at a top medical school).
2. Documented success rate.
3. Willingness to work with the applicant at all stages of the application, including at short notice (things change quickly throughout the process!).

## 21.4 Summary

A decision to apply to medical school should only occur after assessing your application strength. The foundation of that strength begins with technical requirements (did you take all the prerequisites?), your stats (are your GPA and MCAT high enough?), and your integrity (do you have any documented history of ethical or professional transgressions?). These are the deal breakers. After that, the strength of your application can be assessed on a more individualized level (did you complete significant and meaningful volunteering, research, or shadowing, etc., and are your letters of recommendation strong?). There is reasonable data on where the average applicant stands in regard to these metrics, and you should be frequently assessing how you measure up before you invest and dedicate your time and effort in this process.

---

[14] Dampier C. Chris Connolly is a brilliant medical student. He's also a quadriplegic—and the person who may change the way we think about doctors. Available at: https://www.chicagotribune.com/lifestyles/ct-life-quadriplegic-med-student-connolly-0917-story.html. Accessed July 8, 2022.

# 22 Before You Begin: Application Cycle Prophylaxis

*Phillip Wagner and Ray Funahashi*

As they say: an ounce of prevention is worth a pound of cure.

Before you begin your medical school applications, you should take these steps to prevent potential complications before they can even happen. We highly suggest the following steps for a better application experience.

We live in a digital age, and—like it or not—information found on the Internet can affect our chances of employment and medical school admissions. You can bet that there will be an ADCOM member who will Google you or look you up on a social site at some point in your application cycle. As such, it makes sense for you to know what information can be found about you and to manage that information in the best way possible.

Every student should assume that admissions committees do look up applicants online and can stumble upon information that can hurt a candidate.

While it isn't the job description per se of ADCOM members to search the Internet about their applicants, it does happen. Based on the number of people who review your application at the 20 or so schools to which you apply, you should assume that people will be looking for your unofficial, "unfiltered" resume. Here, you will find basic steps to protect yourself against this practice.

## 22.1 Personal Social Media Cleanup: Assess the Damage

Take stock of your Internet presence with an Internet search of your name and a review of your social media profiles.
- Search your name (all permutations) and hometown/school/major/identifying features across multiple search engines (e.g., Google, Bing, DuckDuckGo, Yahoo, and AskJeeves if it still exists—just for fun).
- Review Facebook, LinkedIn, Instagram, Twitter, Researchgate, Quora, YouTube, Pinterest, Tumblr, Twitch, TikTok, Reddit, dating applications and every other platform in which you participate, including online blogs, etc. Ideally, your online presence is *absolutely anonymous* (e.g., no Reddit posts/comments referencing your school, major, unique series of extracurricular activities, intention to apply to medical school, and unseemly political rants). Don't forget about comments/posts on news articles under your real name.

Once you are aware of what your presence is, you should be aware that this collection comprises your unofficial resume. Medical schools, and later on—employers—will use this as a means of seeing who you are when you think the professional world isn't watching.
- **Image cleanup:** Review the aforementioned sources for any information that might be harmful to your admission chances. While there isn't any hard-and-fast rule for what constitutes unprofessional contact, it generally is the wise decision to play it safe. If you are questioning whether or not something is fit for a professional online presence, you should just remove it; if you are questioning what it says about you, others may not be as kind. If it's a difficult decision, weigh the options: what is the upside of keeping that material out there? It's almost certain it isn't worth the downside of being rejected by an admissions committee. Remember: anything that you can be seen doing should be put through this test: **would the average person want to see their doctor doing that?**
- **Playing defense:** Protecting your online presence is about more than getting rid of unflattering content. You should do what you can to make your settings as private and restrictive as possible, viewable to your friends alone. Require that tags in photos have your approval before they post. Some medical students when applying to medical school change their profile names to something that could not be traceable back to them.
- **Politics:** Parties and solo cups and objectionable photos are one thing, you say, but your politics are another. You aren't trying to be unprofessional, just passionate. While that may, in fact, be true, it bears repeating that ADCOM members can and do come from different parts of the political spectrum. While we would never endorse altering your beliefs to promote your career, it's important to be mindful that how you discuss and promote your beliefs can affect how others perceive you professionally. As a doctor, you will work with many colleagues and patients that do not share your views, and a large part

about being a good colleague is respect for others (read: not agreement), and a large part of being a good doctor is patient's not feeling judged. There is a time and a place to discuss politics and other things you are passionate about, and you should be mindful to do it respectfully (or at least try).

- **Going forward:** If you feel restricted by this, it's going to get a lot harder. The further you advance in medical training, the more you will be expected to act in accord with the cultural standards of the profession (for better or worse). This will be very—and increasingly—restrictive for some of you. If it means anything, it does get easier for most of us. Success in working with patients is predicated on their trust in you, and the further you progress in your career, the less you may want to jeopardize that.

The overall rule is this: If you don't think the average person wants to see their doctor doing something, then they shouldn't be able to see you doing it.

## 22.2 Email Preparation: This Email System Setup Will Keep You Sane Throughout the Application Cycle

1. Create a separate professional-appearing (e.g., first name, last name, ± numbers) email (e.g., Gmail) account to be used only for medical school applications and correspondences. This keeps everything you need in one place. Use this email for your primary application. It should be the one you use to email programs, and should be the one listed on your resume.
2. Sync this email account to your phone and—ideally—smartwatch so that you have a unique alert for admissions correspondences. Alternatively, you can set your Gmail to immediately forward all emails to text messages. This way, you will be able to pick interview dates immediately (interview invites are often sent in batches with applicants choosing among available dates and times on a first-come, first-serve basis).

## 22.3 Store All of Your Application Files and Notes on the Cloud in a Single Space

- Create a cloud account if you don't have one already. We're most familiar with Google Drive. Therefore, we will be discussing Google products throughout this section, but be aware that any cloud service with calendar and spreadsheet functionality will work. Keep everything you need for your application here: headshots, resume/CV, published papers (along with succinct summaries of your research activities), information about schools, interview answer fodder, and drafts of your personal statement as well as secondary essays, thank you letters, and everything else there.
- Use Google Calendar to keep track of travel arrangements and interview dates.
- Use a Google Excel spreadsheet to tabulate the following information about your schools: name, location (e.g., geographical region, state), date primary application submitted, date secondary application submitted, outcome (e.g., rejected, interview accepted vs. invited vs. attended, accepted, wait-listed).
  - Update this continually throughout the application cycle, as it is easy to become overwhelmed and miss to-dos without tracking.
  - Keep a running budget in another sheet of the spreadsheet, as expenses can spiral out of control if you're not actively paying attention!

## 22.4 Look into Travel Credit Cards and Loyalty Programs 5 to 6 Months before Interviews Begin

This tip is for you if you are a responsible credit card user! If you anticipate heavy travel (e.g., flying), consider applying for a credit card with generous travel rewards. You can save hundreds of dollars doing this and even have access to luxurious perks such as complimentary airport lounge access. Overall, there is no single best card, and your anticipated expenses will dictate which card will make the most financial sense. We also recommend looking into Loyalty Programs with hotels and airlines if you plan on preferentially using a service to quickly obtain perks. Reviews by Nerdwallet, Wallethub, and ThePointsGuy are good starting points for assessing the pros and cons of cards and Loyalty Programs, and the landscape of available options changes over time.

Keep in mind that you may want to qualify for a card with an annual fee that ultimately ends up being financially worth it during the application year. You can then "downgrade" to a credit card with the same carrier that does not have an annual fee for subsequent years, if you desire.

## 22.5  Be Ready to Manage Your Stress

Learn to manage stress well and to patiently wait amid a backdrop of low-to-moderate grade stress. One of the most frustrating aspects of the application process is that you will spend weeks to months waiting in dead silence after spending countless hours distilling years of hard work into a competitive application. You will understandably be frustrated by this. We recommend hitting the gym hard, taking up a new hobby or two, excelling in your classes/job, and maximizing time with friends and family to stay mentally healthy. This also has the added benefit of giving you great talking points for your interviews.

## 22.6  Summary

This chapter is all about playing professionalism defense by curating your online presence. Applicants can occasionally find this practice restricting, as if they are muting their personalities, especially since they have to be constantly adding a professional filter to deciding whether or not something goes online. Adding this filter is the opposite of spontaneity, and feels like your professional life is overshadowing your personal time. While it is certainly understandable to be upset by this, the only point it is essential to make is this: there can be consequences to how you portray yourself. While that used to mean how you dressed and acted in an interview only, now your digital footprint or resume is much more present and accessible. You don't need us to tell you that there are consequences to actions, but it's a fact that some people have trouble applying this to their online presence. You can be passionate about politics and open about your advocacy as well, but consider and assess whether or not you are being respectful and professional when you do it. Professionalism is something that shouldn't globally dictate every aspect of your life, but it is something about which you should be at least intermittently mindful.

In terms of preparing organizationally for the application process, setting yourself up for success beforehand is key. Creating a dedicated email account, setting aside a portion of a Google Drive (or some other remotely accessible resource), and utilizing a calendar will help ensure you are hitting deadlines and planning effectively. Keeping track of the different variables that matter to you about schools in a spreadsheet can allow you to decide between them systematically and more rationally (rather than just seeing the entire application cycle as a blur).

# 23 Letters of Recommendation

*Phillip Wagner*

Having people professionally vouch for your credentials is an important part of the admissions process. Since getting letters of recommendation may not be something you experienced when you applied to college, we will spell out the basics.

## 23.1 How to Maximize Your Odds of Getting a Strong, Positive Letter of Recommendation

Going into college, you should consider every professor, mentor, and advisor a potential letter writer. Building off of Chapter 19, Finding Mentors, you should:
- Strive to attend most classes, at least early on in a course, especially if you have a strong feeling that you might want this professor to write a letter for you.
- Participate and sit where the professor can see you (some science classes can be large).
- Try to talk to the professor before or after the class about the material. Ask frequent questions about the content and possible connections to outside material.
- Follow up with the professor after tests about questions you don't understand.
- Attend occasional office hours; many professors are not overwhelmed in office hours unless there is a test on the near horizon.
- Keep in touch after the class; consider taking other classes offered by that professor (many teach two or more classes at different difficulty levels).

An added benefit: building a relationship with a professor can have other benefits, including learning about their research and opening up potential research opportunities for you by working on their projects. It's easier to start doing research with a mentor if they already know you.

These things are often a struggle because they are out of most people's comfort zones, especially those who are introverted or find themselves experiencing social anxiety upon asking questions during class, as well as those who would prefer to limit professional interactions to a minimum. Most early science classes also come with the benefit of remote learning and lax or no attendance policies, and some third-party sources are just as good as—if not better—at teaching you the material, making attending a lecture feel like a waste of time. This can be compounded in the science classes, as they tend to be bigger, do not require attendance or participation, issue very few writing or oral assignments, and include very little necessary time for the professor and you to interact. Most often, you will complete one to four multiple choice tests along with a lab component for the course. You can go the entire time without seeing your professor more than a handful of times if you want to, and more importantly, without them seeing you. Make sure to take pains to be present, to be involved, to be inquisitive, and to be the best version of yourself. Keep in mind that mentoring is a two-way street, as many mentors are motivated to learn from their mentees' unique perspectives. Therefore, you should also do your part by staying engaged with your mentors to obtain strong, positive letters of recommendation.

Other professionals can write letters for you. These include academic mentors, employers, research mentors, and advisors. In order to earn the best letter possible from this category of people (whether or not you should focus on letters from these sources is dealt with below), you should follow the same spirit as outlined in the suggestions above. Be punctual, professional, reasonable, and organized. Actively engage in a professional relationship with these people. Remember: to write you a strong letter, they need to understand the full array of your strengths. If they don't have that, they may not be the ideal letter writer.

## 23.2 So How Many Letters Should You Have, and of Which Type?

- First, you should be aware of the general types of letters:
  - Academic:
    - STEM versus Non-STEM.
  - Non-academic.
  - Committee.

- Requirements vary by school, but in general, two STEM and one non-STEM is the bare minimum you should be considering.
  - STEM: Science, Technology, Engineering, Math.
  - Non-STEM: All other disciplines; social sciences such as economics, anthropology, philosophy, psychology, or the humanities, such as English, history, languages, etc. This includes letters from advisors, research mentors, supervisors/bosses, or from any other source.
- Feel free to ask for one extra STEM letter and one extra non-STEM letter. Accidents happen, and it is impossible to predict everything. There are a variety of reasons you should ask for more letters. Here is—by far—the most important and common one:
  - Your professor does not finish your letter on time, or at all: This is more common than you would ever suspect. Your letter of recommendation (LOR) is almost never a professor's priority. Despite it being an established part of their job, it neither earns them a paycheck (like teaching or research) nor does it increase their prestige (like teaching or research), nor keep their department head off their back, nor increase their chances at tenure, and so on. If things come up, your letter will be deprioritized, put off, or forgotten about. Thus, if you only get three letters of recommendation, and one professor—for any number of reasons—neglects your letter, medical schools will not review your application until you have the required number of letters. And, as we all know, applying late in the cycle is a dangerous game. Losing a month to ask for a new letter is something no one wants to do.
- Get at least those three letters above from academic sources, meaning professors who have given you a grade for a course. If they haven't given you a grade, they fall into a generally less impressive group of letter writers known as nonacademic letter writers.
- That said, we also recommend having at least one mentor who can write you a strong, positive nonacademic LOR(s). Acceptable sources include:
  - A research advisor.
  - An academic mentor, generally assigned by the school.
  - A supervisor or employer.
  - A volunteer coordinator.
  - A doctor with whom you have shadowed.
  - A person who is not a family member that has known you for a significant period of time (e.g., clergy). **Note:** Only use this one if you absolutely need to.
    - These last four should generally only be used as letters of last resort, or if you have significant, long-term, relationships with these people who can comment extensively on who you are and your strength as an applicant, and this letter is significantly stronger than an academic letter (professor who has given you a grade for something).
- Letters from research mentors and certain employers can be very strong, and are the exception in this generally weaker category. If a research mentor has worked with you on at least one successful project, can vouch for your professional qualities, and can speak glowingly about your intellectual rigor, curiosity, and potential as a researcher, then his/her letter can be *very* helpful—even stronger than an academic letter in certain contexts.
  - As an aside, if you do dedicated research with someone for a prolonged period of time, i.e., > 1 year, you would do well to have them write you a letter as it may be a potential red flag if they are not willing.

## 23.3 Committee Letters

How does this factor into your school's pre-med committee?
- If you have a pre-med committee, you should do everything you can to use it.
- If your school doesn't have a pre-med committee, don't worry, you are not at a disadvantage.
- However, if you don't use one when your school has one, this is an extremely suspicious move. Schools will either assume (a) you had some issues with your school, or vice versa, that prevents this; (b) you didn't have the skills to prioritize your responsibilities, (c) you are oblivious, or haven't wanted to be a doctor as long as you have claimed.
- Here is the most important thing to keep in mind about your pre-med committee: deadlines. Your pre-med committee application deadline does not line up closely with your application to medical school. Many times, you need to send your application and LORs as much as a year ahead of time to the committee. Even more complicated, most pre-med committees do not accept applications year-round.

So, if you miss the deadline, which is often a very narrow window, you will not be able to use your school's pre-med committee. Then, you will have to explain to certain schools—and this is common—why you elected not to use your school's committee. This isn't the death knell of your doctor-dreams, but it does raise suspicions. You want application admissions officers focused on your good qualities, not on your excuses for why you could not abide by your school's pre-med committee criteria.

## 23.4 "I Have a Lot of Options. Who Should Write My Letters?"

The most important thing is that you choose letter writers who will write a GLOWING letter for you. If you can imagine your letter writer saying things like "I would trust this person to be my doctor" and "best student I've had for x, y, z reasons," etc., you are on the right track. Make sure this person is also strongly advocating for you in your pursuit to go to medical school.

### 23.4.1 Academic

- Professors in whose class you earned an A or an A-; you can get away with a B+, but only under extenuating circumstances or if no better options exist.
- Professors who know you well; you have gone to their class consistently, made your presence known by participating, and possibly have attended their office hours or kept in touch with them. This is easier in non-STEM classes; they tend to be smaller, require participation and attendance, and tend to include writing assignments that allow your professor to get to know you easier.
- Professors who can comment not just on your academic performance, but who you are as a person. Again, easier in non-STEM classes.
- Remember: you can satisfy the letter requirement with only academic letters; you should only use nonacademic letters as part of your top three if you absolutely need to, or as described above, this would be a stronger letter than a professor from whom you received a grade (very rare).
- Minimum: two STEM, one non-STEM (but you can ask for one extra of each as a backup).

### 23.4.2 Nonacademic

- Someone who has known you for a significant period of time.
- Someone with whom you have worked closely.
- Someone who can comment on your good qualities.
- Someone who has seen what you are like professionally; since we don't have grades to go on.
- Can also be tacked on after your three academic letters and committee letter for schools that accept more than three letters.

## 23.5 When Do I Ask for the Letter?

To ensure success, 10 to 12 weeks before you need them. You can certainly ask earlier when your performance is fresher in their mind, but asking too early might hurt you if they will be able to write a stronger letter for you in the future (e.g., you will be doing 6 more months of research with them, you will be taking another of their classes, etc.).

## 23.6 How to Actually Ask

Send an email to the professor covering the following bases:
- Review your relationship ("You taught my Bio 101, 203, and 411 classes).
- Letting them know you will be applying to medical school.
- Ask if they, based on your performance in the class(s) (hopefully A, A, A) and what the professor has seen regarding your dedication, hard work, professionalism, etc., would be willing to write you a **"strong, positive"** LOR.
- Fodder: You can attach your resume/CV at this time, as well as your personal statement (or a more informal blurb about what you hope to do with your life)—they need content!

If you sense any hesitancy or reservation when you talk to your potential letter writer, DO NOT continue to ask them for the letter. No matter what they say, some of that hesitancy will transfer to your letter. Consider it bad juju. Even a slightly negative LOR can be a red flag on your application. You also waive the right to see the LOR, so you may be going into the application cycle doomed to fail without even knowing why. Save yourself the mental anguish of wondering *whether* that lukewarm response from your professor means "meh" LOR that will tank your application.

## 23.7 How to Follow-up

- Don't hesitate to check in on the status of the letter as you get closer to the deadline (e.g., 4 weeks away, 2 weeks away, 1 week away) if it hasn't been submitted yet.
- Ask if they require anything else in order to complete the letter, or if they have any questions.
- If they have submitted your letter, send them a personalized letter thanking them for their efforts.
- When you get good news, such as an acceptance, LET THEM KNOW AND THANK THEM. Many of them will be very happy that they were a part of your success.

## 23.8 What If Someone Asks You to Write a Letter for Yourself?

- Do some serious self-reflection about your strengths and write about them with *specific, concrete examples*. Yes, it's awkward to write an LOR for yourself, and you'll probably be worrying about the supposed writer exclaiming, "Seriously? They think *this* about himself?" Specific examples close the loop here.

## 23.9 Summary

Remember, just like everything else in your application, it comes down to quality over quantity. Three perfect letters and a committee letter are going to beat 10 good letters every time. Academic letters are generally stronger than nonacademic letters, but there are some exceptions. Make sure you set your letter writers up for success by giving them adequate content, and checking in regularly to make sure they are aware of your deadlines. Always ask more letter writers for letters than you need (at least 5). And, when the process is done, remember to thank your letter writers with a thank you letter of your own.

# 24 DO, MD, and International Schools

*Joel Thomas*

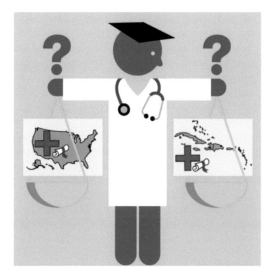

We've been talking about applying to "medical school" a lot so far. You should know, however, that there are two types of US medical schools that offer two different degrees. These two degrees are the Doctor of Medicine (MD) and Doctor of Osteopathic Medicine (DO). Medical schools that give MD degrees are referred to commonly as *allopathic* medical schools. Medical schools that give DO degrees are referred to as *osteopathic* medical schools.

Despite the different names, because licensing exams tightly regulate the path to becoming a physician in the United States, the basic curriculum and clinical training across these types of schools are generally the same.

However, there *are* important differences you should know. Here, we will delve into osteopathic medical schools and International/Caribbean medical schools that confer the MD degree.

## 24.1 Doctor of Osteopathic Medicine (DO)

Many people have never heard of the term "osteopathic medicine," even though they may have been treated by an osteopathic physician. Overall, osteopathic physicians are considered the equivalent of MDs: they are licensed to practice medicine in every state with identical privileges and earning potentials. They also learn the same information as MDs and must pass similar—if not the same—exams for licensing. However, they hold a different degree: Doctor of Osteopathic Medicine (DO) versus the MD, Doctor of ("allopathic") Medicine.

The curriculum at DO schools also includes 300 to 500 hours of physical manipulative techniques ("osteopathic manipulative treatment") and emphasizes—to variable degrees—a different philosophical view of medicine. Lastly, DO schools are *on average* easier to gain admission compared to MD schools; however, this comes at the cost of being less competitive for certain residency programs.

## 24.1.1 History of the DO Degree

You might be wondering why this degree even exists when it sounds like MDs and DOs are virtually identical. To understand, we'll need to take a trip back through time. In the late 19th century, physician A.T. Still founded osteopathic medicine as a countermovement against contemporary medical practices. Dr. Still believed that medicine at the time narrowly focused on the effects of disease rather than their causes. He also aimed to emphasize holistic treatment centered around musculoskeletal manipulation of the patient, believing that seemingly unrelated diseases (e.g., bronchitis, constipation) were manifestations of a dysfunctional musculoskeletal system.[1] Hence, "osteopathy" emerged from the Greek roots for bone ("*osteon*") and suffering ("*-pathos*"). In the proper historical context, his views seem reasonable; many chronic diseases were treated with dangerous drugs such as arsenic, opium, and whiskey aimed at the obvious symptoms, and unsanitary surgical practices at the time often led to overwhelming infection and death.[2]

Fortunately, our understanding of medicine has evolved exponentially, and we now better understand the causes of many diseases; swelling of the legs, for example, may suggest heart failure, and our treatment will be aimed at heart dysfunction rather than the legs themselves. Moreover, the concept of an "osteopathic philosophy" that leads to significant practice-changing behavior is controversial, even within the osteopathic medical community.[3] Like osteopathic medicine, modern allopathic medicine freely acknowledges that all organ systems are interconnected, that medicine and surgery should only be offered if the benefits outweigh the harms, and that complementary and alternative therapies such as acupuncture and chiropractic manipulation may provide symptomatic relief and improve quality of life for patients with chronic, debilitating diseases. In addition, the vast majority of DOs do not regularly use osteopathic manipulative treatment in their practices, and its use appears to decline with more recent graduation from a DO school.[4]

So what are the existing differences between MD and DO schools you should be concerned with? First, all DO schools include education in osteopathic manipulative treatment, which is a hands-on physical treatment that involves stretching and manipulating muscles and joints.

This treatment is based on the principle that every part of the body is interconnected by a continuous layer of connective tissue and muscle (the "myofascial continuity") that can be strategically manipulated to provide relief from disease. The evidence base for this is mixed but ranges from very promising, high-quality data for chronic, nonspecific low back pain[5] to *potentially dangerous pseudoscience* for cranial manipulation.[6,7] However, these problems in evidence-based medicine are not unique to DOs, as allopathic medicine also has examples of treatments that are commonly offered despite limited evidence,

[1] The philosophy and mechanical principles of osteopathy. Available at: https://archive.org/stream/philosophymechan00-stiliala/philosophymechan00stiliala_djvu.txt. Accessed July 8, 2022.

[2] Stark JE. Quoting A.T. Still with rigor: an historical and academic review. J Am Osteopath Assoc 2012;112(6):366–73. Available at: https://pubmed.ncbi.nlm.nih.gov/22707646/. Accessed July 8, 2022.

[3] Kasiri-Martino H, Bright P. Osteopathic educators' attitudes towards osteopathic principles and their application in clinical practice: A qualitative inquiry. Manual Therapy 2016;21:233–240. Available at: https://www.sciencedirect.com/science/article/abs/pii/S1356689X15001770. Accessed July 8, 2022.

[4] Johnson SM, Kurtz ME, Kurtz JC. Variables influencing the use of osteopathic manipulative treatment in family practice. J Am Osteopath Assoc 1997;97(2):80–87. Available at: https://www.ncbi.nlm.nih.gov/pubmed/9059002?dopt=Abstract. Accessed July 8, 2022.

[5] Franke H, Franke J-D, Fryer G. Osteopathic manipulative treatment for nonspecific low back pain: a systematic review and meta-analysis. BMC Musculoskelet Disord 2014;15:286. Available at: https://www.ncbi.nlm.nih.gov/pmc/articles/PMC4159549/. Accessed July 8, 2022.

[6] Hartman SE. Cranial osteopathy: its fate seems clear. Chiropr Osteopat 2006;14:10. Available at: https://www.ncbi.nlm.nih.gov/pmc/articles/PMC1564028/. Accessed July 8, 2022.

[7] Atwood IV KC. Naturopathy, Pseudoscience, and Medicine: Myths and Fallacies vs Truth. MedGenMed. 2004; 6(1): 33. Available at: https://www.ncbi.nlm.nih.gov/pmc/articles/PMC1140750/. Accessed July 8, 2022.

such as vertebral augmentation (e.g., kyphoplasty, vertebroplasty) for osteoporotic vertebral compression fractures.[8] While the majority of DOs do not regularly use osteopathic manipulative treatment,[9] if you have interests in fields such as physical medicine and rehabilitation, sports medicine, or orthopaedic surgery, then you may be able to integrate this additional training into your practice. The alternative would be obtaining an MD degree and pursuing additional training in osteopathic manipulative treatment available to MDs[10] (however—per our understanding—this is rarely, if ever, done).

Secondly, osteopathic medical schools have a reputation for having some emphasis on primary care. As of 2019, nearly 57% of DOs practiced in primary care, compared to <30% of MDs.[11] This does not—of course—necessitate that you pursue primary care if you attend a DO school, but you may want to keep this reputation in mind if you have strong feelings *against* pursuing primary care down the line. If your ultimate goal is to become an academic plastic surgery chief, then DO schools as a whole may not be the best fit for you compared to many academic MD programs.

Another important difference is that historically, acceptance has been less competitive at DO schools compared to allopathic schools in the United States. In 2016, the average undergraduate GPA for MD programs was a 3.70 versus a 3.54 for DO programs, and the average MCAT was a 508.7 for MD programs versus 502.2 for DO programs.[12,13] Keep in mind that there is significant variation between individual DO schools compared to individual MD schools. For example, the average science GPA at Michigan State University College of Osteopathic Medicine for 2019 was a 3.7, with an average MCAT of 507,[14] which is higher than that of several MD programs. DO schools, like MD schools, vary in their admission requirements and competitiveness, and we recommend due diligence in researching the admissions criteria, academic resources, and overall culture of individual schools then applying (▶ Fig. 24.1).[15] The easier access to admission, however, contributes to some stigma against DOs in residency admissions, despite their status as professional equivalents to MDs.

Let's briefly go over the residency application process (more on this in "A Peek at the Residency Application Process and Residency Experience"). Traditionally, MD students applied to "allopathic" residency programs in their 4th year of medical school using the National Resident Matching Program (NRMP). DO students were also able to apply to these programs using the NRMP, but they would often take the standard USMLE Board exams in addition to the DO-specific licensing exams (COMLEX, or "Comprehensive Osteopathic Medical Licensing Examination"). Virtually all of the most "prestigious," academic programs, e.g., Massachusetts General Hospital, Mayo Clinic, participate in the NRMP. DO students also had the option of applying to programs that participate in the American Osteopathic Association (AOA) Match, which was exclusive to DO students. However, the Accreditation Council for Graduate Medical Education (ACGME), American Association of Colleges of Osteopathic Medicine (AACOM), and AOA merged in 2020, allowing MD and DO students alike to apply to programs participating in both services. As of 2021, it is still not totally clear what impact this has had for DO applicants (as well as international applicants). The big-picture data is reassuring, however. The overall match rates for DOs did not change substantially from 2019 (premerger) to 2020 (postmerger), including in competitive specialties like dermatology

8   Buchbinder R, Johnston RV, Rischin KJ, Homik J, Jones CA, Golmohammadi K, Kallmes DF. Percutaneous vertebroplasty for osteoporotic vertebral compression fracture. Cochrane Database Syst Rev 2018;4(4):CD006349. Available at: https://www.ncbi.nlm.nih.gov/pubmed/29618171. Accessed July 8, 2022.

9   Johnson SM , Kurtz ME. Diminished use of osteopathic manipulative treatment and its impact on the uniqueness of the osteopathic profession. Acad Med 2001;76(8):821-8. Available at: https://pubmed.ncbi.nlm.nih.gov/11500286/. Accessed July 8, 2022.

10  Teaching Osteopathic Medicine to MDs. Available at: https://www.fammed.wisc.edu/teaching-osteopathic-medicine-mds/. Accessed July 8, 2022.

11  Murphy B. DO vs. MD: How much does the medical school degree type matter? Available at: https://www.ama-assn.org/residents-students/preparing-medical-school/do-vs-md-how-much-does-medical-school-degree-type#most-dos-choose-primary-care. Accessed July 8, 2022.

12  Table A-16: MCAT Scores and GPAs for Applicants and Matriculants to U.S. MD-Granting Medical Schools, 2018-2019 through 2021-2022. Available at: https://www.aamc.org/download/321494/data/factstablea16.pdf. Accessed July 8, 2022.

13  AACOMAS Profile: Applicant & Matriculant Summary Report. Available at: http://www.aacom.org/docs/default-source/data-and-trends/2016-aacomas-applicant-amp-matriculant-profile-summary-report.pdf?sfvrsn=10. Accessed July 8, 2022.

14  https://com.msu.edu/future-students/applying/profile-successful-applicant

15  Average GPA and MCAT Score for Every Medical School (2022). Available at: Source: https://www.shemmassianconsulting.com/blog/average-gpa-and-mcat-score-for-every-medical-school; plot created in R Version 4.0.3. Accessed July 8, 2022.

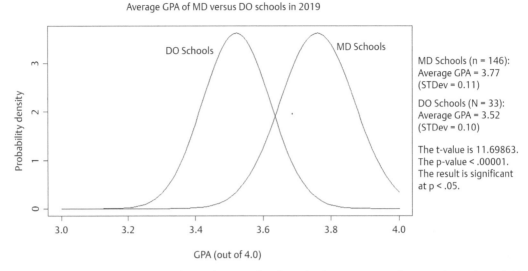

Fig. 24.1 Average grade point average (GPA) of Doctor of Medicine (MD) versus Doctor of Osteopathic Medicine (DO) schools in 2019.

and orthopaedic surgery.[16] That said, this data doesn't capture some of the more granular findings that may have been impacted. For example, MD applicants can now apply to programs in competitive specialties such as dermatology and orthopaedic surgery that had originally been exclusively reserved to DO applicants. It's unclear what impact the merger has had on DO applicants' success rate to these programs.

Every 2 years, program directors at residency programs that participate in the NRMP fill out the "Program Director Survey," which plainly states the variables most important to residency program admission.[17] For "All Specialties Combined," "graduate of a highly-regarded U.S. medical school" was an important factor for nearly half of residency program directors with an average rating of 3.6/5. To put things into context, US News and World Report ranks all US medical schools by residency director assessment score (requires a paid subscription to view), and the top schools are *overwhelmingly* MD schools; the first DO school does not appear until #96 (Edward Via College of Osteopathic Medicine) in the 2022 rankings.[18]

In addition, the most competitive specialties desire research productivity.[19] The average number of abstracts, presentations, and publications in 2020 for successful US MD 4th year applicants in neurosurgery, radiation oncology, dermatology, and plastic surgery were 23.4, 18.3, 19.0, and 19.1, respectively. As a whole, MD programs are more frequently associated with well-funded academic medical centers that give medical students ample opportunities to get involved with productive research. In fact, MD programs

[16] Results and Data. Available at: https://www.nrmp.org/wp-content/uploads/2019/04/NRMP-Results-and-Data-2019_04112019_final.pdf, https://www.nrmp.org/wp-content/uploads/2020/05/MM_Results_and_Data_2020.pdf. Accessed July 8, 2022.
[17] Results of the 2020 NRMP Program Director Survey. Available at: https://www.nrmp.org/wp-content/uploads/2020/08/2020-PD-Survey.pdf. Accessed July 8, 2022.
[18] 2023 Best Medical Schools: Research. Available at: https://www.usnews.com/best-graduate-schools/top-medical-schools/research-rankings. Accessed July 8, 2022.
[19] Charting Outcomes in the Match: Senior Students of U.S. MD Medical Schools. Available at: https://mk0nrmp3oyqui6wqfm.kinstacdn.com/wp-content/uploads/2020/07/Charting-Outcomes-in-the-Match-2020_MD-Senior_final.pdf. Accessed July 8, 2022.

received *800 times* as much research funding in 2011 compared to DO programs.[20] As an extreme example, many DO schools are not even affiliated with a radiation oncology or integrated plastic surgery residency program. While options still exist for DO students to achieve similar research productivity as their MD counterparts before applying to residency programs, these may be cumbersome, (e.g., taking a dedicated research year) often without funding—at another institution.

It's also important to consider the academic atmosphere and emphasis put forth by DO programs. The majority of DO programs openly state in their mission statements that they aim to produce primary care physicians, and more than one-third of DO graduates pursue careers in primary care fields such as internal medicine, pediatrics, and family medicine.[21] While no specialty is off-limits with a DO degree, students' professional careers are strongly influenced by their environments. Perhaps the drive to go to the lab after a busy day on rotations will come more easily when the hallways are adorned with portraits of Nobel laureates. On the other hand, you may find yourself more at ease with the idea of becoming a family physician after attending home health visits hosted by the family medicine interest group at your school.

Of note, there is evidence that the emphasis on primary care at DO schools may not be received well by some students, suggesting some misalignment between attitudes and actual practice in the osteopathic community.[22] Our interpretation is that some students simply attend DO schools because they are — on average — easier to get into compared to MD medical schools with respect to hard academic metrics. Many of these students likely have no strong inclinations towards primary care and intend to practice whatever sub-specialty they want. Altogether, if you're seriously interested in an academic career in a very competitive specialty or just want to keep all doors as open as possible, it may be prudent to defer your application to medical school by 1 or 2 years to make yourself more competitive to MD programs. Of course, this comes with the financial and psychological costs of delaying the road to being an attending. However, if you'd truly be happy practicing virtually any specialty—and this is a very difficult thing to determine before starting medical school—then you are likely to succeed in a DO program, as 89% of 4th year DO students in 2021 matched to a US residency program—a comparable statistic to their MD counterparts' 93%.[23] In addition, the overall match rate between MD and DO applicants appears to be converging over time (▶ Fig. 24.2).

Lastly, there are differences in the scope of international work. While DOs can practice freely in all 50 states in the United States, only 66 countries abroad granted DOs full medical practice rights as of 2014;[24] this may be a consideration if you're strongly interested in international work, particularly in Africa where only a minority of countries allow unrestricted practice to DOs. Fortunately, the outlook for this appears to be improving. In the past decade, more countries have expanded full scope of medical practice to DO physicians, and that number is likely to increase by the time you finish medical school and residency close to 10 years down the line.

## 24.1.2 How to Apply to DO Programs

In most respects, the process of applying to DO programs is identical to applying to MD programs. You try your best in the same prerequisite courses, aim to ace the MCAT, and accumulate meaningful experiences in clinical settings and other extracurriculars. However, you will also need to shadow and obtain a recommendation letter from a DO physician.

The online application portal you will use to apply will, however, be the AACOMAS, rather than the AMCAS (used by the allopathic/MD medical schools).

---

[20] Clark BC, Blazyk J. Research in the Osteopathic Medical Profession: Roadmap to Recovery. Journal of Osteopathic Medicine. Available at: https://www.degruyter.com/document/doi/10.7556/jaoa.2014.124/html "Research in the Osteopathic Medical Profession: Roadmap to Recovery". Accessed July 8, 2022.

[21] What is Osteopathic Medicine? Available at: https://www.aacom.org/become-a-doctor/about-om. Accessed July 8, 2022.

[22] Peters AS, Clark-Chiarelli N, Block SD. Comparison of osteopathic and allopathic medical Schools' support for primary care. J Gen Intern Med 1999;14(12):730–739. Available at: https://www.ncbi.nlm.nih.gov/pubmed/10632817. Accessed July 8, 2022.

[23] National Resident Matching Program, Results and Data: 2021 Main Residency Match®. National Resident Matching Program, Washington, DC. 2021. Available at: https://www.nrmp.org/wp-content/uploads/2021/05/MRM-Results_and_Data_2021.pdf. Accessed July 8, 2022.

[24] https://oialliance.org/the-oia-global-report-global-review-of-osteopathic-medicine-and-osteopathy-2020/.

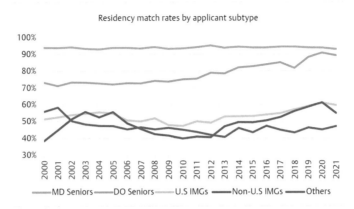

**Fig. 24.2** Residency Match Rates by applicant subtype. Source: Results and Data 2021 Main Residency Match, NRMP.

In your application and interview, you will need to elaborate on why you want to study osteopathic medicine over allopathic medicine. Many students struggle with this aspect, as others have argued that there is no clinically meaningful difference in practice patterns among MD and DO practitioners and that the philosophical differences are relics of a distant past. Nonetheless, the core tenets of the DO philosophy are admirable, and we encourage applicants to emphasize treating the patient as a whole, avoiding overtreatment with unnecessary drugs and interventions, and the utility of having an additional clinical tool to treat patients with at your disposal. **Nonetheless, we cannot—in good faith—recommend picking any DO school over an MD school unless there are seriously compelling reasons otherwise**, e.g., tremendous difference in cost of attendance and you're *sure* you don't want to go into a competitive specialty,[25] or you have highly restrictive geographic circumstances, etc. You may also experience additional professional bias, although —fortunately — this has declined over time to become essentially non-existent in many circles. It's also unclear how much the historical philosophical differences in MD vs. DO approaches to treatment actually matter for contemporary practice. In the worst-case scenario, you can take on additional training in osteopathic manipulative treatment as an MD if you genuinely feel that you're missing out on a crucial treatment philosophy and modality.

Find out more about the DO degree and osteopathic medicine here: http://www.osteopathic.org/osteopathic-health/about-dos/what-is-a-do/Pages/default.aspx

## 24.2 International/Caribbean Medical Schools

International medical schools are a very mixed group, but they broadly refer to medical degree programs (e.g., MD, MBBS) outside of the United States. Of note, Canadian and Puerto Rican medical schools are classified as US MD schools for admission to US residency programs.

Overall, we do *not* recommend applying to non-US medical schools because graduates face significant challenges when applying to US residency programs, and the stigma against these graduates continues to increase each year. For example, in 2021, only 57% of international medical graduates gained admission to residency on their first attempt, compared to 93% for US MD graduates and 89% for US DO graduates.[26] Counterexamples to this generalization, however, include prestigious universities abroad such as the Universities of Oxford and Cambridge or the American University of Beirut Faculty of Medicine.

You're probably most familiar with Caribbean Medical Schools, as they're known for aggressive direct-to-student marketing at undergraduate campuses. To clarify, we're *not* referring to schools in the Caribbean that aim to recruit Caribbean students to practice medicine within their countries. Instead,

---

[25] Which is a virtually impossible decision to make coming into medical school, as *many* medical students discover that they like another field after exposure to it in medical school.

[26] Results and Data. Available at: https://www.nrmp.org/wp-content/uploads/2021/05/MRM-Results_and_Data_2021.pdf. Accessed July 8, 2022.

You're probably most familiar with Caribbean Medical Schools, as they're known for aggressive direct-to-student marketing at undergraduate campuses. To clarify, we're *not* referring to schools in the Caribbean that aim to recruit Caribbean students to practice medicine within their countries. Instead, we mean the medical schools in the Caribbean that recruit American undergraduates who hope to practice medicine in the United States (e.g., St. George's University, Ross University, American University of the Caribbean School of Medicine, and Saba University School of Medicine). On the whole, these schools are for-profit institutions; this doesn't necessarily suggest that they're only out for your tuition dollars, but it's an important fact about their overall priorities and likely explains some of the push for aggressive marketing. These schools are generally more expensive than their US counterparts, especially compared to in-state tuition at public medical schools; in 2016, the average tuition and fees for 4 years at a public medical school was $138,368[27] versus approximately $265,000 at St. George's and $238,000 at Ross University.[28] Admittedly, the average tuition and fees for 4 years at a private medical school is comparable at $234,672, but recognize that the bargain of a high-quality US MD at a public institution doesn't exist in the Caribbean. In addition, those numbers do not include administrative fees and cost of living such as housing, groceries, and travel on and away from the islands, which are known to be quite expensive.[29] Moreover, the outcomes at these schools are highly variable, with first-attempt pass rates on the USMLE Step 1 ranging from 19 to 84%.[30] However, that 84% may be misleading, as several of these schools have zero tolerance policies for failure in the preclinical years. That is, students whom they believe are unlikely to pass Step 1 are dismissed from the schools before they take the exams, artificially inflating the reported pass rate.[31]

Of course, the importance of Step 1 scores has changed dramatically now that the exam is moving to pass/fail. Statistics about Step 2 CK scores are harder to come by, but we anticipate similar trends because Step 1 score has historically strongly correlated with Step 2 CK scores.[32]

It's also somewhat difficult to assess specifics about the quality of education and professional outcomes at these schools, as hard data isn't centralized in databases as with MD and DO schools in the AAMC and AACOM. The higher quality schools, e.g., St. George's University and Ross University School of Medicine, participate with US financial aid programs through the Department of Education, however, and are thus required to share statistics about their classes. The realities are sobering; in 2012, about 50% of graduates from Ross University failed to graduate on time, almost 33% of the class at American University of Antigua, and close to 20% at St. George's. These statistics also do not account for students who left the program for one reason or another; among students who started at St. George's University in Fall 2009, 10% dropped out and 1% transferred, leaving only 65% of the class that graduated in 4 years.[33]

The academic atmosphere at Caribbean schools is also markedly different from that of US MD and DO programs. We will continue to use St. George's University as a comparison, as it is generally considered to be the best Caribbean MD program; it's reasonable to conclude that whatever shortcomings they have are magnified at less renowned institutions. First, many of these schools have extremely large class sizes (up to 800 students per class) that may markedly detract from the intimate academic experience available to US MD and DO students.[34] This may seem like a relatively minor point, but our experience has been that

[27] Tuition and Student Fees Reports. Available at: https://www.aamc.org/data/tuitionandstudentfees/. Accessed July 8, 2022.

[28] Tuition Fees. Available at: https://www.sjsm.org/tuition-fees/. Accessed July 8, 2022.

[29] Larkin M. Crunching the numbers. Available at: https://www.avma.org/News/JAVMANews/Pages/150601a.aspx. Accessed July 8, 2022.

[30] van Zanten M, Boulet JR. Medical Education in the Caribbean: Variability in Medical School Programs and Performance of Students. Academic Medicine 2008;83(10):S33–S36. Available at: https://journals.lww.com/academicmedicine/Fulltext/2008/10001/Medical_Education_in_the_Caribbean__Variability_in.9.aspx. Accessed July 8, 2022.

[31] McFarling UL. Why the United States is no longer turning up its nose at Caribbean medical schools. Available at: https://www.statnews.com/2017/02/17/caribbean-medical-schools/. Accessed July 8, 2022.

[32] Monteiro KA, George P, Dollase R, Dumenco L. Predicting United States Medical Licensure Examination Step 2 clinical knowledge scores from previous academic indicators. Adv Med Educ Pract 2017;8:385–391. Available at: https://www.ncbi.nlm.nih.gov/pmc/articles/PMC5482402/. Accessed July 8, 2022.

[33] Second-chance med school. Available at: https://www.nytimes.com/2014/08/03/education/edlife/second-chance-med-school.html. Accessed July 8, 2022.

[34] World-class Medical education at one of the top Caribbean medical schools - UMHS School of Medicine. Available at: https://www.umhs-sk.org/blog/caribbean-medical-schools-definitive-guide/#Class_Size. Accessed July 8, 2022.

the camaraderie and sense of community at smaller US programs directly contributes to well-being during the stresses of medical school. There's just something extremely reassuring about being able to randomly stop by a professor's office to chat about an exam, for example. The level of approval/accreditation at Caribbean schools also varies widely, as some schools are affiliated with clinical sites that aren't accredited by the ACGME.

We will not spend much time discussing international medical schools beyond the Caribbean, as these represent such a heterogenous group that it's hard to draw general conclusions. For example, you'd probably guess that your chances of getting a residency spot in the United States are dramatically different if you went to the University of Cambridge versus a for-profit degree mill with outdated facilities elsewhere. Keep in mind that many of these schools are not aiming to produce graduates that plan to practice in the United States. For example, medical schools in India are (understandably) more focused on producing graduates who pass the board exams and practice medicine in India. As such, if you choose to attend a school that is not focused on passing the American licensing exams, you may have to do significant self-studying to pass these exams *in addition to* whatever academic and licensing requirements are present in your country of study.

So why do students apply to these schools? The obvious reason is that it's easier to get in (average undergraduate GPA of 3.3 and average MCAT of 498 at St. George's, widely considered the best Caribbean medical school)[35] and that there is still *some* chance of becoming a physician in the United States. However, it's critically important to do some self-reflection. Becoming a physician at a US MD program—where the first-time match rate has historically been over 90%—is arduous to begin with. By going to these schools, you will be embarking on a highly stressful academic journey at an institution where the odds are stacked against you to begin with. Even if you *do* gain acceptance to a residency program, there is a much greater likelihood of training at a less-renowned residency program or even not entering the field you originally wanted to do. You will likely be paying much more tuition, and if you don't go to a school that participates in federal US loans, you may have to take out private loans with higher interest rates that don't offer as many of the repayment or forgiveness options available to US borrowers. You will likely be one of *thousands* of students on campus and possibly miss out on the intimate academic experience seen at US programs. Everyone who enrolls at these programs believes that they will beat the odds and be the exception to the rule. However, the statistical reality is bleak, and no one ever plans to be the student who can't keep up. Failing or dropping out is always something that happens to someone else, but the reality is that we're all just "someone else" to someone else.

Our final recommendation on international MD programs—particularly Caribbean programs—is to do some serious self-reflection on what you want out of your life. Could you see yourself achieving similar satisfaction from becoming a physician assistant, biomedical researcher, pharmacist, or nurse practitioner? Could you see yourself taking a few years off to strengthen your application to apply again to MD and DO programs to maximize your odds at success as a physician? Keep in mind that many medical students apply to Caribbean programs because they did not meet the academic standards demanded by US programs. While there's certainly more to becoming an excellent physician than book-smarts and test-taking ability, there are legitimate reasons why US programs favor academic excellence. Unless you truly had extenuating, one-off circumstances that kept you from excelling in college, your academic performance thus far *does* predict your success in medical school and beyond,[36] and it is much more likely that you will struggle in a Caribbean school if you already struggled academically in college.

At the end of the day, if you *only* see yourself happy as physician—no matter what the trials and tribulations you face—*and* you have failed at least one application cycle to US MD and DO schools, then we

---

[35] Frequently Asked Questions. Available at: https://www.sgu.edu/academic-programs/school-of-medicine/faq/#toggle-id-6. Accessed July 8, 2022.

[36] Agahi F, Speicher MR, Cisek G. Association Between Undergraduate Performance Predictors and Academic and Clinical Performance of Osteopathic Medical Students. J Am Osteopath Assoc 2018;118(2):106–114. Available at: https://www.ncbi.nlm.nih.gov/pubmed/29379965. Accessed July 8, 2022.

Table 24.1 Differences in admissions selectivity as well as match outcomes for the different types of schools in 2020

|  | MD programs | DO programs | International programs |
|---|---|---|---|
| Average GPA | 3.77 | 3.52 | 3.3 (at best—this is for St. George's, one of the most competitive international programs) |
| Average MCAT | 508.7 | 502.2 | 498 (at best—this is for St. George's, one of the most competitive international programs) |
| Percentage of graduates in the most competitive specialties, i.e., dermatology, orthopaedic surgery, plastic surgery, and neurosurgery, who attended such a program for medical school | 88 | 9.2 | 2.8 |

Abbreviations: GPA, grade point average; MCAT, Medical College Admission Test.

recommend reaching out to current and former students at international MD programs and asking them honest questions about their experiences and regrets. Ask about what struggles they may have faced in achieving a residency spot and what resources their school offered. We also recommend reading blogs by students who personally attended Caribbean medical schools: "My Medical Journey,"[37] "Adventures in Caribbean Medical School,"[38] "Million $ Mistake,"[39] and "MD and Beyond"[40] are particularly well-written. However, you should take these first-hand accounts with a grain of salt, as they may not necessarily be representative of everyone's experience. Moving forward, it's ultimately your decision, but you should absolutely have all the hard facts available to you, including the ones that the schools themselves don't freely share.

Ultimately, we recommend that you attend a US MD program over a DO program in almost all scenarios, and that you attend a DO program over an international program in almost all scenarios. ▶ Table 24.1 illustrates the differences in admissions selectivity as well as match outcomes for the different types of schools in 2020.

## 24.3 Summary

Two medical doctorate degrees exist: MD and DO. While these two degrees used to be different in training and philosophy, they are becoming more similar every year to the point of being largely identical in function and scope of practice. DO is generally a less competitive application process, requiring specifically a lower GPA and MCAT score, and graduates tend to disproportionately go into primary care. DOs can now match into MD residency spots and take the same licensing exams. While in general they have been historically less competitive in the residency match, that gap is also closing. Exceptional applicants from DO schools outperform MD counterparts every year, and are matching into increasingly competitive specialties. As of 2022, we generally recommend trying to attend MD schools over DO schools—unless there are extenuating reasons. This recommendation may become out of date soon, however.

---

[37] My Medical Journey. Available at: https://nearlytheremd.wordpress.com/. Accessed July 8, 2022.
[38] Adventures in Caribbean Medical School. Available at: https://medschooll8y-thelongjourneyhome.blogspot.com/. Accessed July 8, 2022.
[39] Caribbean Med School. Available at: https://milliondollarmistake.wordpress.com/. Accessed July 8, 2022.
[40] MD and Beyond. Available at: http://mdandbeyond.weebly.com/. Accessed July 8, 2022.

For those that are not competitive enough to get into an MD program, we recommend either improving your application or making the best of it at a DO program. If the prestige difference bothers you to the point you would rather not go at all, consider this: a DO can do everything an MD can do. If being a medical doctor is your dream job, and you are only willing to consider being an MD, then ask yourself: is being a doctor your dream job or just your dream title?

For the Caribbean schools, they should be viewed as schools of last resort. Talented people overcome the challenges there, and match successfully into US residencies every year, but the risk is exceptional. You should make certain to be honest with yourself about your chances of success there and be OK with the prospect of (expensive) failure. In virtually all cases, we recommend attending a DO program over a Caribbean MD program.

# 25 Dual-Degree Programs: MD/PhD, MPH, MBA, JD, and Others

*Jorna Sojati and Ray Funahashi*

While getting ready to apply to medical school, you might come across some intimidating terms like "MD/PhD," "MD/JD," or "MD/MPH." These are MD dual-degree programs (sometimes referred to as joint-degree or combined degrees programs).

A dual-degree program is when two (or more) schools or departments within a university partner to enable a student to earn two degrees in a back-to-back or integrated way.

An MD (or DO) dual-degree program is one where medical students earn a second degree (i.e., Master's, JD, or PhD) in addition to their MD or DO degree.

In this chapter, we'll talk about how dual-degree programs work, and give you the low down on the common types of dual degrees US medical schools offer: MD/Ph.D., MD/JD, MD/MPH, MD/MBA, MD/MPP, and MD/MS programs.[1] We'll also touch on how to decide whether a dual-degree program is for you, the application process for these programs, and the types of careers that graduates of these programs have.

Before the 1950s, medical schools offering additional degrees to the MD or DO were rare. But in 1964 the National Institutes of Health (NIH) launched the Medical Scientist Training Program (MSTP) that expanded funding and greatly increased the number of MD/PhD dual-degree programs, especially at research-centric medical schools. MD/PhD program students traditionally would complete the first 2 years of medical school and then do an accelerated PhD program (which on average took 3 years to complete), and return to finish the last 2 years of medical school to finish their MD degree.

Then from the early 2000s, other MD dual-degree programs proliferated rapidly across medical schools, following the paradigm that future medical leaders should influence domains complementary to and beyond clinical practice and medicine. Besides the MD/PhD, many schools started to offer the MD/MPH (Master's in Public Health), MD/MBA (Master's in Business Administration), and even MD/JD (Law) dual-degree programs.

In the recent decade, the variety of dual degrees continued to rapidly expand, exemplified by medical schools such as Harvard, Stanford, Duke, and Michigan, each of whom now offers at least 11 different MD/Master's dual degrees.

## 25.1 Why Are Schools Offering More MD Dual Degrees?

The explosion of healthcare data and technology is accelerating change in medicine and creating cross-disciplinary fields. These new fields are not adjacent to medicine. Instead, they are beginning to integrate into the very core of medicine. The coming integration of AI and medicine is one example that will significantly change clinical practice in the coming decades.

Unfortunately, preparing medical students to become physician leaders in the rapidly changing (especially technological) medical landscape and emerging fields is a tremendous challenge for medical school curriculums due to the existing strain of the clinical curricular volume.

As a result, many of the top medical schools are encouraging graduates to train in cross-disciplinary and emerging fields by structuring their MD curriculum to enable students to enroll in dual-degree programs.

Dual-degree programs also benefit medical schools and partner schools. Schools enhance their production of future cross-disciplinary leaders and increase the diversity, experience, and knowledge of their school cohorts. The cross-student flow between schools leads to more extraordinary collaborative projects and impact.

The push for establishing dual degrees is also being driven by medical student interest and demand. Medical students are completing dual-degree programs to pursue cross-disciplinary career goals and in order to become innovators and leaders.

From 2010 to 2018, there has been a 434% increase in students pursuing a dual MD-MPH degree. At the University of Michigan, at least 15% of medical students pursue a dual degree.[2]

---

[1] Note that many DO schools offer similar programs, e.g., DO/PhD, DO/JD, etc.
[2] Dual Degrees. Available at: https://medicine.umich.edu/medschool/education/md-program/opportunities/dual-degrees. Accessed July 8, 2022.

At #3 US News–ranked Duke Medical School, 40% of students now graduate with a second degree.[3]

For some students, the prospect of extending their academic years with an additional degree doesn't seem worth it.

Whether dual-degree programs are beneficial depends on your personal career goals. However, increasingly more students are considering doing dual degrees due to the following benefits.

## 25.1.1 Students Obtain Cross-Disciplinary Education, Training, and Networking with a Second Degree

- Specific interests such as public health, healthcare business, bioinformatics, policy are very difficult to learn in significant depth with the standard medical school curriculum.
- Formal classes give the time to establish a solid foundation in the subject, especially if the student doesn't have previous background.
- Students learn not only didactic material but also how other smart individuals think about solving problems.
- Students will establish and expand your network in the field of interest, which will help you kick-start your career in the field. You will have a framework that encourages interfacing with accomplished professionals who you would otherwise have difficulty encountering otherwise.
- Many Master's programs will require a capstone project or internship experience that will help you get your foot in the door in the field.

For example, an MD/MBA medical student taking the summer to intern at a healthcare venture capital firm (a field that is notoriously difficult to get into) can potentially open doors for more roles in venture capital as a resident or after residency.

Similarly, an MD/MPP (Master's in Public Policy) medical student can intern at a think tank or nongovernmental organization (NGO) to gain real-world experience in health policy work.

## 25.1.2 Master's Dual Degrees Are Accelerated So They Can be Earned Together with the MD in 5 Combined Years

- Two-year Master's programs are often stripped to their core and curriculum compromises are made between the medical school and partner school to make a combined 5-year dual degree possible.
- This results in tremendous time and money savings. For example, an MBA or MPH, which are traditionally 2-year degrees, can be earned in a single-year timeframe.

## 25.1.3 Medical Students May Get Admissions Benefits

Having taken the Medical College Admission Test (MCAT) and been admitted to medical school, as a medical student you may be viewed by some partnering dual-degree programs as a strong academic applicant.

Because of this, some schools may waive standardized tests normally required for admissions, such as the Graduate Record Examinations (GRE) and Graduate Management Admissions Test (GMAT), for medical student applicants. This again saves time and money.

While some dual-degree programs have a reputation of nearly assured admission for medical students, other schools maintain very independent admissions for each dual-degree program. Unless explicitly stated, you should not assume guaranteed admissions into any dual degree as a medical student.

## 25.2 What Kinds of Dual Degrees Are Medical Schools Currently Offering?

The most common dual-degree programs across the top 30 medical schools per US News are shown in ▶ Fig. 25.1.

---

[3] Dual Degree Programs. Available at: https://medschool.duke.edu/education/health-professions-education-programs/doctor-medicine-md-program/curriculum/third-year-51. Accessed July 8, 2022.

- MPH — 93%
- MBA — 77%
- Clinical research (Master's) — 63%
- Biomedical informatics (Master's) — 37%
- Bioethics (Master's) — 30%
- MPP (Public policy) — 30%
- Healthcare management (Master's) — 27%
- JD (Law) — 23%
- Bioengineering (Master's) — 23%
- M.Ed (Medical education) — 17%
- Basic (Master's) — 10%

Percentage of schools offering MD dual degree

Mean # programs **7.9** at Top 10 schools

**5.3** at Top 30 schools

Median # programs **4.5** at Top 30 schools

**Fig. 25.1** The most common dual-degree programs across the top 30 medical schools per US News. Source: Pitt Med Dual Degrees Report 2021.

## 25.3 How Do Dual Degrees Work?

### 25.3.1 Students Generally Complete Their Additional Degree after Their Core Clerkship Year

Generally, medical students leave to begin their additional (dual) degree after completing their core clerkship rotations. At many medical schools, this would be after MS3 year, while at Duke Medical School, for example, this is after MS2 year.

### 25.3.2 MD Dual Degrees Vary Widely Partnership Level, Curriculum Integration, and Accommodation

In contrast to MD/PhD dual-degree programs, which are similarly structured across medical schools, levels of partnership for other MD dual degrees vary widely between schools.

Partnership levels determine schedules' conflicts between the timeline of the two degrees, the number of shared credits, scholarship funding, and joint subject classes.

Now let's dive into more details about the types of dual-degree programs!

## 25.4 The Physician-Scientist (MD/PhD)

The combined MD/PhD program is historically the most established of programs (as described above) and it's the one you've likely heard the most about. They are typically 7- to 8-year programs and for students who are interested in having a very research-focused career, perhaps leading a research lab as a principal investigator (PI). You can be a PI without a PhD but the graduate degree gives you 3 to 4 extra years of dedicated classes, time, experience, and mentorship in research to help you toward your research aspirations.

## 25.4.1 Why Do an MD/PhD Program?

Given that the MD/PhD program has the greatest length and the commitment out of the dual-degree programs, it's important to make sure that the career path of a physician-scientist is right for you. These programs are designed for students who have a passion for medical[4] research and specifically want to become physicians that incorporate research into their clinical careers.

There are many MD-only physician-scientists who are every bit as capable as their MD/PhD counterparts when it comes to research. What it truly comes down to, however, is the amount of autonomy that you want in your career. Most MD physicians who conduct research do so in the context of larger clinical studies or as part of a bigger lab, rather than being a PI. Moreover, PhD training provides specialized intensive training, especially when it comes to basic science or computational research, which puts MD/PhD graduates at a significant advantage compared to their MD-only counterparts.

MD-only physicians who are invested in research, who take positions as academic faculty members and do become PIs (and there are many), often don't feel prepared enough to pursue an independent research career immediately after their training and tend to complete extended post-doc fellowships to gain experience. And so, in considering MD/PhD programs, you should truly think about what research means to you. If it's something that you hope to integrate into your everyday career, and cannot imagine having a medical career that doesn't allow you to both see patients and study their diseases, then we recommend you apply to MD/PhD programs and begin both your clinical and scientific training as early as possible! If you're not entirely committed to the idea of a physician-scientist career, then doing an MD program (with the option to further your research training down the road, if it suits you) may be a better idea. At the same time, if you have a passion for research and appreciate the clinical impact that medical research has, but don't know if you want to practice medicine, then consider doing a standalone PhD program instead. Many medical schools offer an array of PhD programs that graduate top-notch medical scientists prepared to do groundbreaking work in the field of healthcare.

Ultimately, this is not a decision you should make lightly, but if you are ready to commit to a rewarding career that integrates research and medicine, then MD/PhD programs can provide a wonderful environment to build your scientific and clinical skills. You can read more about MD/PhD programs in the 2018 Association of American Medical Colleges (AAMC) National MD/PhD Outcomes Study.[5]

## 25.4.2 How Are MSTPs Different from MD/PhD programs?

You may have heard the term MSTP (Medical Scientist Training Programs) used interchangeably with MD/PhD programs, but there is a difference between the two. MSTPs are a subset of MD/PhD programs that are either partially or fully funded by the National Institutes of Health (NIH). Non-MSTP programs may not be NIH-funded, but they often are stably funded by other federal organizations or by the school itself.

This should not deter you from applying to non-MSTP MD/PhD programs, nor should it mean that your applications should be MSTP-specific. While the NIH affiliation certainly adds some value, you should recognize that different MD/PhD programs (regardless of their funding source) have their own unique sets of objectives that promote vastly different learning environments. In the same way that you research medical schools, you should also research their MD/PhD programs and see whether their mission statements and curriculum align with your interests. This is much more important than where they get their funding from. It's valuable for the application process to recognize the differences between MSTP and non-MSTP programs, but certainly not to let it negatively cloud your judgment and bias your application.

---

[4] Typically basic or translational research, although there are notable MD/PhDs who focus on scholarly work in the social sciences, humanities, and clinical research.

[5] National MD-PhD Program Outcomes Study. Available at: https://store.aamc.org/downloadable/download/sample/sample_id/162/. Accessed July 8, 2022.

### 25.4.3 What Is the Timeline for MD/PhD Programs?

Just so you're aware, you won't be working on both your MD and PhD degrees at the same time in most cases. Most programs recognize the dedication it takes to each individual program in order to become both an effective clinician and researcher, and will actually actively discourage students from trying to focus on both at the same time. Instead, most programs are run on the "2- 3/4 -2 track." This means that they start with the first 2 years of medical school (which is the didactic portion in most medical school programs), followed by 3 to 4 years of graduate school that culminates into a thesis, and then a return to medical school for their last 2 years of clinical work. An example of this type of curriculum in the Johns Hopkins MD/PhD program is shown in ▶ Fig. 25.2.[6]

There is great variation among MD/PhD programs on when the PhD lab rotations are actually done. Most schools tend to have students commit at least two of their summers (the incoming summer prior to MS1, and the summer between MS1 and MS2) to research rotations so that they can hit the ground running once the PhD years come around. Others choose to follow the traditional PhD curriculum and have students do lab rotation in their first year of graduate school.

Another important thing to note (and definitely a good question to ask during the interview process) is what curricular components are in place for mediating the difficulty in transitioning from graduate school back to medical school. This is by far the trickiest part of the MD/PhD curriculum, and the way that this transition is navigated is very school-specific. Some programs offer longitudinal clinical experiences during graduate school (usually a half-day every few weeks) that offer students continuous clinical exposure during their PhD years. Others offer a class toward the end of the PhD years geared toward reintroducing clinical components and making sure that MD/PhD candidates feel comfortable going back into the clinic.

Most of these programs take 7 to 8 years to complete, depending on the length of the PhD training. Although finishing in 3 years is certainly ideal, one personal piece of advice I would offer is to be wary of schools that strongly push for their PhD students to be finished in 3 years. Over time, 4 years has proven to be an ideal length of time for conducting PhD work that manifests in a valuable and productive thesis, and—while it certainly can be done—trying to finish a PhD in 3 years can put a lot of pressure on students, contribute to a hectic work environment that doesn't effectively foster learning, and significantly limit the scope of the research.

Although most programs are structured similarly, every candidate's research focuses and clinical interests will be different. Be sure to find a program that provides flexibility within this timeline, so that you can tailor the curriculum to work best for you.

### 25.4.4 How Does Financial Aid for MD/PhD Programs Work?

Fortunately, most MD/PhD programs minimize the financial toll that 4 extra years of school puts on a student. In addition, programs offer full or partial financial support for their students. The majority of MD/PhD programs, as well as all MSTPs, do offer full tuition remission for both medical and graduate school, along with a living stipend that typically averages ~$30,000/year. During medical school, these costs are covered by the program. During graduate school, however, your stipend is typically provided either from the laboratory that you are working in, from training grants within that graduate program, or from federal grants that MD/PhD students individually apply for, such as the NIH F30.

That said, while free medical school with a living stipend does sound enticing, consider the fact that—assuming the same age of retirement—**you could be losing 4 years of attending physician salary (several hundred thousand dollars to over a million dollars, yearly, depending on your specialty)** because of the extra years spent on the PhD. Moreover, most MD/PhD graduates enter academia, where typical compensation is much lower on average. As such, it's possible that the financial benefits of an MD/PhD program are not as great as they appear at face value.

### 25.4.5 How Does the MD/PhD Application Process Work?

Although this can differ between schools (and you should always check the school-specific requirements listed on a medical school's website), most MD/PhD programs have a similar application process as regular

---

[6] https://mdphd.johnshopkins.edu/curriculum/

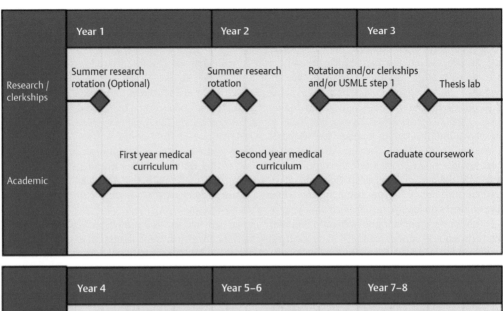

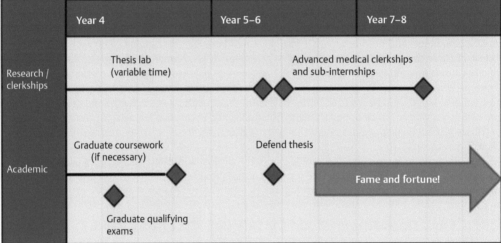

**Fig. 25.2** Johns Hopkins MD/PhD program sample timeline.

MD admissions via the American Medical College Application Service (AMCAS). As you fill out the AMCAS form, you'll see the option to designate your application as MD-only or MD/PhD. The only difference between the two is that an MD/PhD application will require two extra essays: one MD/PhD-specific essay detailing why you'd like to pursue this career path, and a "Significant Research Experiences" essay that details the research experiences you've had thus far, the institutions and supervisors that you've worked under, the length of your research experiences, the specific projects you've worked on and your contributions, and how each of these experiences have shaped you overall. You will also be asked to document the total number of hours you've committed to research, so it would be helpful to start keeping track of your research time throughout your undergraduate training.

One unique aspect of the MD/PhD application process is that you can also designate applications to individual schools as either MD/PhD or MD-only. What this means is that for each school you add to your application list, you can choose to send the entire MD/PhD application or apply solely to their MD program. This means that they won't see your MD/PhD essays as part of the application, nor will they know that you've applied MD/PhD to other schools. That said, it's not traditionally very common to send a combination of both MD/PhD and MD-only applications, as most programs that choose not to consider someone for an MD/PhD position will automatically defer them to MD-only admissions. However, I do know a few applicants who submitted MD-only applications to schools ranked highly on their list that did not offer MD/PhD programs, or to schools with more competitive MD/PhD program statistics that they didn't feel they met the requirements of.

From there, the application process is very similar to that of regular MD admissions. Upon screening of your primary application, most schools will send you secondaries. Depending on the school, you may be asked to fill out the same secondary application as all MD applicants, an MD/PhD-specific secondary, or both. After submitting your thoughtfully-written secondary applications, you'll hopefully be offered interviews. Although the interview process is known to be particularly pricy as a whole, MD/PhD interviews can be especially expensive as they typically end up being a 2- to 3-day stay at each institution. Although this can vary by institution, the typical interview setup is as follows:

- You usually fly in the day before and the school will host a preinterview dinner/social event with current MD/PhD students at that school.
- The next 2 days will be full of interviews, with one day dedicated to your PhD interviews and another to your MD interviews.

A few schools will offer to reimburse you for your flights and lodging, but many will not. As such, students are often limited to the number of schools they apply to and interview at based on their budget.[7] The average applicant usually applies to ~15 to 20 programs (with a good mix of both "reach schools" and "safety schools"), and the general rule of thumb is to expect interviews from ~½ of the schools you apply to. I ended up applying to 15 MD/PhD programs, and the interview process alone ended up costing me ~$6,000 for the eight interviews that I went to.

Most schools offer MD/PhD-specific second-look weekends where you get to find out a lot more about individual programs and meet with faculty members in your research area(s) of interest.

### Special Feature: NIH Oxford-Cambridge Scholars Program[8]

The NIH Oxford-Cambridge Scholars Program (OxCam) is an MD/PhD program that allows students to do their MD curriculum at any medical school in the United States and their PhD at both the NIH and the University of Oxford **or** Cambridge in the United Kingdom. Aside from the multicultural experience and networking opportunities associated with the three institutions, students also learn under the British doctoral system in which formal courses are not taken during the PhD program.

## 25.4.6 Are GPA and MCAT Requirements Different for MD/PhD Programs?

Yes. Matriculants to MD/PhD programs have higher GPAs and MCAT scores than matriculants to MD-only programs. This is not surprising because the programs select strongly for applicants with significant academic aptitude who can extend their knowledge to generate and test novel scientific hypotheses. ► Table 25.1 and ► Table 25.2 provide the average GPA and MCAT data for matriculants recorded by the AAMC for MD-only versus MD/PhD admissions. Note the average total GPA and MCAT of 3.73 and 511.5 for MD-only versus 3.80 versus 516.2 for MD/PhD ($p < 0.0001$ for both—an extremely statistically significant difference).

Another nuance to note, however—while most schools only require the MCAT for medical school admissions, some graduate programs may make the GRE an additional requirement. For this reason,

---

[7] That said, and as emphasized in Chapter 35, Interview Trail Travel and Attire, we encourage you to spend more money for more opportunity. You don't want to spend the rest of your life wondering "what if" because you didn't spend an additional $1,000 to $2,000 for the opportunity to potentially attend a dream school. That cost is a drop in the bucket in the grand scheme of things.

[8] Welcome to the NIH Oxford-Cambridge Scholars Program. Available at: https://oxcam.gpp.nih.gov/. Accessed July 8, 2022.

**Table 25.1** MCAT scores and GPAs for applicants and matriculants to U.S. medical schools, 2017–2018 through 2020–2021

| | Matriculants | 2017–2018 | 2018–2019 | 2019–2020 | 2020–2021 |
|---|---|---|---|---|---|
| MCAT CPBS | Mean | 127.6 | 127.7 | 127.8 | 127.8 |
| | SD | 2.2 | 2.1 | 2.2 | 2.2 |
| MCAT CARS | Mean | 126.9 | 127.1 | 127.1 | 127.0 |
| | SD | 2.3 | 2.3 | 2.3 | 2.3 |
| MCAT BBLS | Mean | 127.9 | 128 | 128.1 | 128.1 |
| | SD | 2.1 | 2.1 | 2.1 | 2.0 |
| MCAT PSBB | Mean | 128 | 128.3 | 128.5 | 128.6 |
| | SD | 2.1 | 2.1 | 2 | 2.0 |
| Total MCAT | Mean | 510.4 | 511.2 | 511.5 | 511.5 |
| | SD | 6.6 | 6.5 | 6.5 | 6.5 |
| GPA Science | Mean | 3.64 | 3.65 | 3.66 | 3.66 |
| | SD | 0.31 | 0.3 | 0.30 | 0.31 |
| GPA Non-Science | Mean | 3.79 | 3.8 | 3.81 | 3.82 |
| | SD | 0.22 | 0.21 | 0.22 | 0.21 |
| GPA Total | Mean | 3.71 | 3.72 | 3.73 | 3.73 |
| | SD | 0.25 | 0.24 | 0.24 | 0.24 |
| Total Matriculants | | 21,338 | 21,622 | 21,869 | 22,239 |

This table displays MCAT scores and GPAs for applicants and matriculants from 2017–2018 through 2020–2021 by mean and standard deviation (SD). Please email datarequest@aamc.org if you need further assistance or have additional inquiries.

it's important to look into the requirements of not only the MD/PhD program itself but also of the graduate program that you hope to join.

## 25.4.7  What Type of Research Can You Do as an MD/PhD Student?

While this can vary between institutions, most established research institutions will offer this basic cluster of graduate programs: Biochemistry/Molecular Biology, Genetics, Cellular/Developmental Biology, Microbiology & Immunology, Chemistry/Pharmacology, Bioengineering, Neuroscience, Public Health/Epidemiology, Computational Biology/Biostatistics, Biophysics/Structural Biology. Other popular graduate research fields include Bioethics/Philosophy, Anthropology, Health Policy, and Translational Sciences, which are offered by quite a few institutions but not all. Finding a graduate program and research faculty that suit your scientific interests is arguably the most important factor when choosing the right MD/PhD program for you.

## 25.4.8  What Careers Do MD/PhD Graduates Have?

The career path of a physician-scientist has traditionally been described as the "80–20 split," meaning that 80% of their time is dedicated to research while 20% is spent practicing/seeing patients. However, an

**Table 25.2** MCAT® scores and GPAs for MD-PhD applicants and matriculants to U.S. medical schools, 2017–2018 through 2020–2021

| MD-PhD Matriculants | | 2017–2018 | 2018–2019 | 2019–2020 | 2020–2021 |
|---|---|---|---|---|---|
| MCAT CPBS | Mean | 129.2 | 129.0 | 129.0 | 129.2 |
| | SD | 1.9 | 2.0 | 1.9 | 1.9 |
| | Minimum | 123.0 | 123.0 | 122.0 | 123.0 |
| | Maximum | 132.0 | 132.0 | 132.0 | 132.0 |
| MCAT CARS | Mean | 128.0 | 128.2 | 128.2 | 128.1 |
| | SD | 2.2 | 2.1 | 2.2 | 2.1 |
| | Minimum | 122.0 | 121.0 | 121.0 | 122.0 |
| | Maximum | 132.0 | 132.0 | 132.0 | 132.0 |
| MCAT BBLS | Mean | 129.3 | 129.4 | 129.5 | 129.5 |
| | SD | 1.9 | 1.8 | 1.8 | 1.7 |
| | Minimum | 123.0 | 123.0 | 123.0 | 122.0 |
| | Maximum | 132.0 | 132.0 | 132.0 | 132.0 |
| MCAT PSBB | Mean | 128.9 | 129.0 | 129.4 | 129.5 |
| | SD | 2.0 | 1.9 | 1.7 | 1.7 |
| | Minimum | 123.0 | 123.0 | 124.0 | 123.0 |
| | Maximum | 132.0 | 132.0 | 132.0 | 132.0 |
| Total MCAT | Mean | 515.4 | 515.6 | 516.1 | 516.2 |
| | SD | 5.9 | 5.6 | 5.4 | 5.2 |
| | Minimum | 495.0 | 497.0 | 501.0 | 495.0 |
| | Maximum | 528.0 | 528.0 | 528.0 | 528.0 |
| GPA Science | Mean | 3.76 | 3.76 | 3.77 | 3.77 |
| | SD | 0.24 | 0.23 | 0.22 | 0.24 |
| | Minimum | 2.50 | 2.49 | 2.43 | 2.35 |
| | Maximum | 4.00 | 4.00 | 4.00 | 4.00 |
| GPA Non-Science | Mean | 3.84 | 3.84 | 3.84 | 3.85 |
| | SD | 0.19 | 0.18 | 0.16 | 0.17 |
| | Minimum | 2.49 | 2.83 | 2.98 | 3.03 |
| | Maximum | 4.00 | 4.00 | 4.00 | 4.00 |
| GPA Total | Mean | 3.79 | 3.79 | 3.80 | 3.80 |
| | SD | 0.20 | 0.19 | 0.18 | 0.19 |

*(Continued)*

**Table 25.2** (*Continued*) MCAT® scores and GPAs for MD-PhD applicants and matriculants to U.S. medical schools, 2017–2018 through 2020–2021

| MD-PhD Matriculants | | 2017–2018 | 2018–2019 | 2019–2020 | 2020–2021 |
|---|---|---|---|---|---|
| | Minimum | 2.75 | 2.68 | 2.77 | 2.87 |
| | Maximum | 4.00 | 4.00 | 4.00 | 4.00 |
| Total MD-PhD Matriculants | | 646 | 672 | 708 | 701 |

The following table displays MCAT scores and GPAs for MD-PhD applicants and MDI-PhD matriculants to U.S. medical schools from 2017–2018 through 2020–2021. MCAT scores and GPAs are displayed by mean and standard deviation (SD). Please email datarequest@aamc.org if you need further assistance or have additional inquiries.

analysis done by the AAMC in April 2018 focused on MD/PhD graduate career trajectory showed that there is much more heterogeneity in career trajectories. While a few MD/PhD graduates have committed to research-only or clinical-only careers, the majority have split their time between research and medicine in a variety of different ways (▶ Fig. 25.3).

This study also revealed that many more MD/PhD graduates are veering away from traditional bench research and are instead using their training to better integrate clinical medicine with other research types, including translational, patient-oriented, or health services/outcomes research.

With this, we hope you've gotten a better idea of what it means to become a physician-scientist, how MD/PhD programs work, and what to consider when applying for these types of programs. Unfortunately, there is no "cookie-cutter" career path as an MD/PhD. Instead, clinician-scientists continue to find unique and innovative integrations of medicine and research that allow them to study the topics they are passionate about, treat the patient groups they are interested in, and change medicine for the better.

## 25.5 Other Dual-Degree Programs

Let's learn more about the other dual-degree programs. Ten percent of medical students in 2017 pursued a dual degree, up from 7.7% in 2011.[9] While many students use these additional degrees to make themselves more competitive for specific, niche careers, others end up obtaining them while making themselves more competitive for extremely competitive residency programs (e.g., Master's degree while doing dermatology research).[10]

### 25.5.1 Should You Consider Non-MD/PhD Dual Degrees?

Our main recommendation for dual degrees is to *seriously evaluate your specific career goals and whether a dual degree is necessary or adds a significant return on investment.*

We've previously mentioned the training, experience, and networking benefits of doing a dual degree.

But there are significant costs to pursuing a dual degree. Many MD dual-degree Master's programs require you to self-fund it. Even if your school heavily subsidizes the additional degree, you incur a significant opportunity cost by losing one year's worth of attending physician salary per additional year spent on a second degree (i.e., a loss of hundreds of thousands of dollars).

In addition, the quality and opportunities afforded by these programs vary tremendously from school to school. The best thing would be to contact the specific programs, as well as current students and alumni of the programs.

For some students the return on investment of dual degrees may be low for their career goals, while for others, it will be necessary to gain access to extremely competitive career paths.

---

9  Pitt Med Dual Degrees Report 2021.
10  While many of these research years don't confer a formal degree, some do: https://www.icre.pitt.edu/cstp/index.html

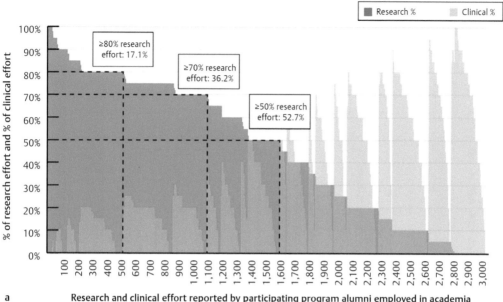

a      Research and clinical effort reported by participating program alumni employed in academia

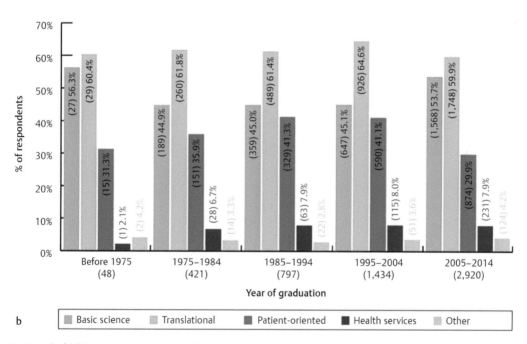

b

**Fig. 25.3 (a, b) (a)** Research and clinical effort reported by participating program alumni employed in academia. **(b)** Types of research being conducted by participating program alumni. Source: 2018 AAMC National MD-PhD Program Outcomes Study.

We would like to highlight that students who don't plan on entering clinical medicine out of medical school are *strongly* encouraged to consider a dual degree to make themselves more competitive for jobs, as much of a physician's value to employers comes from extensive clinical experience gained through residency.

With all that said, let's explore the most popular dual-degree programs!

## 25.6  Public Health

### 25.6.1  MD/MPH

The MPH has historically been the most popular dual degree among medical students due to its high versatility and complementary aspect to the MD. The MD/MPH physician may research and identify public health issues and implement an evidence-based approach to health improvement. Depending on the coursework and concentrations offered, students can pursue career interests in population health, biostatistics, public and health policy, clinical research, global health, environmental health, or health education. Notably, the great majority of CDC leaders hold the MPH degree. Earning the MPH as a dual degree halves the MPH program duration from 2 years to 1 year, and the GRE admissions requirement is usually also waived, so you save considerable time and cost.

### Potential Career Areas

- Public Health Researcher.
- NGO director or founder.
- Academic faculty.
- Government institutions (i.e., CDC leadership, Health Commissioner).
- Think Tank Consultant.

### Example Thesis Projects

- Adiposity in Infancy: Anthropometric Models.
- Prevalence and Health Burden of Cardiovascular Disease in Older US Veterans.
- Health Care Utilization and Costs for Dementia Patients in China.
- Utilizing Covid-19 Models in Humanitarian Crisis Settings.
- Developing a Framework for Civilian-Military Public Health Operations Involving Non-State Armed Groups.
- Global Routine Immunization Policies for Refugees.
- The Relationship Between Health Insurance Literacy, Health Insurance Coverage, and Health Insurance Utilization in the United States.
- Birth Characteristics and Risk of Early-Onset Ovarian Cancer.

### Program Structure Length

With a dual-degree program it is roughly one year in duration. Some light coursework or thesis project requirements may "spill over" into the fourth year of medical school.

### Application Timing

There are some programs you get "admitted" to as you begin medical school, but most programs enroll medical students between the third and fourth year of medical school. (After core clinical rotations are completed.)

### Admission Requirements

Commonly the GRE, but this requirement is frequently waived for medical students.

### Our Recommendation

If you have aspirations for a public health career (e.g., CDC director, NGO founder), then an MPH may give you an advantage. Interestingly, the majority of CDC leadership have MPH degrees. If your interest is primarily in biostatistics or clinical trial design, there are opportunities to learn without enrolling in a degree (i.e., research apprenticeship, online courses). In addition, some residency programs may help their residents pay for their MPH, so that might be worth researching.

# 25.7 Business

## 25.7.1 MD/MBA

The MBA degree is a highly versatile and complementary dual degree for students who have career interests in the business of healthcare, administration, consulting, finance, startups, drug or medical device development, and/or innovation.

The degree can better prepare the student for eventually starting or running a private medical practice. Earning the degree through the dual degree halves the program duration from 2 years to 1 year, and the GMAT admissions requirement is sometimes also waived, so you save considerable time and cost.

### Potential Career Areas

- Hospital administrator.
- Academic dean.
- Consultant (i.e., business strategy/management, insurance, venture capital).
- Startup founder.
- Tech transfer expert.

### Example Thesis Projects

- Increasing Preventative Care through Employee Benefits.
- Correlation Between Patient Care and Ability to Pay in Local Community.
- Healthcare Medical Talent Acquisition and Retention.
- Safety and Privacy Regulation Compliance of Hospital Systems.
- Benefits and Problems with US News Hospital Ratings.
- Improving Health Services for Veterans.
- Seamless EMR/EHR Adoption.
- Streamlining of Disaster Drill Procedures.
- Improving ER Incident Reporting Systems.
- Increasing Hospital Nurse Retention.

### Program Structure Length

With a dual-degree program it is roughly one year in duration. Some light coursework or thesis project requirements may "spill over" into the fourth year of medical school.

### Application Timing

There are some programs you get "admitted" to as you begin medical school, but most programs enroll medical students between the third and fourth year of medical school. (After core clinical rotations are completed.)

### Admission Requirements

Commonly the GMAT, and this requirement is sometimes but not always waived by the business school.

### Our Recommendation

This degree would be good to consider if you have significant interest in healthcare management (e.g., hospital administration, entrepreneurship, healthcare economics, healthcare consulting), or doesn't plan on going into clinical medicine.

One of the greatest values you get from an MBA program is the networking/alumni base.[11] Most of the technical knowledge can be self-studied so you may want to carefully consider the opportunity + financial cost.

---

[11] https://mba.wharton.upenn.edu/value-wharton-mba/: "The value of an MBA in today's market can be hard to calculate, but the greatest value of a Wharton MBA is the network you inherit."

However for the student who plans on entering business immediately out of medical school, we *strongly* advise you to consider MD/MBA programs. The MBA gives medical students a "hard" skill to lean on for jobs, so it is especially useful to the student who does not plan on going to a residency program out of medical school.

**Note:** The **MD/MHA** (Master's in Health Administration) dual degree, which is similar to an MBA but focused on the specifics of health administration, sometimes at the expense of general business principles. *If you're interested in the MD/MHA, you may want to consider the MD/MBA instead, as the MD/MBA is more widely recognized in industry and more versatile compared to the MD/MHA.*[12]

## 25.8  Law

### 25.8.1  MD/JD

The JD dual degree is for students with career interests in health law, health policy, biotechnology, or bioethics; in academia, government, or the private sector. MDs will be able to apply their clinical experience and knowledge to assist high-level policy decisions in a variety of environments.

The JD degree helps students:
- Expand their knowledge of the US Legal System specific to healthcare.
- Understand the rule of law through reading and analyzing previous case laws, statutes, and regulations.
- Enhance their ability to communicate with colleagues and peers regarding legal issues that affect the health workplace.
- Gain familiarity with contemporary legal issues facing the United States and the world both in general and in healthcare.

Earning the degree through the dual degree shortens the obtaining of both degrees independently from 7 years (4 years for MD, 3 years for JD) to 6 years, depending on the program.

Most MD/JD's are practicing physicians and some are practicing lawyers.

## Work May Be Related to
- Health policy and healthcare system development.
- Medical malpractice consulting.
- Medical staff privilege matters.
- Medical board disciplinary actions.
- Managed care contracts and disputes.
- Medical business transactions.
- Healthcare employment agreements.

## Example Thesis Projects
- Constitutional Privacy Issues Regarding Vaccines.
- Surrogate Decision-Makers in End-of-Life Care.
- Analysis of Historical Malpractice Cases in Radiology.
- Impact of Patient Protection and Affordable Care Act on Patient Care.

## Program Structure Length

The JD is a 3-year degree as a standalone but with a dual-degree program and it is frequently accelerated to roughly 2 years in duration. Some light coursework or thesis project requirements may "spill over" into the fourth year of medical school.

---

[12]  Pitt Med Dual Degrees Report 2021.

## A Note about Law School Summer Semesters

Generally, the first two summer semester (breaks) are devoted typically for internships. Many students spend their 1 L (first-year law school) summer in an unpaid internship or unpaid judicial clerkship. The 1 L summer is more about gaining exposure to the legal field in general. The 2 L summer is different, in that students spend time in a paid position at a place where they eventually hope to work, whether that's at a law firm, a district attorney's office or public defender's office, a government agency, or a public interest legal organization.

## Application Timing

There are some programs you get "admitted" to as you begin medical school, but most programs enroll medical students between the third and fourth year of medical school. (After core clinical rotations are completed.)

## Admission Requirements

Commonly the LSAT, and this requirement is often NOT waived for medical students.

## Our Recommendation

The MD/JD is typically a self-funded 2-year commitment, so we recommend speaking to advisors in the program and alumni of the program to gain more information about whether their program is right for you.

## 25.9 Public Policy

### 25.9.1 MD/MPP

The MPP Master's in Public Policy degree is for students who wish to combine their clinical knowledge with the study of policies or administer programs involving healthcare issues of public concern. Graduates of this dual degree will be prepared to assume leadership positions in international, federal, state, and local governments, global organizations, nonprofit institutions, large service delivery organizations, or research centers.

## Potential Career Areas

- Physician Policy Consultant.
- Management Consultant.
- Think Tank Researcher.
- Policy Director.
- Various positions at NGOs, government.

## Example Thesis Projects

- Shifting Federally Funded Research into Pasteur's Quadrant: A Case Study of the SBIR Program at NIH.
- Interstate Equity in Health Policy.
- Medical Records: The Role of Advocacy Coalitions in Policy Change.
- The Effects of Core Divestments on Innovations in the Pharmaceutical Industry: A Public Policy Analysis.
- Professionalism and Self-Regulatory Standards: Responsiveness of Medical Licensure and Certification.
- Machine Tractable Human Tissue: Policy Implications for Medical Privacy.
- Policy Intersections or Policy Chasms: State Elder Mobility Policy, Practice, and Long-Term Care Reform.

## How Does MPP Differ from the MPH?

An MPH is suited for working closely with the community on solving and preventing public health problems.
An MPP is suited for engaging in the political process to influence policy outcomes.

Example questions appropriate for the MPP include:

- How can business and government work together to create economic policies that are strong and sustainable?
- How can policymakers provide good, affordable housing?
- How can schools and educators cut down on childhood obesity and improve graduation rates?
- How can the local government do a better job of engaging with members of the community to make better policy?

## Program Structure Length

With a dual-degree program it is roughly one year in duration. Some light coursework or thesis project requirements may "spill over" into the fourth year of medical school.

## Application Timing

There are some programs you get "admitted" to as you begin medical school, but most programs enroll medical students between the third and fourth year of medical school. (After core clinical rotations are completed.)

## Admission Requirements

Commonly the GRE, but this requirement is frequently waived for medical students.

## Our Recommendation

If your primary interest is working in government and/or affecting legislative or health policy, the MPP may be a better choice compared to the MPH.

# 25.10 Biomedical or Clinical Informatics

## 25.10.1 MD/MSc

The MS Biomedical Informatics degree is for students who envision solving research questions or real-world problems at the intersection of health, medical, and biology using computational tools and data. Depending on the coursework and concentrations offered, students will learn about data science, data analytics, and human-centered design and systems. In addition, students can pursue career interests in academia or industry (pharmaceutical, healthcare technology) using this increasingly in-demand skillset.

## Potential Career Areas

- Physician Scientist.
- Informaticist.
- Chief Data/Information Officer.
- Consultant.

## Example Thesis Projects

- The Use of Sequential Pattern Mining to Predict Next Prescribed Medications.
- Reducing Respiratory Virus Testing in Hospitalized Children with Machine.
- Learning and Text Mining.
- Using Electronic Health Records to Identify Incarceration History Among Veterans.
- Adherence to Prospective Registration Policy and Implications for Clinical Trial Endpoint Integrity.
- Inter-Rater Reliability of Physical Abuse Determinations and Abusive Fracture Incidence at a Level 1 Pediatric Trauma Center.
- Strategic Genome Mining for Novel Antimicrobial Compounds.

## Program Structure Length

With a dual-degree program it is roughly one year in duration. Some light coursework or thesis project requirements may "spill over" into the fourth year of medical school.

## Application Timing

There are some programs you get "admitted" to as you begin medical school, but most programs enroll medical students between the third and fourth year of medical school. (After core clinical rotations are completed.)

## Admission Requirements

Commonly the GRE, but this requirement is frequently waived for medical students.

## Our Recommendation

This dual degree may be worth considering if you're interested in computational research and especially if you don't have a background in computer science. You will likely need to take some remedial courses to qualify for the admissions so inquire about this with the school's program as soon as possible. This degree, like the MBA, gives medical students a "hard" skill to lean on for jobs, so it is especially useful to the student who does not plan on going to a residency program out of medical school. For example, a medical degree combined with a rigorous background in informatics is very appealing to think-tanks and other consulting organizations.

# 25.11  Bioengineering

## 25.11.1  MD/MSc

The MS Biomedical Engineering degree bridges the gap between medicine and technology, enabling future physicians to apply high-tech research and solutions to improve health and healthcare. Typical programs focus on medical devices, biomaterials, and cell-based innovations. Examples of projects include the design of surgical robotics tools, implantable medical devices, prosthetics, hospital equipment, 3D printing for organs, and novel drug delivery methods. In addition, some programs may extend their focus to pharmaceuticals and biologics.

## Potential Career Areas

• Physician Researcher.

Physician Innovator/Engineer/Inventor.
• Entrepreneur.
• Consultant.

## Example Thesis Projects

• Element Modeling of Biodegradable Magnesium Stents.
• Development of a Planning Tool for Robot-Assisted Partial Nephrectomy Surgery based on 3D Reconstructions of Kidneys.
• Targeted Drug Delivery for Liver Cancer: Modeling the Impact of Cancer Burden on the Particle Distribution in a Patient.
• 2-Oxazoline-Based Plasma Coatings for Antifouling Application.
• Chip-Based Raman Sensors for Disease Diagnosis and Drug Monitoring.
• Monte Carlo Simulations on Dosimetry and Image Quality for Pediatric Imaging in Total Body PET.

## Program Structure Length

With a dual-degree program it is roughly one year in duration. Some light coursework or thesis project requirements may "spill over" into the fourth year of medical school.

## Application Timing

There are some programs you get "admitted" to as you begin medical school, but most programs enroll medical students between the third and fourth year of medical school. (After core clinical rotations are completed.)

## Admission Requirements

Commonly the GRE, but this requirement is frequently waived for medical students.

## Our Recommendation

This dual degree may be worth considering if you're interested in medical devices, robotics, cell engineering, etc. You may need to take some remedial courses to qualify for the admissions so inquire about this with the school's program as soon as possible. This degree, like the MBA, gives medical students a "hard" skill to lean on for jobs, so it is especially useful to the student who does not plan on going to a residency program out of medical school.

# 25.12  Clinical Education

## 25.12.1  MD/MSc

The M.Ed. Master's in Clinical (or Medical) Education degree is for students who, as future clinicians, aim to transform health professions education and advance the health sciences and healthcare nationally and internationally. The trainee will combine medical training with an understanding of effective teaching practices, individual lesson plans, and how different students learn. The focus of research can be centered on medical school, residency, or continuing education, in addition to medical subspecialties.

## Potential Career Areas

- Clinician Instructor/Educator.
- Public Health Educator.

## Example Thesis Projects

- How Resident Resilience and Tolerance of Ambiguity Impact Burnout, Medical Error, and Clinical Competence.
- Assessing Awareness and Use of Evidence-Based Learning Strategies.
- Real Event Learning and Analysis (REAL): Assessing and Improving Surgical Team Performance.
- Understanding Internal Medicine Residents' Knowledge and Comfort in Caring for Patients with Opioid Use Disorders.
- Improving the In-clinic Teaching of Junior Residents.
- Clinical Pedagogical Methods and Outcomes in the Hospital.
- Design an eLearning Program.

## Program Structure Length

With a dual-degree program it is roughly one year in duration. Some light coursework or thesis project requirements may "spill over" into the fourth year of medical school.

## Application Timing

There are some programs you get "admitted" to as you begin medical school, but most programs enroll medical students between the third and fourth year of medical school. (After core clinical rotations are completed.)

## Admission Requirements

Commonly the GRE, but this requirement is frequently waived for medical students.

## Our Recommendation

Many medical schools offer electives in clinical pedagogy. Mileage may vary on the return on investment for this degree.

# 26 Medical School Rankings

*Phillip Wagner*

## Student Perspective

When I was deciding between medical schools, I asked both my research mentor and my academic mentor their opinions on the schools to which I was accepted. I was legitimately having trouble with the decision. Having gone through all my interviews, studied numerous resources both formal and informal, and done everything a judicious applicant could do to be informed about what many consider to be a very important decision, I was shocked by the response I received. Having explained the various pros and cons as I saw them, I received a nearly identical response from both mentors that amounted to this: "What do the rankings say?"

## 26.1 Ranking Overview

Medical school rankings are ordered lists released by various third-party groups that attempt to quantify complex quality differences in medical schools for the supposed purpose of helping prospective applicants decide between them. These lists are presented to consumers in a best-to-worst order.

### 26.1.1 Who Does the Ranking?

An ever-growing number of entities have gotten into the ranking business for medical schools, a list currently including The Princeton Review, Top Universities QS, and Student Doctor Network, among many others, but by far the most notable, popular, and prolific are those rankings released annually by US News and World Report (USN). When the mentors in the above student perspective box were talking about rankings, when medical schools present their respective ranks to visiting applicants, when applicants are deciding between the prestige of various medical schools to which they have been accepted, it was the USN rankings to which they were referring. As the USN rankings and their methodology are the current industry standard, we will be focusing heavily on their system, its benefits and flaws, and how it can be used.

### 26.1.2 Who Ranks the Rankers? A Historical Perspective

There was a time when US News was a popular magazine company that contained the product of real journalism, and competed with the likes of *Time* and *Newsweek* in its scope of circulation. As a small offshoot of its journalistic enterprise, US News started publishing rankings of various schools, hospitals, and automobiles, among other things. It is the oldest and most widely consumed ranking list of academic institutions in the country.[1] For reasons outside the scope of this text, journalistic businesses including US News experienced economic hardship over the past several decades, and US News was forced to delay, and eventually cease releasing its magazine in print. Electronic issues continued to be released for several years until those too proved unprofitable. The company's financial saving grace, ultimately bringing it back to profitability, was its pursuit of service journalism, which in this case means rating and ranking consumable goods.[2] While there are other ranking systems put forth by this company, the Best Colleges Rankings are its flagship product, and its predominant source of revenue and survival. When asking yourself "Do the rankings matter?" the answer is almost certainly "yes," but remember that the entity to which they matter most is not you, your future employers, the

---

[1] U.S. News college rankings are denounced but not ignored. Available at: https://www.washingtonpost.com/local/education/us-news-college-rankings-are-denounced-but-not-ignored/2011/09/02/glQAn6Bzz]_story.html. Accessed July 8, 2022.

[2] Value Added: U.S. News & World Report returns to the ranks of profitability. Available at: https://www.washingtonpost.com/business/economy/value-added-us-news-and-world-report-returns-to-the-ranks-of-profitability/2013/04/27/2e16c306-ae05-11e2-a986-eec837b1888b_story.html. Accessed July 8, 2022.

National Institutes of Health (NIH) department assessing your grant proposals, or those evaluating you for competitive residency spots. **The entity to which the US News rankings matter the most is US News.** Keep that in mind while using them, and when assessing how helpful they are for your decisions.

It goes without saying that rankings matter to schools and their bottom line as well. **For undergraduate schools, researchers have found that an increase in 1 spot in the rankings leads to 1 to 2% increase in the number of applicants to that school.**[3]

## 26.2 The Methodology: What Goes into Ranking a Medical School?

To US News' credit, its ranking methodology is readily accessible and easy to understand, giving you the ability to judge and determine what the rankings mean to you. The two main subcategory rankings that US News releases for medical schools are rankings for Research and Primary Care.

For each subcategory, USN determines what quality measures should factor into a school's rank, and assigns each school a numerical factor based on how they perform with regard to that metric. These measures are proxies for quality. They do not directly represent quality, something that is hard to quantify for organizations as complex as medical schools. These proxy scores in each category are then themselves assigned a numerical value (weighted) for how much it matters relative to other proxy quality measures. These numbers are then added, and an entity as complicated and multifaceted as educational experience is distilled to one number. The schools are then ranked according to this one total number.

Do you remember how you were graded in middle school, high school, or college for a certain class? The teacher evaluated your performance based on tests, quizzes, homework assignments, class participation, and a class project. Each was assigned a different percentage weight to indicate its importance. These areas were being used as proxies for the quality of your work in different metrics. The teacher added up these points, and you received one final grade. If the teacher then decided to create a ranked list based on final grade—a practice that still happens at some institutions—that would be your "class rank." That is exactly what is happening with medical school rankings. More often, these final grades are used to assign you a tiered rank, grades A through F, each representing a different tier. The only difference with US News' rankings is unlike your graded assignments and test scores, their weighted metrics are almost never based on performance.

### 26.2.1 The Rankings Algorithm: Research versus Primary Care

USN ranks nearly every type of school, undergraduate and graduate, and is consistently adding subgroup rankings to its catalogue. To be clear, its ranking algorithm—the equation used to determine the final ranking—is different for each type of educational and professional system it is reviewing. High-schools are ranked by a different algorithm than medical schools, and law schools are ranked differently from MBA programs. Below, you can find the rough algorithm from the previous iteration and the updated changes from the most recent tweak.[4]

The chart in ▶ Table 0.1 breaks down the quality proxies and their relative weights used in generating the USN rankings. Those quality proxies highlighted in blue are the main proxies, and are composed of the proxies below it that are white. Their weights in the respective rankings are given by percentages.

## 26.3 Contextualizing These Quality Proxies: What Are They?

### 26.3.1 Quality Assessment

#### Peer Assessment

Deans of medical schools, Directors of Admission, and Heads of Internal Medicine Departments rate the quality of education/reputation of competing medical schools.

---

[3] Luca M, Smith J. Salience in Quality Disclosure: Evidence from the U.S. News College Rankings. Available at: https://web.archive.org/web/20131010062004/http://www.hbs.edu/faculty/Publication%20Files/12-014.pdf. Accessed July 8, 2022.

[4] Morse R, Brooks E, Hines K, Lara-Agudelo D. Methodology: 2023 Best Medical Schools Rankings. Available at: https://www.usnews.com/education/best-graduate-schools/articles/medical-schools-methodology. Accessed July 8, 2022.

**Table 26.1** Ranking criteria and weight

| Criteria | Research ranking weight | Primary care ranking weight |
| --- | --- | --- |
| Quality Assessment | 40%→30% | 40%→30% |
| Peer Assessment Score | 20%→15% | 25%→15% |
| Residency Director Score | 20%→15% | 15%–>15% |
| Research Activity | 30%→40% | 0% |
| Total Research Activity | 15%→25% | 0% |
| Avg. Research Activity/faculty member | 15% | 0% |
| Primary Care Production (previously primary care rate) | 0% | 30%→40% |
| Graduates (currently/still) Practicing in Primary Care Setting(new) | 0% | 0%→30% |
| Graduates going into Primary Care | 0% | 30%→10% |
| Student Selectivity | 20% | 15% |
| Median MCAT Score | 13% | 9.75% |
| Median Undergraduate GPA | 6% | 4.5% |
| Acceptance Rate | 1% | .75% |
| Faculty Resources | 10% | 15% |

## Residency Director Score

If you aren't familiar with what a residency director does, you should be. They deal with the ranking and eventual hiring of medical school graduates into residency spots at their program, and often have years of experience assessing candidates sent to them by different medical schools.

## Limitations

These two rankings make up the "quality score" aspect of the rankings. One can see several limitations of this measurement initially. Chief among them are (1) Peer Assessment Score is more reputation/perception-based than quality-based, and Deans of Medical Schools have a conflict of interest in ranking their competitors in a system where they stand to benefit from ranking them poorly, and (2) an imperfect quality assessment—but a quality assessment nonetheless—already complicated by a strong conflict of interest, makes up almost half of the criteria that claims to judge which medical schools are the best—40% to be exact.

## 26.3.2 Research Activity

### Total Research Activity

The amount of NIH funding a school receives to perform research. This is academic grant funding from the federal government directly given to faculty members for their research endeavors.

### Average Research Activity per Faculty Member

Total dollars given per teaching faculty at the medical school.

## Limitations and Context

Total Research Activity is probably an adequate predictor of how easy it is to get involved in research while enrolled at that particular medical school—and how easy it will be to have your research funded while there. Participating in research while in medical school is an incredible boost to your residency application, and is even expected for more competitive fields, so this statistic can be useful as well. Great researchers bringing in big dollars, however, do not indicate that those researchers are excellent teachers. If you don't plan on doing research, these numbers aren't as helpful for you. Not really worth considering from an applicant's perspective, as you generally shouldn't be selecting a school based on who has slightly more research money, but something to consider when judging the quality of these rankings.

## 26.3.3 Primary Care Production Rate

### Primary Care Rate

This criterion makes up 10% of the primary care rankings, and could therefore be a valid measure of a school's ability to produce amazing primary care physicians. However, this criteria is only the proportion of a school's graduates that end up going into primary care specialties—general internal medicine, family medicine, and general pediatrics. This is, perhaps, the most flawed measurement in the entire ranking system as it only shares an outcome measure that is not universally desirable, yet treats it as such by awarding points for it. It has become more flawed in recent years due to the fact that many internal medicine graduates (a primary care field) have been delaying fellowship, but practice as a "primary care doctor" right out of residency, but only for a year or two. This was recently lowered from a massive 30% weight to 10% to make room for an arguably better, newer metric below.

### Graduate Practicing in Primary Care (Still)

Shows what proportion of a school's graduates from the 2013–14 graduating class are STILL practicing in primary care.

## 26.3.4 In Defense of This Ranking Criteria

It may indicate a school's attitude toward the primary care specialties. A high proportion of graduates entering these fields may indicate that if you are interested in primary care and attend this institution, you may find yourself surrounded by other like-minded matriculants that were both selected and self-selected for going to a place that focuses on training primary care physicians. You may not be pressured by the administration to participate in heavy research activities, and thus have more time to shadow or volunteer in the clinic. You may have ready access to primary care mentors as well, or more electives focused on primary care.

## 26.4 On the Other Hand

This also may indicate that a high percentage of the students at this school do not, in general, have competitive enough academic profiles to successfully match into the more competitive specialties, and were thus relegated, by poor board scores or third and fourth year clinical grades, to pursue these less competitive specialties, primary care included. In general, primary care specialties are relatively noncompetitive, pay relatively poorly (relative to other fields of medicine), and are universally regarded as less prestigious (whether that should be the case is an entirely different discussion). The issue with this ranking system is that it does not allow you to differentiate between a school with a high percentage of very competitive applicants that actually want to pursue a primary care specialty, and a school where a high percentage of students are forced to pursue a less competitive specialty. A high percentage of students going into primary care specialties are excellent for the health of the country, but not helpful for an applicant interested in assessing educational quality.

### 26.4.1 Student Selectivity

#### MCAT Score

This is an important criterion, as it allows for some measure of standardization for comparison among applicants that attended different colleges and had varying extracurricular experiences. At the same time, it should be noted that this ranking system used to value the Medical College Admission Test (MCAT) at around 6% of research rankings rather than 13%. Schools that don't value the MCAT as much as grade point average (GPA) or clinical experiences when selecting applicants took a ranking hit upon this change, even though nothing really changed at all. This brings up an important accessory point: **the criteria are always changing in the ranking algorithm, making it hard to compare schools over time—often, the schools haven't changed when their rankings do; it is the algorithm that has changed.**

#### GPA

While this may seem like an essential ranking to include, it is problematic, bordering on preposterous, to compare the GPAs of two students who went to different colleges with different majors—different colleges grade on different scales, and grade inflation is more rampant at some places than at others—and not all students received the same degree. How do you compare a 3.9 GPA in an English degree at a noncompetitive school with a 3.6 GPA in a Chemistry/Physics double major from a notoriously rigorous college? These things, while both under the heading of GPA, are largely incomparable. Judging a school's ability to educate doctors based on this metric is an additional level of problematic reasoning.

#### Acceptance Rate

This metric, if weighted any higher, would be very dangerous and misleading when factored into school quality. For instance, some of the least competitive schools have some of the lowest acceptance rates. Throughout 2010 to 2019, Harvard Medical College received less than half the applications than Albany Medical College did. Compare the top five schools in USN Research rankings to those ranked in the 70s (the midway point in the rankings). The trend is the same. Because the latter of these schools are respected mid-tier schools that hold admissions criteria of average competitiveness relative to the rest of accredited medical schools, they are the reach schools for applicants in the lowest competitive third of applicants, prime targets for those in the middle competitive third, and safety schools (not that this is often a term with much applicability to medical schools) for those in the top third. So, many people apply to these schools. Harvard's reputation, on the other hand, factored in with the high average GPA and MCATs among previous classes, causes many applicants to self-screen themselves away from applying there, especially when application costs vary around $150 a school, and not too many people want to throw away that amount of money. Thus, for medical schools, at least, a low acceptance rate sometimes indicates a less competitive institution, but is viewed positively in the rankings.

### 26.4.2 Faculty Resources

This is the ratio of full- and part-time faculty to medical school class. Like some of the other measures, it is an indicator of the wealth of the institution rather than the quality of the schooling. While there are compelling academic arguments out there for why this ratio improves schooling, it is undisclosed why it is weighted heavier in the primary care model than in the research model.

## 26.5 Overall Limitations and Criticism

Given their popularity and influence, the backlash to these and other rankings systems has been well documented. The themes of the criticism are consistent, and while they haven't (and likely will not) be able to unseat the rankings and rankers from educational prominence, they provide helpful perspectives on how to use the information they provide without relying on it. Below is a sampling of those criticisms and their sources.

- **USN ranks colleges when it probably should just rate them:** There is a lot of intellectual dishonesty when you collect a bunch of poor proxies, assign them arbitrary values and relative weights, and then reduce the complexity artificially to a single number. It might be more valuable, perhaps, to rate them on certain specific characteristics, and leave it at that. (The opinion of Ted Fiske, a competitor of USN and creator of an alternate rating system).[5,6]
- **The rankings don't have a single measure of educational success:** As you go through the medical school rankings, you might notice not one of them tracks a single measure of how well the school educates. They encompass stats of those admitted, money available for teaching, but never step scores, success in residency placement, etc.[7]
- **The rankings never change the current prestige hierarchy:** Those who were at the top before the rankings started are still at the top. There is very little mobility, and when there is, it is often because the algorithm changed, and not the school. Allegations have piled up over the years that USN throws out algorithm changes because they don't keep the established "top" schools at the top of the rankings.[8,9]
- **Most of the proxies measure wealth and not education:** Categories like faculty resources, endowment, alumni giving, research funding are actually just measuring one thing.
- **The rankings are a self-fulfilling prophecy.** Peer Assessment rankings, weighted quite heavily for medical schools, is a proxy for reputation, a part of which is based on current USN rankings.[10]
- **Schools that don't play along are punished:** USN depends upon schools submitting data to rank them. Back in 1995, Reed College decided it did not want to submit any more information to USN, and consequently saw its ranking drop significantly. A group of students at Reed College used statistics to prove that their school was being penalized. When schools stopped submitting info, USN had still been ranking them, but did so by artificially loading the algorithm against them by giving them completely made up—and artificially low—test scores.[11]
- **No Tiers:** While a classmate may have gotten a 96, and you got a 94, the only thing that survives is your letter grade. It's not hard to see why a tiered system, especially with all the flaws inherent in the exact ranking of medical school quality, is superior for conveying information to consumers. You may have received a 94 instead of a 96 in your class, but your classmate's class rank may be 4 out of 50, and yours might be 12th. While you may have the twelfth highest grade, is there really that much difference in performance between you and your classmate, or any of the students in between for that matter? No—you all get As. While one school is higher than another, will that matter if you consider them to be the same tier?
- **Ranking changes are often due to algorithm changes, not changes in educational prowess:** Not only does the ranking methodology that USN and other companies use change from time to time, but so do other factors in ways for which the rankings algorithm cannot adequately compensate. For example, occasionally medical schools receive large grants isolated to one year from a significant donor. Did the students matriculating at that school receive a better education? Did their perceived reputation among residency programs dramatically change? Likely not.

---

5  U.S. News changed the way it ranks colleges. It's still ridiculous. Available at: https://www.washingtonpost.com/education/2018/09/12/us-news-changed-way-it-ranks-colleges-its-still-ridiculous/. Accessed July 8, 2022.

6  Why College Ratings Are Better Than Rankings: A Wiser Way To A College Choice. Available at: https://www.forbes.com/sites/christeare/2015/08/30/college-guidebook-guru-ted-fiske-answer-our-questions/?sh=31e0008952ef. Accessed July 8, 2022.

7  Same as note 3.

8  Thompson N. Playing With Numbers. Available at: https://washingtonmonthly.com/2000/09/01/playing-with-numbers/. Accessed July 8, 2022.

9  U.S. News changed the way it ranks colleges. It's still ridiculous. Available at: https://www.washingtonpost.com/education/2018/09/12/us-news-changed-way-it-ranks-colleges-its-still-ridiculous/. Accessed July 8, 2022.

10  Breslow S. The Case Against Being (Ranked) the Best. Available at: https://web.archive.org/web/20170225045251/https://tsl.news/opinions/4182/. Accessed July 8, 2022.

11  Lydgate C. Students Find Glaring Discrepancy in US News Rankings. Available at: https://www.reed.edu/reed-magazine/articles/2019/usnews-discrepancy.html. Accessed July 8, 2022.

## 26.6 Summary

Medical school rankings are hard to extricate from the typical applicant's decision-making process. It's important to understand their numerous and significant limitations and outright methodological flaws. You can consider the rankings themselves as flawed proxies for prestige, which should be a factor (among many others) you consider when ultimately deciding on a program. However, when you consider them, treat them as tiers and not a linear progression. Ultimately, this will factor into, but should not come close to dictating, your final decision.

# 27 Making Your List: What Schools Do I Apply To?

*Joel Thomas*

Once you've gotten the housekeeping out of the way, you will need to decide *how many* and *which* medical schools to apply to. This is not a trivial decision. A carefully calculated list of schools could mean the difference between jump-starting a fulfilling career in medicine and failing to gain admission, paying exorbitantly high tuition at School X when better-value options were available, or—perhaps worst of all—hating your life at a medical school that is a poor fit for you.

As of 2020, there are ~140 US Doctor of Medicine (MD) schools and ~35 Doctor of Osteopathic Medicine (DO) schools in the United States. The average MD applicant applies to 16 MD schools, and the average DO applicant applies to 9 DO schools.[1,2]

You should apply to 25 to 35 schools at most. It's true that there's an element of luck to the whole process (e.g., whether it's raining on the day you interviewed[3]), and—all things equal—applying to more schools increases your odds of acceptance. However, if there are serious shortcomings in your application to begin with (e.g., grade point average [GPA] <3.0), applying to more schools will not give you any significant advantage. Moreover, you may become fatigued with completing the enormous number of secondary applications, leading to lower quality essays. Lastly, there are probably diminishing returns on the marginal advantage you gain beyond 35 schools.

To begin the process of deciding *which* schools to apply to, you should assess how competitive you are as an applicant. We recommend **WedgeDawg's Applicant Rating System** developed by "WedgeDawg," a high-profile poster on Student Doctor Network. This is an algorithm that weighs your GPA, Medical College Admission Test (MCAT), research, clinical experience, shadowing, volunteering, leadership and teaching, undergraduate school, under-represented minority (URM) status, upward GPA trend, and "miscellaneous factors" to generate a score to compare your overall competitiveness to that of specific medical schools. Medical schools are stratified into competitiveness categories, (e.g., "top," "high," "mid," and "low."). WedgeDawg also identifies "low-yield" schools, or schools that receive an enormous number of applications relative to their class size; your odds of getting into these schools are lower compared to schools with similar stats unless you have specific, compelling reasons for attending. Limitations of this method, however, include lumping all DO schools into a single category and subjective, imperfect assessment of extracurricular activities.[4] Nonetheless, this is the best "objective" method of assessing your competitiveness we have thus found.[5]

After getting a sense of your application's competitiveness, you can begin to create your school list. You should create an excel spreadsheet—preferably on the Cloud that you can update on-the-go—that you can update in real time with additions, removals, and important dates, (e.g., secondary application received versus submitted), interview invite received, date of interview, acceptance versus wait-list versus rejection status, etc. Once that's done, we can begin the process of creating a school list.

- Apply to *all* of the public medical schools in your state of residence, regardless of whether you are competitive. You should also consider in-state private schools that have preferences for in-state students; you may want to inquire about these schools with your pre-med office.
  - Note that your "state of residence" may differ from where you live, work, or attend school. Roughly speaking, state of residence is the state of your permanent address and/or vehicle registration. However, you should discuss with your school's financial aid office if you are in doubt.

---

[1] Note that you can apply to a combination of MD and DO schools. We recommend this strategy if your MCAT and GPA are borderline for MD schools (see Chapter 24, DO, MD, and International Schools).

[2] aacom®. Available at: https://www.aacom.org/docs/default-source/data-and-trends/2020-aacomas-applicant-matriculant-profile-summary-report.pdf?sfvrsn=d870497_20. Accessed July 8, 2022.

[3] Redelmeier DA, Baxter SD. Rainy weather and medical school admission interviews CMAJ 2009;181(12):933. Available at: https://www.ncbi.nlm.nih.gov/pmc/articles/PMC2789141/. Accessed July 8, 2022.

[4] If you'd like more information about specific DO schools to gauge your competitiveness, you can refer to this user-submitted list containing all DO (and MD) schools with average GPA and MCAT: https://themedicalschooldirectory.com

[5] Another method is the "LizzyM" score, which simply assigns you a score based on your GPA and MCAT score. Schools are also assigned LizzyM scores based on their average GPA and MCAT. https://www.studentdoctor.net/schools/lizzym-score will allow you to calculate your LizzyM score and find medical schools within a specific percentage of your score.

- You have a comparative advantage at your state schools compared to out-of-state applicants. This *may* be sufficient to overcome relatively low stats as well.
- Your state schools are likely to be cheaper than private schools and out-of-state public schools. Note that *some* state public schools allow students to obtain in-state residency after attending the school for one year. For example, the University of North Carolina does this, but University of Colorado at Denver does not.[6]
- Also consider "personal ties" to a region, which can give you an advantage to schools in that region. For example, you may be a resident of Maine, but your closest support system may be in New York. If you emphasize this in your application, you may gain an extra glance when applying to New York schools.
- Some states (i.e., states with few or none public medical schools) have interstate agreements with medical schools that give their students in-state status. For example:
  - The **Western Interstate Commission for Higher Education** allows students from select Western states (e.g., Montana, Wyoming) and the Northern Mariana Islands to attend certain public medical schools with in-state status.
  - The **University of Washington School of Medicine** gives in-state status to applicants from Washington, Wyoming, Alaska, Montana, and Idaho. *We do not recommend applying to this school if you are not a resident of these states, as they only accepted 0.14% of out-of-state applicants (i.e., applicants not from the aforementioned states).*
  - **Finance Authority of Maine's Access to Medical Education Program** gives in-state status to Maine residents at Dartmouth, University of Vermont, and UNECOM.
  - **Delaware Institute of Medical Education and Research** gives in-state status to Delaware residents at Jefferson Medical College.

## Student Perspective

While your state medical school is likely to be cheaper than private schools and out-of-state public schools, this is not always the case. The sticker price at a private medical school I had gotten into was dramatically higher than that of my state school. I also didn't expect any financial aid because I didn't receive any need-based aid from the undergraduate schools that had accepted me. You can imagine the look on my face when my top-choice non-state school gave me enough need-based aid to make attendance dramatically cheaper than my state school!

- Even if you're not a Texas resident, you should still consider applying to *Texas schools*. While it's true that ~10% of matriculants at Texas schools are out-of-state students,[7] only about 25% of applicants to these schools are from out-of-state; in 2018, *close to 33% of out-of-state applicants matriculated* at a Texas school. Texas schools also give in-state tuition to virtually every out-of-state applicant. Finally, Texas Medical and Dental Application Service (TMDSAS) is relatively easy (and inexpensive) to complete in addition to American Medical College Application Service (AMCAS) or American Association of Colleges of Osteopathic Medicine Application Services (AACOMAS), and only half of the schools require secondaries. However, you should review the timeline for submitting TMDSAS, as the Texas cycle runs slightly earlier than AMCAS/AACOMAS.
- Use the MSAR + /– ChooseDO + /– online research (e.g., official school websites, virtual fairs, forums with a grain of salt) to learn more about the schools. Ideally, you will want to choose schools you're competitive at that are also **good "fits"**.

---

[6] Student Affairs. Available at: http://www.ucdenver.edu/anschutz/studentresources/Registrar/StudentServices/Residency/Pages/Residency-prospect.aspx. Accessed July 8, 2022.

[7] Texas actually limits the number of out-of-state matriculants in exchange for state subsidies for medical education—hence the low tuition.

- A school is a good fit for you if your personal and professional interests and experiences align with the school's mission statement. *For the vast majority of applicants, this will be a nonissue.* Most medical schools have essentially the same mission: to create compassionate physicians who are leaders in patient care +/− research (more so if the school is well known for research output). That said, some schools do have niche mission statements that may be more appealing to certain students.
  - For example, Loma Linda School of Medicine states, "The mission of the School of Medicine is to continue the teaching and healing ministry of Jesus Christ." If you are a devout scientologist, this may not be the school for you.
- Other interests and experiences that warrant discerning among specific schools include:
  - Strong desire to work with *certain patient populations* (e.g., urban vs. rural, immigrants and refugees, Spanish-speaking patients—consider Florida, NYC, Texas, and California in particular).
  - Specific *extracurricular interests:* Interning at the CDC, White House, or United Nations may be easier with physical proximity in Atlanta, DC, or NYC, respectively.
  - *Dual-degree* options.
  - Unique *curriculum:* These include the accelerated preclinical at Duke with a research year,[8] required research thesis at Yale,[9] longitudinal research project at Pitt,[10] paid research years at many schools, required EMT training at Hofstra,[11] and free tuition with an extra fifth research year and small class size at Cleveland Clinic Lerner College of Medicine.[12] *See the list at the end of this chapter for additional unique curricular features.*
  - Specific *research* interests (particularly for MD/PhD applicants).
  - If you're interested in a *specific field of medicine* (e.g., radiation oncology, integrated plastic surgery, dermatology), and your school does not have a residency program in that field, you *will be at a disadvantage* for getting into that field.
    1. At minimum, you will lose the advantage of having a "home program" to apply to. Generally speaking, residency applicants have the best chance of gaining acceptance to their home programs, or programs at their own medical schools.
    2. Lack of a residency program often suggests lack of high-quality research and teaching faculty who would be able to write strong letters of recommendation for residency applications.
- In general, we recommend *avoiding schools with graded (e.g., "honors, high pass, pass, low pass, fail") preclinical courses* unless you have an otherwise compelling reason to apply (e.g., strong school reputation, in-state status, you are an international applicant, etc.). It can be, however, hard to do this as a lot of the pass/fail schools tend to be more prestigious—you may be leaving some less competitive schools on the table. Obviously pass/fail is far better, but not better than not getting in.
  - Residency programs generally do not care about your preclinical grades.[13] As such, many medical schools have transitioned to pass/fail grades in the preclinical years to minimize needless competition among students, as well as to probably assuage students' personal sense of perfectionism.
  - That said, this may change in the wake of the decision to make United States Medical Licensing Exam (USMLE) Step 1 pass/fail.

---

[8] Curriculum. Available at: https://medschool.duke.edu/education/student-services/office-curricular-affairs/about-duke-curriculum. Accessed July 8, 2022.

[9] https://medicine.yale.edu/md-program/research/medresearch/

[10] School of Medicine's Longitudinal Research Project (LRP). Available at: https://scholarlyproject.medschool.pitt.edu/. Accessed July 8, 2022.

[11] Emergency Medical Technician Training. Available at: https://medicine.hofstra.edu/education/md/md-emt.html. Accessed July 8, 2022.

[12] About. Available at: https://portals.clevelandclinic.org/cclcm/About-the-College. Accessed July 8, 2022.

[13] Results of the 2018 NRMP Program Director Survey. Available at: https://www.nrmp.org/wp-content/uploads/2018/07/NRMP-2018-Program-Director-Survey-for-WWW.pdf. Accessed July 8, 2022.

## USMLE Step 1

The United States Medical Licensing Exam (USMLE) is a three-part exam (Steps 1, 2, and 3) taken by anyone wishing to obtain a US medical license. Step 1 tests the basic science of medicine and is typically taken immediately after the preclinical years of medical school. Some foreign medical graduates, however, take it years after practicing as a physician in their home countries, as they need to take all three steps to obtain licensure in the United States. In addition, some medical schools allow their students to take Step 1 after clinical rotations, and some evidence suggests that this leads to higher scores (with MD/PhD students at the same school serving as internal controls, as they take Step 1 immediately after preclinical years).[14]

Historically, Step 1 was intended to be a minimal competency test that one simply had to pass to demonstrate mastery of the basic sciences of medicine. Because this exam is one of the few standardized tests one takes at *all* medical schools, residency programs began to evaluate one's score as one of the most—if not *the* most—important variables for resident selection.[15] Average scores on the exam increased over time, and the amount of content tested on the exam grew dramatically. This raised significant concern, as much of the material tested was of questionable clinical relevance (e.g., highly specific gene mutations for rare diseases). Moreover, a significant market for test preparation erupted, and many students at medical schools emphasized Step 1 preparation over studying for their own schools' courses. Lastly, the exam contributed to a significant amount of student stress, as one's chances for competitive residency programs were almost entirely determined by performance on a single 8-hour exam testing *all* of the material absorbed in the first 2 years of medical school. Memorizing every factoid in the 800-page review book for the exam, daily flashcard preparation for *years* leading up to the exam, and 14-hour study days in the months preceding the exam became the gold standard for aspiring dermatologists and orthopaedic surgeons, much to the exasperation of the National Board of Medical Examiners (NBME).

In February 2020, the NBME made the controversial decision to make Step 1 a pass/fail exam, to begin no earlier than January 2022. While studying for Step 1 was—in fact—a highly stressful ordeal that potentially emphasized material of questionable clinical relevance, it provided one of the few standardized metrics across medical schools. A high score on Step 1 leveled the playing field and allowed applicants from less prestigious medical schools to gain similar footing for residency applications. While it is too early to assess the downstream effects of this change, some unsavory scenarios have been hypothesized.[16,17]

First, the *prestige* of one's medical school may become substantially more important for competitive residency programs. Strong students tend to perform consistently well, and thus it is unlikely that residency directors will immediately come to believe that a "pass" from a DO school will be equivalent to a "pass" from Harvard Medical School. Again, while it is too early to tell, we recommend being mindful of particular medical schools' reputations among residency program directors per US News. Next, *pass/fail preclinical grading* may become less common as schools may feel compelled to provide grades to further stratify students for residency programs. *Extracurricular* activities in medical school (mainly research) may become more important to further distinguish strong applicants, and one's numerical grade on *USMLE Step 2 CK* (which tests clinical knowledge and is taken after rotations, i.e., *immediately* before residency applications) may replace the role that Step 1 previously held.

[14] Daniel M, Fleming A, O'Conner Grochowski C, et al. Why Not Wait? Eight Institutions Share Their Experiences Moving United States Medical Licensing Examination Step 1 After Core Clinical Clerkships. Acad Med 2017;92(11):1515-1524. Available at: https://www.ncbi.nlm.nih.gov/pubmed/28422816. Accessed July 8, 2022.

[15] Results of the 2018 NRMP Program Director Survey. Available at: https://www.nrmp.org/wp-content/uploads/2018/07/NRMP-2018-Program-Director-Survey-for-WWW.pdf. Accessed July 8, 2022.

[16] Nolen LS, Goshua A, Farber ON, Tiako MJN. Cheers and jeers as med school's Step 1 test becomes pass/fail. Available at: https://www.statnews.com/2020/02/14/cheers-and-jeers-as-med-schools-step-1-test-becomes-pass-fail/. Accessed July 8, 2022.

[17] Nolen LST. Why Pass/Fail Step 1 is Really Only Step 1. Available at: https://www.thecrimson.com/article/2020/2/18/nolen-pass-fail-step-1/. Accessed July 8, 2022.

- After adding all of the schools with in-state preferences, you will evenly distribute the rest of your list with a healthy mix of "reach," "match," and "safety"[18] schools. For a typical applicant, we recommend 25% reach schools, 50% match schools, and 25% safety schools.
  - "Reach" schools are those where your average GPA and/or MCAT are lower than 1 standard deviation (SD) of the school's average. "Match" schools are those where your GPA and/or MCAT are within 1 SD of the school's averages. "Safety" schools are those where your GPA and/or MCAT are greater than 1 SD of the school's averages.
  - That being said, if you *really* want to attend specific reach schools, feel free to add more as long as you have the minimum number of match and safety schools. Just keep in mind that you will need additional time to produce high-quality secondary essays.
  - Consider speaking with your school's pre-med office to learn which schools have *historically admitted applicants from your school.* This is most useful if you're a "typical applicant" from your school. If your stats or extracurriculars are significant deviations, you should adjust accordingly, e.g., with counsel from your pre-med office.
    - You may also want to get feedback from Internet forums (e.g., SDN, reddit.com/r/premed) on your tentative school list. Obviously, take the advice with a grain of salt, but these forums often have helpful medical students and admissions faculty willing to give free advice. Moreover, the turnaround time tends to be fantastic—you may get detailed responses within hours of asking!
  - For example, a New York State resident will add SUNY Upstate, SUNY Downstate, SUNY Buffalo, and SUNY Stony Brook (fur schools) to her list. She feels apprehensive about her chances of admission and would like to apply to 24 schools in total. She recognizes that this will be more time-consuming than applying to 15 schools, and she budgets time for secondary applications earlier than most applicants. She notes that all four of the SUNY schools are "safety" schools for her in terms of GPA and MCAT. Thus, she adds 2 more safety schools, 12 match schools, and 6 reach schools.
- And that's it! While the decision is important, we don't recommend stressing *too* much about it. While there can be significant differences between medical schools, your future will ultimately be in your own hands. Ultimately, you should be adaptable and open to attending any of the medical schools to which you apply.

### Historically Black Medical Schools

Historically Black medical schools are institutions that aim to recruit Black students and foster learning environments addressing the specific challenges and cultural contexts of the Black community.[19] Students at these schools may gain additional insight into health issues and social contexts that disproportionately affect people of color, as well as more mentorship opportunities with Black faculty. Moreover, students may be relatively shielded from microaggressions experienced by Black students at predominantly non-Black medical schools. Note that non-Black students can gain admission to these schools if they have significant experience working with underserved populations.

## 27.1  Should I Apply Early Decision?

As discussed in Chapter 20, The Big Picture, early decision allows you to initially apply to one and only one school, from which you will hear your admission status no later than **October 1** the year before matriculation. If accepted, you are required to attend this school. You cannot apply to any other medical schools unless you receive a rejection from this school. Again, we generally do not recommend this strategy unless you are a very competitive applicant with strong ties to that school, and the school has made it very clear that you are likely to be accepted.

In this case, you would save money and time spent applying to other schools. In the grand scheme of your medical career, however, that investment would be a drop in the bucket. If you are rejected by this

---

[18]  This is a misnomer. No medical school is a safety school for anyone, as you can easily be rejected for unpredictable reasons.

[19]  Gasman M, Smith T, Ye C, Nguyen T-H. HBCUs and the Production of Doctors. AIMS Public Health. 2017; 4(6): 579–589. Available at: https://www.ncbi.nlm.nih.gov/pmc/articles/PMC6111265/. Accessed July 8, 2022.

school, you will be at a significant disadvantage in applying to other schools because your application will not be submitted until October 1, which is extremely late in the rolling admissions schedule.

An example of an applicant who may benefit from this is a New York local who wants to go to SUNY Upstate College of Medicine. They did several summers of research there as an undergraduate, and already volunteer at the school's free clinic as an interpreter. The applicant wants to stay locally because they want to stay close to their aging grandmother who lives in Syracuse. Their research mentor is part of the medical school leadership, and has been actively recruiting the applicant to stay. They also have a competitive GPA and MCAT for the school.

Even in this fortuitous scenario, *admissions are highly unpredictable.* There is still the possibility of rejection, and we think it's a safer move to spend the time and money applying to a full list of medical schools to avoid the significant hit to your application and spend *even more* time and money applying to medical school again next year (as well as the opportunity cost of losing a full year of attending physician salary—$300,000–$700,000 compared to around $500–$4,000 for schools). There is very little to be gained by knowing where you will go a few months before everyone else, but a lot more to lose if you don't get accepted.

## 27.2 Medical Schools with Unique Features

We researched every medical school in the United States and identified schools with unique features (as of 2020) that may interest applicants. In alphabetical order:

- **California Northstate University College of Medicine:** This is a for-profit medical school, and you are unable to use federal student loans to finance your education. However, the school offers private loans with competitive options (fixed interest rate comparable to federal loans, income-based repayment plans, payment deferment during residency, 3-year interest-free grace period after residency). You should discuss with your school's financial aid office the pros and cons of applying and attending.
- **Case Western Reserve University School of Medicine:** Students have access to "HoloLens," a headset-based hologram simulation for gross anatomy.
- **Charles R. Drew University:** Historically Black medical school.
- **Cleveland Clinic Lerner College of Medicine:** 5-year tuition-free program with a required research year (with an option for a Master's degree) and heavy emphasis on research. It has a small class size of 32 students with an emphasis on small-group problem-based learning sessions. There is also no traditional gross anatomy dissection; students observe and learn from physicians' leading dissection.
- **Duke University:** Extremely lengthy secondary application that has historically changed yearly. The curriculum features an accelerated 1-year preclinical curriculum that may be difficult for some students. The third year of medical school is spent on a research project.
- **East Carolina University Brody School of Medicine:** North Carolina public school that does not accept out-of-state applicants: "No out-of-state applicants have been considered or admitted in over 25 years."[20]
- **Emory School of Medicine:** World-renowned MPH program with physical proximity to the CDC. The curriculum also includes a 5-month "Discovery Phase" during clerkships that allows students to work on research full-time. This may be extremely helpful if you become interested in a competitive specialty after clinical rotations but lack the field-specific research that most students obtained in their preclinical years.
- **George Washington School of Medicine:** If you have taken the MCAT multiple times, the school will take the highest score for each subsection across multiple takes.[21]
- **Hofstra University:** All incoming medical students are EMT trained. Lectures are mandatory and not recorded for remote access. Gross anatomy lab also has pre-prepared bodies with corresponding radiographic imaging.
- **Howard University College of Medicine:** Historically Black medical school that graduates the largest number of Black physicians.

---

[20] Selection Factors. Available at: https://medicine.ecu.edu/admissions/selection-factors/. Accessed July 8, 2022.
[21] MD Program Frequently Asked Questions. Available at: https://smhs.gwu.edu/academics/md-program/admissions/faqs#mcat –this is called superscoring! . Accessed July 8, 2022.

- **Loma Linda University School of Medicine:** Seventh-Day Adventist medical school with a strong emphasis on Christian principles. Consider the following recommendations from their student handbook:[22]
  - Premarital/extramarital sex: "Faculty, staff, students, administrators, and trustees of Loma Linda University Health are expected to respect and honor Christian sexual standards as held by the Seventh-day Adventist Church. We believe that God's ideal for sexuality is achieved when premarital and extramarital sexual expression and conduct are chaste and behaviors that suggest otherwise are avoided."
  - Regular chapel attendance: "In keeping with the commitment of the University's mission, students must meet special expectations, such as attendance at required Chapel services in the University Church… More than two absences per quarter may jeopardize your status in school."
  - Tobacco and alcohol: "The University holds that a lifestyle that is free of alcohol, tobacco, marijuana, and recreational/illegal drugs is essential for achieving this goal. University policy is that all students are expected to refrain from the use of tobacco, alcohol, and other recreational or unlawful drugs during the period of their enrollment at the University… The University reserves the right to investigate any student where reasonable suspicion exists of drug or alcohol involvement. This includes the right to search a personal office, locker, on-campus vehicle or residence hall room, or personal property."
- **Mayo Medical School:** Significant financial aid, with an average scholarship of $35,000 in 2018 toward the tuition of $57,170.[23] Students can also rotate at all three Mayo Clinic locations (Minnesota, Florida, Arizona) for clerkships with subsidized travel.
- **Meharry Medical College:** Historically Black medical school.
- **Midwestern University Chicago College of Osteopathic Medicine:** Yearly cost of attendance is >$100,000.[24]
- **Morehouse School of Medicine:** Historically Black medical school.
- **Mount Sinai School of Medicine:** Offers affordable (~$600/month) subsidized housing within walking distance of the medical school in Manhattan. Also offers take-home exams that may be completed over the weekend during the preclinical years.
- **New York University School of Medicine:** Every student receives a full-tuition scholarship. The school also offers a 3-year MD program that allows students to fast-track into residency at NYU in the field of their choice. The 3-year MD program is also available to students who have completed a PhD elsewhere, as well as to MD/PhD students at NYU and students with early commitment to a particular specialty. The school also offers subsidized Manhattan housing.
- **Oakland University William Beaumont School of Medicine:** All admitted students get a "free"[25] MacBook Pro. The school is also very generous with scholarships, giving aid to close to 33% of the matriculating class in some years.
- **Southern Illinois University School of Medicine:** Illinois medical school that only accepts Illinois residents.[26]
- **Tufts University Maine Track:** Collaboration between Tufts School of Medicine and Maine Medical Center that allows students to spend 2 years in Boston and 2 years in Maine for clinical rotations. The program has a heavy emphasis on rural medicine in Maine, and Maine residents have significant scholarship opportunities that lower the cost of attendance to "in-state" levels. The program also emphasizes primary care. You will likely need a car to get to rotation sites.
- **Uniformed Services University of the Health Sciences:** US federal government-run medical school that aims to produce physicians who will serve in the military and US Public Health Service. In exchange, students do not pay tuition. You do not need military experience to apply, and the majority of admitted students have no prior military experience.

---

[22] Student Handbook. Available at: https://home.llu.edu/sites/home.llu.edu/files/docs/student-handbook.pdf. Accessed July 8, 2022.

[23] Tuition and Aid. Available at: https://college.mayo.edu/academics/school-of-medicine/md-program/tuition-and-aid/. Accessed July 8, 2022.

[24] Downers Grove Tuition and Fees. Available at: https://www.midwestern.edu/downers-grove-il-campus-catalog/downers-grove-overview/office-of-student-financial-services/downers-grove-tuition-and-fees.xml. Accessed July 8, 2022.

[25] Likely included in tuition costs.

[26] FAQ. Available at: https://www.siumed.edu/studentaffairs/faq.html. Accessed July 8, 2022.

- **University of Chicago School of Medicine:** Known for merit scholarships, particularly for applicants with *very* high stats. The curriculum also includes a mandatory research project.
- **University of Illinois College of Medicine:** Significant emphasis on social justice. The school has a very diverse student population and highlights its role in producing a significant number of Black and Hispanic physicians.[27] Annual *cost of attendance* is also >$100,000 for out-of-state students,[28] and students cannot establish state residency for tuition purposes by simply attending school.
- **University of Miami:** Known for merit scholarships, and reserves ~50 class spots for the MD/MPH program.
- **University of North Carolina:** Extremely difficult to gain admission as an out-of-state applicant. The school is limited to enrolling 20 out-of-state students per year, and the vast majority of applicants are from out-of-state.[29] However, admitted out-of-state students get extremely affordable in-state tuition after 1 year of school.
- **University of Pennsylvania:** Known for merit scholarships, particularly for applicants with *very* high stats.
- **University of Pittsburgh School of Medicine:** Known for merit scholarships, particularly for applicants with *very* high stats. The curriculum also includes a mandatory research project.
- **Vanderbilt University:** Known for merit scholarships, particularly for applicants with *very* high stats.
- **Washington University in St. Louis:** Extremely high average GPA and MCAT for the matriculating class. Also known for merit scholarships, particularly for applicants with near-perfect stats.
- **Yale School of Medicine:** Mandatory research thesis that often takes students 5 years to graduate.[30]

## 27.3 Summary

Your list of schools to apply to is critically important; choosing poorly can easily result in a failed application cycle or not getting into the school that would be the best fit for you. First, you should critically evaluate your competitiveness as an applicant. Second, you should apply to all public schools in your state of residence, as well as nonpublic schools that have preferences for in-state students; also consider schools in states to which you have strong personal ties. You should also strongly consider applying to Texas schools, even if not a Texas resident. Next, you should use public resources (e.g., MSAR, ChooseDO) to identify schools that are good "fits" based on your narrative and personal interests/values. After adding all public schools and schools with in-state preferences (+/− Texas schools and other schools in areas with personal ties), you should distribute the other schools that would be good fits in a distribution of 25% reach schools, 50% match schools, and 25% safety schools. We generally advise against applying early decision. We also recommend looking through our list of schools with unique features.

27 Diversity and Inclusion. Available at: https://chicago.medicine.uic.edu/education/md-student-life/diversity/. Accessed July 8, 2022.
28 Financial Aid Federal Loan Offer Letter Cost of Attendance (COA). Available at: https://medicine.uic.edu/financial-aid/cost/. Accessed July 8, 2022.
29 The Syllabus Getting Into Med School (cont.). Available at: https://www.greensboro.com/blogs/the_syllabus/the-syllabus-getting-into-med-school-cont/article_50aedf88-f777-5d51-b3f4-adc30a4860f4.html. Accessed July 8, 2022.
30 Med school on the five-year plan. Available at: https://medicine.yale.edu/news/yale-medicine-magazine/med-school-on-the-fiveyear-plan/. Accessed July 8, 2022.

# 28 Primary Application: AMCAS, AACOMAS, and TMDSAS

*Joel Thomas*

In Chapter 20, The Big Picture we discussed the *primary application*, the component of your application sent to every school. Different types of schools have different primary applications. US MD schools accept the AMCAS (American Medical College Application Service), DO schools the AACOMAS (American Association of Colleges of Osteopathic Medicine Application Service), and Texas medical schools the TMDSAS (Texas Medical and Dental Schools Application Service). Broadly speaking, these applications ask for your personal background and demographics (including any history of criminal or institutional infractions), grades, Medical College Admission Test (MCAT) score, extracurricular activities, letters of recommendation, and personal statement.

This chapter and the ones to follow (Chapter 29, Transcript Review; Chapter 30, Activities and Meaningful Experiences; and Chapter 31, Personal Statement) discuss primary application components. Here, we will discuss how to start your primary application, as well as basic demographic information, what materials you should have ready for the upcoming sections, and the logistics of submitting and making changes to your primary application. Before you start filling out *any* of these primary applications, you should have physical copies of your official transcripts for *all* college courses. This may require requesting official transcripts from institutions abroad (i.e., study abroad programs), your high school, or community college depending on which application service you're using and how your school reports credit in these scenarios. You should also carefully read the official guidelines for each application service and regularly refer to them when filling out the application, as the primary applications have had significant changes in the past. If you have even the slightest doubt about any application component, consult with your prehealth advisor as well as the official guidelines for your application service.

You should also brainstorm acceptable answers to a variety of narrative prompts that are common to all of the primary applications. For most applicants, this will largely be questions asking you to expand on your extracurricular activities. However, other prompts that may be applicable to certain applicants include:

- **MD/PhD and DO/PhD applicants:** "Why MD/PhD?" and "Discuss your research experience in detail."
- **Previous matriculation at a medical school (or any other health profession program):** You will need to explain why your medical education was stopped and why you're reapplying for matriculation at different institutions. "Previous matriculation" includes medical schools outside of the United States, as well.
- **Institutional/criminal record or dishonorable military discharge:** You will need to take full responsibility for the event, explain that it was an isolated lapse of character that is not representative of your general behavior, and provide evidence of prolonged good behavior and/or what you have learned from the incident.
  - For example, a satisfactory answer to institutional action for underage possession of alcohol would be, "In October of my freshman year, I was caught in possession of several bottles of beer in my dorm. I took courses on the dangers of underage drinking and have served as a peer counselor on campus for alcohol abuse since then. The experience was a wake-up call to the risks of underage drinking, and I have maintained good behavior since then."
  - Recall from Chapter 2, What Medical Schools Look For that institutional/criminal action is not necessarily the kiss of death. Depending on the severity of the infraction, you may be able to overcome your history and gain admission to a medical school. These scenarios are evaluated on a case-by-case basis, and sufficiently severe actions against you may render a medical career virtually impossible. In addition, if your institutional record was expunged or forgiven in some way, consult with your prehealth advisor to determine whether you need to disclose the action on your primary application. Likewise, if your criminal or military history has been modified by the court, you should consult with an attorney to determine whether you're obligated to disclose to medical schools (if it's not apparent per the official guidelines of the application service).

Assuming you already have a polished personal statement and have brainstormed answers for the narrative prompts, the primary application should take you several hours to complete. Most of the application is fairly straightforward, but because this component of your application is scrutinized by all of the schools you apply to, you should be extremely careful when filling it out. Moreover, some sections—particularly referring to legal and institutional action taken against you—may include questions requiring nuanced answers that can dramatically impact your overall application. Hastily answering these questions may lead to needlessly hurting your application up front *or* being forced to contact many different schools at a later time to inform them that you incorrectly filled out the application *or* having your acceptance rescinded down the line. *Again, if you have* any *doubt about an application section, refer to the official guide for that primary application and consult with your prehealth advisor.*

Because different types of medical schools use different primary applications (i.e., AMCAS for US MD schools, AACOMAS for US DO schools, and TMDSAS for Texas MD and DO schools), we will discuss each type of primary application separately.

## 28.1 AMCAS

For Fall 2020 Admissions, applicants can begin filling out AMCAS on May 1, 2019 (with the first date of submission being May 30, 2019). To begin, simply create an account on the AAMC website and use your account to fill out AMCAS.

Upon logging in, you will be taken to your "Dashboard," when you can see all application cycles you have applied to (if applicable). Select the relevant application cycle to return to (or begin) your AMCAS application for that cycle.

The AMCAS Application Page (▶ Fig. 28.1) contains four sections: your Identifying Information, the AMCAS Application components (with options to print forms), Quick Links, and Document Status. The AMCAS Application itself contains nine major components: identifying information, schools attended, biographic information, course work, work/activities, letters of evaluation, medical schools, essays, and standardized tests.

- **Identifying Information**—This is straightforward.
- **Schools Attended**—This section asks about your high school, undergraduate institution, and *all* other institutions where you have an official record of having taken a course. This may include:
  - Specific circumstances that require a careful reading of the AMCAS Guidelines include:
    ○ Study abroad.
    ○ College courses taken in high school.
    ○ Post-baccalaureate programs.
    ○ Dual degrees (e.g., BA and BS from different undergraduate schools within the same university OR bachelor + master programs).

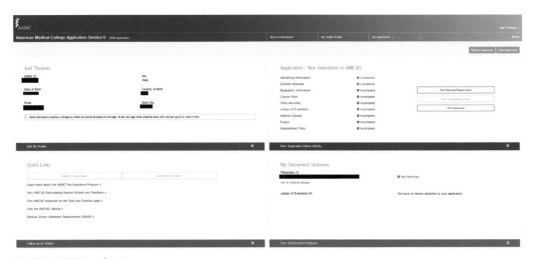

**Fig. 28.1** AMCAS application.

- **Previous medical school matriculation**—This section asks if you have ever attended or matriculated at any medical school (*in any country*) for a medical degree. If you select "yes," you are given 1,325 characters (including spaces) to explain the circumstances that led you to apply to medical school again in the United States.
- **Institutional action**—This section asks if you ever received any institutional action from a college or medical school for "unacceptable academic performance" or "conduct violation," *even if such an action does not appear on or has been removed/expunged from official transcripts.*
  - If you select "yes," you will have 1,325 characters (including spaces) to explain the incident and date of occurrence.
- You should select "yes" to whether your AMCAS information will be released to your prehealth advisors.
- **Biographic Information:** This is mostly straightforward. Triple-check your "preferred address," as the AAMC will use this information to communicate with you.
  - **Languages:** Do not exaggerate your language proficiency. Be prepared to speak in whatever language you report at your stated level of proficiency—interviewers have been known to test applicants on this.
  - **Childhood information:** This section collects information that helps admissions determine if you grew up in a low-income or medically underserved area (e.g., "income level of your family during the majority of your life from birth to age eighteen," "Were you required to contribute to the overall family income?", Pell Grant Recipient).
  - **Military discharge:** This section asks if you were discharged by the Armed Forces of the United States and whether this was a dishonorable discharge.
    - If you select "yes," you will have 1,325 characters (including spaces) to explain the incident, period of service, and rank at time of discharge.
  - **Criminal history (felony and misdemeanor):** This section asks whether you have been convicted of, or pleaded guilty/no contest to, a felony or misdemeanor.
    - *Read the instructions on the AMCAS Guidelines very carefully.* They list certain circumstances that allow you to select "no" for these questions, even if you have a history (e.g., juvenile status at the time, expunged or sealed record, state specific provisions, executive pardon). If in doubt, you may need to consult with an attorney.
    - If you select "yes," you will have 1,325 characters (including spaces) to explain the conviction(s), the sentence imposed, and the subsequent rehabilitation.
  - **Disadvantaged status:** This section asks if you would like to be considered a "disadvantaged" applicant." If you select "yes," you will have 1,325 characters (including spaces) to explain your reasoning.
    - Examples of disadvantaged status—per the AAMC—include growing up in a medically underserved or impoverished area, receiving federal benefits as a family, or having a life event affecting your immediate family with significant impacts on social or educational circumstances.
    - *This is distinct from but often related to under-represented minority (URM) status.* For example, a Black applicant whose family income is below the poverty line would qualify as both "disadvantaged" and URM, whereas a Black applicant who grew up in a wealthy, accommodating household should *not* select the "disadvantaged" box.
    - This is an opportunity for applicants to demonstrate that they have overcome and grown from relatively unique obstacles in their lives.
- **Coursework:** See Chapter 29, Transcript Review.
- **Work/Activities:** See Chapter 30, Activities and Meaningful Experiences.
- **Letters of Evaluation:** Refer to Chapter 23, Letters of Recommendation.
- **Medical Schools:** This section allows you to select the individual US MD schools that will receive your primary application.
  - This is where you can select special programs at medical schools (e.g., dual-degree programs, deferred matriculation), as well as the Early Decision Program (see Chapter 20, The Big Picture).
  - This section asks about *reapplicant status.* You are considered a reapplicant to a medical school if that medical school had received your *verified* AMCAS application (or application from another service or directly through the school, e.g., early admission program) in a prior application cycle.

- ○ *Only your "reapplicant schools" will see your reapplicant status.* For example, if you previously applied to New York Medical College but not Albany Medical College, then New York Medical College will note that you are a reapplicant but *not* Albany Medical College. New York Medical College will likely compare your current application to your previous application. Be prepared to explain in your secondary application and/or interview how you have strengthened your application to New York Medical College since then.
    1. That being said, schools are allowed to ask whether you have applied to other medical schools in the past on their secondary applications. This is a relatively uncommon question, however.
  - ○ *This is different from whether you have been accepted by any medical school through AMCAS in the past.* If this is the case and you are reapplying, *every* school will see that you have been accepted in the past and are reapplying. For example, if you have been accepted by *only* New York Medical College through AMCAS in the past and are now reapplying to New York Medical College and Albany Medical College, *both* schools will see that you were accepted in the past and are now reapplying.
  - You can continue to add medical schools to receive your primary application after you have submitted AMCAS.
  - *A small number of US MD schools do not participate in AMCAS (e.g., most Texas schools, CUNY Sophie Davis).*
- **Essays:** This is where you write your personal statement (aka "personal comments"). The prompt is "Use the space provided to explain why you want to go to medical school," and you have 5,300 characters (including spaces) to answer.
  - Refer to Chapter 31, Personal Statement for guidance on *creating* your personal statement. The AAMC recommends expanding on why you have selected medicine, what motivates you to learn more about the field, and aspects of your life that haven't already been discussed in other parts of your application (e.g., unique challenges in your life or large fluctuations in your academic history).
  - ADCOMs will receive your essay as plain text in a PDF. To avoid formatting errors, we recommend writing your polished essay in another word processor (e.g., Microsoft Word) and then *rewriting the same essay in the application.* Indenting, for example, will not be transferred into the AMCAS essay section (the AAMC recommends including an extra space between paragraphs to overcome this limit).
  - MD-PhD applicants will write two additional essays: a "Why MD-PhD?" essay that's limited to 3,000 characters (including spaces) and a description of research experiences limited to 10,000 characters (including spaces). MD-PhD applicants will also be asked to estimate their total hours of research experience.
- **Standardized Tests:** All previously scored (i.e., un-voided) MCAT attempts will be automatically uploaded to this section. Double-check that this is accurate.
  - If you are planning to take the MCAT or haven't received your score yet, answer "yes" to whether medical schools should anticipate a future score and list the date of the recently taken or planned MCAT attempt.
  - *Most medical schools require that your MCAT score is no more than 3 years old (although some accept up to 5 years).* If you are on the border, check the school's website or contact their pre-med office—there is some variance on whether it is 3 years from your application, or from matriculation.
  - Dual-degree programs may require additional test scores. You have the option of manually entering your scores for these tests, but they are *not* verified by AMCAS. As such, you may need to send those scores directly to the individual schools.

After certifying and submitting your AMCAS (with the requisite application fees), you are only allowed to change certain aspects of your identifying information, add additional letters of evaluation (i.e., *not* removing letters that were already sent), add additional medical schools, or choose to release information to your prehealth advisor. You should monitor your application regularly to ensure that submitted documents (e.g., letters of recommendation, transcripts) have been received and processed appropriately.

After receiving an initial, conditional acceptance by any medical school, you will receive an email for a background check by Certiphi Screening. You will pay $71 for this background check. Applicants from specific states may have additional stipulations regarding the background check. Refer to the AMCAS Guide for Applicants for additional details.

## 28.2 AACOMAS

To begin, simply create an account on the AACOM website and use your account to fill out AACOMAS.

The AACOMAS Application Page (▶ Fig. 28.2) contains four main sections: Personal Information, Academic History, Supporting Information, and Program Materials. At the top of the application page is a link to "Add Program," where you will add the individual schools to which you want to apply. "Submit Application" allows you to pay and submit your application, and "Check Status" allows you to check the status of your application at each of your schools.

Each of the main four sections has its own subsections.

- **Personal Information**—Most of this section is straightforward. Some questions at the end will ask about educationally/environmentally disadvantaged status (e.g., high school dropout, public assistance, first-generation college student, English as a secondary language), as well as economically disadvantaged status (*by comparing your family's tax returns to federal poverty guidelines*). Specific subsections of note include:
  - **Release statement:** This section mostly asks you to agree to standard certification and release statements (e.g., your application will be sent to the AACOM and your prehealth advisor). However, you are also asked to agree to allow programs to see that you are applying to them *before you submit* your application so they can send you information and text notifications.
  - **Influences:** You will be asked how you learned about osteopathic medicine.
  - **Other information:** If you have a history of *complicated* institutional, criminal, or military action taken against you in the past (e.g., expunged, revision, court pardon, etc.), you may want to consult with an attorney or your school's prehealth advisor as to whether you can safely omit this history from your AACOMAS.
    - **Language proficiency:** Do not exaggerate your language proficiency. Be prepared to speak in whatever language you report at your stated level of proficiency—interviewers have been known to test applicants on this!
    - **Military discharge:** If you were dishonorably discharged from the military, you will have 500 characters (including spaces) to explain your circumstances.

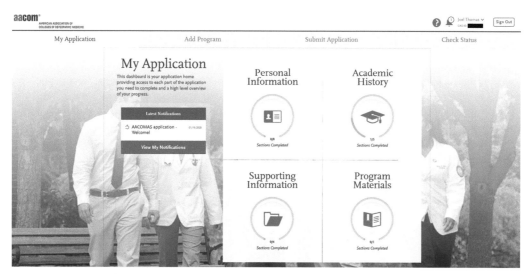

**Fig. 28.2** AACOMAS application.

- o **Criminal history:** If you were convicted of a misdemeanor or felony, you will have 500 characters (including spaces) for each to explain your circumstances, the consequences, and what you have learned from the incident.
    - o **Institutional action:** If you had any institutional action taken against you for academic or student conduct reasons, you will have 500 characters (including spaces) for each type of offense (academic vs. conduct) to explain your circumstances.
    - o **Denied readmission:** If you were denied readmission to any academic program for academic reasons, you will have 500 characters (including spaces) to explain.
    - o **License infraction:** If you had any sort of license, certification, registration infraction or revocation of clinical privileges, you will have 500 characters (including spaces) to explain.
    - o **Prior matriculation at medical or health profession school:** You will have 500 characters (including spaces) to explain.
- **Academic History**—See Chapter 29, Transcript Review.
    - **Standardized tests:** Whereas MCAT scores are automatically sent to AMCAS (as both are under the auspices of the AAMC), you must choose to release your MCAT scores to AACOMAS through the online MCAT score report. You will also have to manually enter your MCAT scores.
- **Supporting Information**
    - **Evaluations:** See Chapter 23, Letters of Recommendation.
        - o Letters of recommendation: waive access, and allow school and AACOMAS to contact them
    - **Experiences:** See Chapter 30, Activities and Meaningful Experiences.
    - **Achievements:** These include awards, honors, presentations, publications, and scholarships. You will have 600 characters (including spaces) to elaborate.
    - **Personal statement:** Refer to Chapter 31, Personal Statement for guidance on *creating* your personal statement. This should *not* be identical to your AMCAS or TMDSAS personal statement (if applicable).
        - o You should specifically emphasize your experiences with osteopathic medicine and how you came to decide that osteopathic medicine best aligns with your personal and professional values. Note that many matriculants to DO schools do *not* feel this way. As discussed in Chapter 24, DO, MD, and International Schools, most practicing osteopathic physicians do *not* use osteopathic manipulation, and the once prominent historical differences between MD and DO practice have largely dissipated. Nonetheless, ADCOM members will want to hear why you are interested in attending a DO school specifically. While it may be the case that the average GPA and MCAT scores at the DO schools that you're considering happen to be lower (and closer to your GPA and MCAT), increased odds of admission is *not* a convincing reason to the ADCOM.
        - o In general, DO schools emphasize primary care and "holistic health" that views the patient as a whole, rather than focusing on disease. You should emphasize any experiences with underserved populations and primary care.
- **Program materials**—Several of the programs you've added will have specific additional requirements such as individual entry of prerequisite courses.

After submitting your application, you can update planned or in-progress courses with final grades during specific time periods. You *must* send an official transcript to AACOMAS *after* hearing that your application was successfully updated (i.e., do *not* send the transcript before updating). You can also update your basic information, add additional programs, edit or delete incomplete letters of recommendation, and add new test scores, experiences, and achievements.

## 28.3 TMDSAS

For Fall 2020 Admissions, applicants can begin filling out (*and submitting*) TMDSAS on **May 1**. However, applicants do not appear to be at any significant disadvantage by submitting in June (▶ Fig. 28.3). Beyond June, however, it seems as though applicants are at a comparative disadvantage in terms of getting interview invites.

To do so, simply create an account on the TMDSAS website (Applicant Login -> "New User? Register Here") and use your account to fill out TMDSAS.

Note that as of 2021, the following Texas MD and DO schools (i.e., *not University of the Incarnate Word School of Osteopathic Medicine)* participate in TMDSAS: Baylor College of Medicine, UT Southwestern, UT

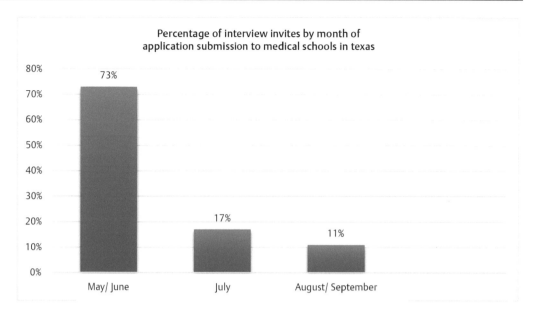

**Fig. 28.3** Interview invites by month of TMDSAS submission. (Adapted from: Tweet[1] by TMDSAS Support.)

Galveston, McGovern Medical School at Long School of Medicine at UT Health San Antonio, Texas A&M, University of North Texas Health Science Center Texas College of Osteopathic Medicine, Texas Tech in Lubbock, Texas Tech in El Paso, University of North Texas–Texas College of Osteopathic Medicine, UT Austin Dell, UT Rio Grande Valley School of Medicine, University of Houston College of Medicine, and Sam Houston State University College of Osteopathic Medicine.

TMDSAS also offers a "**match**" that is *only available to Texas residents.* In this process, applicants that are interviewed at schools participating in TMDSAS rank the schools they interviewed at in order of preference for matriculation. The schools also rank interviewees, and TMDSAS then "matches" applicants to schools based on this data.

From November 15 to December 31, schools may send prematch acceptance offers to interviewees. Accepting an offer reserves the spot but is nonbinding; declining the offer frees it to another interview. *Notify the school as soon as possible with your response to their offer.* During this time, an interviewee may hold multiple offers.

In addition, interviewees must still rank schools according to their preferences and submit a final rank list by January 19. On February 1, interviewees may receive a *single* acceptance offer from the school that they ranked highest *if* that school also ranked the interviewee favorably. This acceptance is *not* binding. Interviewees are still in the running for future potential offers from schools that they ranked higher. However, interviewees are taken out of the running for acceptances from schools *lower* than the highest ranked school that offered an acceptance. In addition, interviewees may receive *no* offers if none of their ranked schools ranked them favorably.[2]

To illustrate, let's say Bill interviewed at five schools: A, B, C, D, and E. He ranks them,

1. School A
2. School B
3. School C
4. School D
5. School E

---

[1] Available at: Did you know that for EY2018, 73% of applicants that were invited to an interview submitted their TMDSAS application in May/June? https://twitter.com/TMDSASSupport/status/961662554983550976/photo/1 02/18/2018. Accessed July 8, 2022.

[2] Refer to the TMDSAS page explaining the match process: https://www.premedpath.com/application-cycle/tmdsas

Schools A and B rank Bill relatively low on *their* rank lists. However, Bill is ranked in the top 5 interviewees for schools C and D. In December, he receives acceptance offers from schools C and D. Come February 1, he is matched to school C. *His application is now withdrawn from schools D and E*, but he does not have to matriculate at school C. If schools B and C choose to offer Bill an acceptance down the line, his application will be withdrawn from the schools on his rank list (i.e., school C if accepted to B, schools C and B if accepted to A). Applicants finally commit to matriculate on April 30, allowing them to weigh their Match offer with schools outside of TMDSAS (e.g., AMCAS, AACOMAS) if relevant.

You should also be aware that some Texas schools require CASPer (see Chapter 32, Altus Suite: CASPer, Snapshot, and Duet). As of 2020, these include Texas A&M University College of Medicine, Texas Tech University HSC School of Medicine, Texas Tech University HSC Paul L. Foster School of Medicine, The University of Texas Medical Branch at Galveston, and Long School of Medicine UT Health San Antonio. If you plan to apply to any of these schools, you should take Altus Suite in March to early July.

Of note, TMDSAS has significantly shorter character limits (300 including spaces) for describing extracurriculars compared to AMCAS (700 including spaces).

We will now review the components of TMDSAS.

- **Select Schools and Application History**—This is mostly straightforward. You are also asked to disclose whether you will be applying to schools through non-TMDSAS services (and provide a list of non-TMDSAS schools to which you are applying).
  - **Application History (i.e., reapplicant status):** You are asked to disclose whether you have had a TMDSAS *transmitted* to schools in the past. If "yes," you must explain where and when you applied, as well as the outcomes of that application.
    - If you are a reapplicant, then certain portions of your prior TMDSAS will be rolled over. However, you should still carefully check each section and make appropriate updates.
- **Personal Information**
  - **General demographic:** This is mostly straightforward. You are asked to explain if "someone other than your biological parent(s) [played] a role in your life."
  - **Socioeconomic info:** This is mostly straightforward.
  - **Military service:** This is mostly straightforward.
  - **Financial info:** This is mostly straightforward.
  - **Criminal history:** The TMDSAS application handbook lists specific circumstances in which you do not need to disclose your criminal history. In addition, if there are changes to your criminal history (e.g., being *charged* with a misdemeanor or felony) AFTER submission of TMDSAS, you must inform the application service *and* the admissions' office of each school you haven't applied to within 10 business days of the charge or conviction.
- **Education History**
  - **High school:** This is mostly straightforward. Note that you are required to self-report your Scholastic Aptitude Test (SAT) and American College Testing (ACT) score. You must pick your single overall best attempt and thus *cannot superscore results of individual sections across multiple test attempts.*
  - **Colleges attended:** You must indicate future coursework. If you are unsure of your future courses, enter placeholder information and *return to update this information after submission.*
    - TMDSAS has specific directions for foreign courses; refer to the application handbook.
    - **Fresh Start:** TMDSAS asks whether applicants participated in the "Academic Fresh Start Provision." If yes, they must provide all transcripts and relevant documentation. Refer to the TMDSAS handbook for additional information.
    - **Release of information:** You're strongly encouraged to select "yes" to allow your Health Professions Advisor to view your application.
- **Transcripts**—See Chapter 29, Transcript Review. Note that the "Colleges attended" section must be completed before sending transcripts.
  - **Terms attended:** This is mostly straightforward. Note that Winter terms are defined by the year in which the term was completed, which may differ from how your institution defines them (e.g., "December 2018–January 2019" would be a Winter 2019 term for TMDSAS).
- **Training History**—Here, you will clarify, if applicable, non-traditional status, interruptions to your education or profession, and institutional action.
  - **Non-traditional applicant status:** If you identify as a non-traditional applicant you will have 1,000 characters to explain your circumstances. Broadly speaking, non-traditional applicants are those who

did not follow the "standard" educational path of "graduate high school -> enroll in college -> apply to medical school during college OR after 1–2 gap years."

- ○ The following would certainly count as non-traditional applications: medicine as a second career, significant educational gap, part-time college student, working full-time during college, and GED instead of high school diploma.
- ○ If you are unsure whether your particular educational path is non-traditional, discuss with your prehealth advisor.
- If you are the subject of any institutional action or state licensure board action AFTER submission of TMDSAS, you must inform the application service *and* the admissions' office of each school you haven applied to within 10 business days.
- **Activities**—See Chapter 30, Activities and Meaningful Experiences.
- **Essays**—See Chapter 31, Personal Statement for help constructing the personal statement. Note that TMDSAS has *multiple* personal statement prompts. As with the AMCAS and TMDSAS essays, you're strongly encouraged to *first* complete your polished essay draft in a word processor (e.g., Microsoft Word) and then manually transcribe into the application service to avoid formatting errors.
  - **Why medicine:** The first prompt "asks you to explain your motivation to seek a career in medicine. You are asked to include the value of your experiences that prepare you to be a physician." You have 5,000 characters (including spaces).
  - **Diversity:** The second prompt asks you to "describe your personal characteristics (background, talents, skills, etc.) or experiences that would add to the educational experience of others." You have 2,500 characters, including spaces. See Chapter 33, Secondary Application for strategies to discuss how you would contribute to diversity.
  - **"Optional" essay:** You have 2,500 characters (including spaces) to discuss anything else relevant to your application that was not already discussed. You are **strongly** encouraged to complete this essay.
  - **DO/PhD and MD/PhD:** You have 5,000 characters (including spaces) to "Explain your motivation to seek a MD/PhD or DO/PhD dual degree... [and] your research interests and career goals..."
- **Proof of Texas Residency**—This section allows you to provide evidence of Texas residency, e.g., for participation in the Match. You should refer to the TMDSAS Handbook for specifics, but this includes Texas high school graduation, permanent residency in Texas, significant gainful employment, property ownership, and ownership of a Texas business entity. Depending on your particular circumstances, you may need to upload supporting documents (e.g., proof of property or business ownership).
  - Applicants with permanent resident, Visa, or DACA (Deferred Action Childhood Arrival) status should refer to the TMDSAS Handbook for specific instructions.
- **Supporting Documents**
  - Upload photo: You must upload a professional photo taken in business attire (i.e., a suit). It must be smaller than 100 kB.
  - MCAT score: You must send your MCAT score(s) to TMDSAS. Refer to the TMDSAS Handbook for instructions.
    - ○ You must also update your application with any changes to planned test dates after submission.
    - ○ Note that MCAT scores up to *5 years old* may be used for TMDSAS, compared to *3 years* for AMCAS.
  - Letters of evaluation: See Chapter 23, Letters of Recommendation. TMDSAS has a strict limit of three individual letters of evaluation *or* a Committee Letter/Packet, with an option to submit one additional letter.
- **Chronology of Activities**—This is a section that is automatically generated from information entered in prior sections. It details your educational/professional career from high school graduation to matriculation at medical school for this application cycle.
  - Click "Show Activities Calendar" to view the generated chronology. If there are gaps greater than 3 months without autopopulated explanations, you must explain what you did during this time.
  - Of note, only the first 50 characters (including spaces) of your extracurricular descriptions will be carried over to your Chronology of Activities. As discussed in Chapter 30, Activities and Meaningful Experiences, you should be mindful in how you describe your extracurriculars to produce a more enticing Chronology of Activities.
- **Payment and Submission**—This is straightforward.

After submitting your TMDSAS, you are only allowed to change certain aspects of your application, e.g., personal info, coursework, MCAT test dates, *letters of evaluation (i.e., changing evaluators)*, proof of residency and residency documents, schools applied to, photograph (*only if the photo is missing or does not meet requirements*), and chronology of activities. You should monitor your application regularly to ensure that submitted documents (e.g., letters of recommendation, transcripts) have been received and processed appropriately. TMDSAS may also make automatic changes to aspects of your application; if you believe any of this is in error, you should immediately contact them through the internal message service. You also need to submit updated transcripts as you receive additional grades at the end of each term, and you should also update your placeholder courses after submission once you finalize your future schedule.

You are also able to submit the secondary application (see Chapter 33, Secondary Application) for certain schools without receiving an invitation. These include UT Southwestern and Texas A&M (per their application portal). The other schools either do not have secondary applications or send you an invitation to complete the secondary.

## 28.4 Summary

Submit your primary application as soon as possible, as accurately as possible. Read the available/official guide that comes with the primary application to make sure you are filling it out correctly; given how these applications are constantly evolving, you *must* cross-check any recommendation made in this book with the official instruction. Consult with your pre-med advisor or another trusted source if you have additional concerns or questions.

# 29 Transcript Review

*Joel Thomas*

Transferring your transcript information to your primary application is a straightforward process for most applicants. First, you manually enter all of your college courses and the grades you received into the primary application. Next, you request for official copies of those transcripts to be sent to the primary application service (e.g., by speaking with your university's registrar). The primary application service will receive your official records and cross-check your manually submitted information with the official records. If there are no discrepancies and your submitted information is consistent with the application service's specifications, then your application will be "verified/validated." *For American Medical College Application System (AMCAS) and American Association of Colleges of Osteopathic Medicine (AACOMAS), only verified applications are sent to the medical schools.*[1] If your submitted information is inconsistent with the official records or does not meet the specifications of the primary application service, you may experience delays to verification that can disadvantage your application.

We chose to devote an entire chapter to this task because even minor discrepancies between the submitted information on your primary application and your official transcript can lead to **application delays** of up to several weeks. As mentioned in Chapter 20, The Big Picture, applications are evaluated on a rolling basis; **having your application evaluated weeks late can thus place you at a significant disadvantage**. In addition, different primary application services have their own requirements for entering specific transcript sections. As such, lack of attention to detail may also lead to an application delay.

Before you proceed with transcript entry, you should obtain a copy of your official transcript from *every* institution where you *attempted* college-level coursework, even if you did not receive credit. This includes community colleges where you may have taken summer courses, registered courses that did not earn credit (e.g., incompletes, audits, withdrawals, failures), home study programs, and military education (among others). All things considered, if you have any doubt about whether you need a transcript from a specific institution, you should contact your prehealth advisor and AMCAS directly.

You do not, however, need your high school transcript; Advanced Placement (AP) and International Baccalaureate (IB) credit per your college transcript should be sufficient *unless you formally took college courses through an institution in middle or high school (even if these courses did not count toward any grade or degree)*.[2] If this is the case, you should request transcripts from those institutions as well.

In addition, the different primary application services have their own instructions for courses taken in other countries, generally distinguishing between (1) credits transferred to a US or Canadian institution (i.e., study abroad), (2) nontransferred credit from a foreign institution, (3) medical degree coursework,[3] and (4) credits taken at an American College Overseas.[4]

Because of the differences in transcript entry instructions, we will now discuss each primary application separately. For each application service, we will discuss the components that are likely to be relevant to the majority of applications. We will flag specific instructions for special circumstances that may apply to a minority of readers: *we urge these readers to refer to the official instructions of the application service to obtain additional, detailed information.*

## 29.1 AMCAS

**Transcript requests to yourself:** Do this *before* the application service opens (~May 1) so that you can accurately enter your courses.

**Transcript requests to AMCAS:** After listing the schools where you *attempted* college courses on AMCAS, you will be able to print a Barcoded Transcript Request Form to send to your registrar(s). This form allows AMCAS to easily file the mailed transcript(s) with your submitted application. Thus, you

---

[1] TMDAS simply updates medical schools with a "validated" status to your application after you have been interviewed at any program.

[2] AP and IB courses taken in high school that did not result in college credit need not be reported.

[3] AMCAS states that DO coursework should be listed under "regular coursework."

[4] 2023 AMCAS® Applicant Guide. Available at: https://students-residents.aamc.org/media/11616/download: 2022 AMCAS Applicant Guide. Accessed July 8, 2022.

should request that the registrar include the Transcript Request Form with your mailed transcript. Alternatively, *some* undergraduate institutions are allowed to submit electronic transcripts; contact your school's registrar to determine if this is the case.[5]

You can request that your official transcripts be sent to AMCAS as soon as it opens (~May 1). This way, they will already have your documents the moment that you submit your application (~May 30), minimizing the time to begin the verification process. However, most institutions will not have Spring grades by then.

As such,

- *If your spring grades are relatively unimportant*: Request your transcripts be sent as soon as AMCAS opens. There won't be any significant changes to your application if your spring grades are largely representative of your academic performance before then.
- *If your spring grades are important*: Check with your institution(s) about the latest date that Spring grades will be entered. If they are before the date that AMCAS opens (May 30), then you are probably fine to wait for spring grades, especially if you can request (i.e., pay extra for) express mailing. "Important" spring grades include a significant increase in grade point average (GPA), 3 + prerequisite courses, etc.

AMCAS will send you regular email notifications between the time of application submission and receipt of all official transcripts; you can also check the status of sent transcripts on the application main menu. In addition, you will be contacted by AMCAS if they believe that they are missing official transcripts.

## 29.1.1 AMCAS Transcript Entry Synopsis

Transcript entry is done in the "Course Entry" section. You must enter your courses in chronological order, exactly as written on the official transcripts. Enter the course name number, credit hours, and grade exactly as they appear on your transcript; refer to the official instructions if you cannot fit the information exactly. You will also classify each course by the subject matter (e.g., biology, chemistry, arts, education, philosophy and religion, etc.) by the *content* of the course, which may differ from the department that administered it per your transcript; **refer to the official guide for an exhaustive list of recommended classifications.** You will also select whether the course included a lab component, as well as whether it was an honors course.

If there is no grade on your transcript because the grade has not been finalized, simply leave "grade" empty. **However, if you had received an official grade at any point (e.g., repeated or removed course), you *must* enter the original grade.** For courses that are pending grades, designate them as "current" or "future" courses accordingly.

If you attended multiple institutions (e.g., university during fall/spring and community college during the summer), you MUST list where the courses were *taken*, even if credit was transferred elsewhere. For example, a summer biology course at your community college should be listed as taken at the community college, even if your main university accepted credit for that course.

Your "year in school" (e.g., high school, freshman, sophomore, junior, senior) is determined by credit hours accumulated thus far; refer to the AMCAS guide for specific instructions (particularly if you came in with significant AP/IB credit OR if you took non-AP/College Level Examination Program (CLEP) college courses in high school).[6] In addition, the AMCAS year starts in summer and ends in spring, so even if your institution counts a summer course in 2019 as part of the 2018–2019 school year, you will enter it in AMCAS as part of the "2019–2020 school year." AMCAS also has specific instructions for applicants who did not complete a college degree in 4 years (e.g., 3 or 5 y), as well as those who completed combined programs (e.g., BA/MS) or post-baccalaureate programs.

---

[5] If your institution does not provide official transcripts, the registrar must send AMCAS an official letter stating this is the case. In addition, if your institution has closed, you must obtain archived records, e.g., from the State Department of Education/Commerce or the National Student Clearinghouse.

[6] AP, CLEP, and Exempt courses for which you received credit should be counted as "Freshman" credit or whatever year your school counted them on your transcript. AP credit should be counted only once, even if multiple institutions gave you credit for the same AP course; use whichever school gave you more credit hours. Refer to the guide for additional instructions on AP and AP-like courses.

After verification, your AMCAS application will contain the following information in the "Coursework" section:

| Symbol | Meaning |
|---|---|
| / | A course verified without correction. |
| X | A course verified with corrections. |
| O | A course listed in the Coursework section but not reflected on an official transcript; format corrections not required. |
| ⊗ | A course listed in the Coursework section but not reflected on an official transcript; format corrections have been made. |
| ≠ | Coursework not intended to be verified by AMCAS. |

AMCAS will also generate its *own GPA* for your application using the verified GPA to create a more standardized GPA across applicants. This includes adding *all* grades from the official transcript (including those not counted toward a degree or your overall GPA per your school) and omitting grades that are not listed on the official transcript (e.g., spring grades that were not yet on the official transcript). AP, IB, and pass/fail credit do not contribute to the AMCAS GPA but are simply reported under "supplemental (credit) hours." While AMCAS GPAs almost always differ from your institutions(s),[7] they rarely do so by a significant amount.

After your transcript is verified, you have the option of disputing changes (e.g., incorrect course classification) with an academic change request in the "Quick Links" section of the main menu. In general, we do not recommend doing this unless there are significant discrepancies that would have a major impact on your application, as you risk delay in verification.

## 29.1.2  AMCAS Course Entry Special Cases

Of note, if your school allows academic forgiveness for repeated courses, AMCAS requires official records of both the original grade (and attempted records) and the new, final grade. Likewise, AMCAS will separately count each attempt of a repeated course, even if your institution only counts the final grade toward your GPA.

Refer to the AMCAS Applicant Guide for specific instructions if the following circumstances apply to you:
- CEGEP/Grade 13 credit.
- Clock hours; Continuing Education Units (CEUs).
- Courses with narrative evaluations.
- Delayed/deferred matriculation to medical school.
- Deferred grade, i.e., course that takes multiple terms to complete before a final grade.
- Foreign coursework (with specific instructions for American colleges overseas).
  - Distinguished from study abroad.
- Full-year courses.
- Incomplete grade.
- Exempt grade.
- Graduate coursework taken as undergraduate (or vice versa).
- Life Experience Credit.
- Medical degree coursework (with specific instructions for "US MD" coursework).
- Military credit.
- Multiple instances of independent study, orchestra, etc.
- No record, i.e., from administrative/logistical error by the institution.
- "Repeating" an AP class, e.g., taking Intro to Biology in college after receiving AP Biology Credit.

---

[7] For example, AMCAS will distinguish between (+) and (−) grades, even if your institution's GPA does not.

- Tiered pass/fail, i.e., high pass, pass, fail.
- USAFI/DANTES credit.
- Withdrawal.

### 29.1.3 AMCAS Concluding Thoughts

Refer to the AMCAS Applicant Guide at all times. *Carefully* read the sections on Course Entry, as they are liable to change since the time this book was written. Lastly, AMCAS is very straightforward about the consequences of inaccurate transcript entry; check again to make sure you have avoided the following errors:

> **Most common reasons for a returned application**
>
> - Failure to include original grades and credit hours for repeated courses.
> - Failure to list 10 or more courses that appear on an official transcript.
> - Failure to list 10 or more credits as they appear on your official transcript(s).
> - Failure to list 10 or more grades as they appear on your official transcript(s).
> - Failure to list coursework in chronological order.

## 29.2 AACOMAS

### 29.2.1 Transcript Requests to Yourself

Do this *before* the application service opens (~May 2) so that you can accurately enter your courses. Don't forget to request transcripts from any institution attended as part of study abroad, as well. AACOMAS distinguishes between study abroad at an overseas US institution (refer to the list on the AACOMAS website) vs. study abroad at a "foreign" institution that does not appear on your official transcript. Refer to the specific AACOMAS instructions.

Of note, AACOMAS has specific instructions for foreign non-English-speaking institutions. That is, while AACOMAS *itself* does not require any documentation for foreign, non-English courses, *individual DO schools* may require a "US equivalency report" by a third-party service that provides a standardized translation of foreign coursework. Refer to specific instructions on the AACOMAS guide, and get into contact with these agencies *as soon as possible*.

### 29.2.2 Transcript Requests to AACOMAS

After listing the schools where you *attempted* college courses on AACOMAS, you will be able to print a Transcript Request Form to send to your registrar(s). This form allows AACOMAS to easily file the mailed transcript(s) with your submitted application. Thus, you should request that the registrar include the Transcript Request Form with your mailed transcript, as well as your AACOMAS ID number. Alternatively, *some* undergraduate institutions are allowed to submit electronic transcripts[8]; contact your school's registrar to determine if this is the case.

You can request that your official transcripts be sent to AACOMAS as soon as it opens (~May 2). This way, they will already have your documents the moment that you submit your application, minimizing the time to begin the verification process. However, most institutions will not have Spring grades by then. As such,

- *If your spring grades are relatively unimportant*: Request your transcripts be sent as soon as AACOMAS opens. There won't be any significant changes to your application if your spring grades are largely representative of your academic performance before then.
- *If your spring grades are important*: Check with your institution(s) about the latest date that Spring grades will be entered. If they are before the date that AACOMAS is sent to schools (June 15), then you are probably fine to wait for spring grades, especially if you can request (i.e., pay extra for) express mailing. "Important" spring grades include a significant increase in GPA, 3 + prerequisite courses, etc.

---

[8] Specifically, if they use Credentials Solutions, Parchment, or National Student Clearinghouse services.

You should regularly monitor the "Check Status" page on AACOMAS to assess the status of your transcript(s).

## 29.2.3 AACOMAS Transcript Entry Synopsis

Transcript entry is the bulk of the "Academic History" section. AACOMAS allows two options for transcript entry.

The first is **Paid Professional Transcript Entry**, through which AACOMAS representatives manually enter the information from your official transcript(s). This essentially ensures that your application will not be delayed as long as they receive all the required documents. It costs $69 for up to three transcripts, $95 for four to six, and $145 for seven or more transcripts. Refer to the Applicant Guide for additional specific instructions on this service.

We do not have strong opinions about Professional Transcript Entry. Consider using it if you can afford it and have a complicated academic history, but be aware that multiple buyers have reported typos in the final product. In addition, for most applicants, transcript entry is straightforward and probably not worth the professional fee.

We will now discuss the second option: manual transcript entry. You must enter your courses in chronological order, exactly as written on the official transcripts. First, specify how your school classifies terms (e.g., semester, quarter, trimester) and enter terms and your academic status (e.g., freshman, sophomore, junior, senior, graduate, post-baccalaureate—refer to AACOMAS instructions). Next, enter the course name, number, credit hours, and grade exactly as they appear on your transcript; refer to the official instructions if you cannot fit the information exactly.[9]

Of note, if your institution uses "credit units," e.g., 1.0 or 0.50 formats, check whether your transcript has a *conversion ratio* to semester hours, e.g., "1 unit is equivalent to 4 semester hours." If not, contact your registrar's office to confirm. If there *is* a conversion ratio, you must *manually* convert the credit units to semester hours and enter the converted semester hours on AACOMAS. For example, 0.50 credit units may be converted to 2.0 credits; you would enter this as 2.0 credits on AACOMAS. Refer to the Applicant Guide for additional guidance.

You will also classify each course by the subject matter (e.g., biology, chemistry, arts, education, philosophy and religion, etc.); refer to "AACOMAS Course Subjects" for an exhaustive list of recommended classifications.[10] You will also select whether the course included a lab component, as well as whether it was an honors course.

Refer to AACOMAS for "Academic Status" (e.g., high school, freshman, sophomore, junior, senior), particularly if you did not complete a college degree in 4 years (e.g., 3 or 5 y), or if you participated in a combined program (e.g., BA/MS) or post-baccalaureate program.

If there is no grade on your transcript because the grade has not been finalized, simply leave "grade" empty. Designate "Planned/In Progress" courses without grades accordingly. Note that any term containing such courses cannot be marked as "complete."

AACOMAS will also generate its *own GPA* for your application using the verified GPA to create a more standardized GPA across applicants. This includes adding *all* grades from the official transcript (including all grades earned for repeated courses—*AACOMAS does not honor institutional grade forgiveness/replacement or academic renewal policies*) and combining GPAs across multiple institutions in the same year. While AACOMAS GPAs almost always differ from your institutions(s), they rarely do so by a significant amount.

After your transcript is verified, you have the option of disputing changes (e.g., incorrect course classification) with an academic change request by emailing AACOMAS with the subject line "Course Subject Correction"; refer to the Applicant Guide for additional instruction. In general, we do not recommend doing this unless there are significant discrepancies that would have a major impact on your application, as you risk delay in verification.

---

[9] Entering credit hours may be confusing. There are two drop-down boxes; the first is the whole number digit for credit hours, and the second is the decimal digit for credit hours. For example, a course awarding 4.0 credits would be entered as "4" in the first box and "0" in the second box.

[10] In contrast to AMCAS, AACOMAS subject assignments are based on the title/department on your official transcript, *not* the content of the course itself.

## 29.2.4  AACOMAS Course Entry Special Cases

Refer to the AACOMAS Guide for specific instructions if the following circumstances apply to you:
• Continuing Education Units (CEUs).
• CLEP credit.
• Courses with narrative evaluations.
• Courses with "suggested" credits and/or grades.
• Foreign coursework (with specific instructions for American colleges overseas):
  - Distinguished from study abroad.
  - Refer to the specific instructions for English vs. French-Canadian Canadian institutions.
• Graduate coursework taken as undergraduate (or vice versa).
• Incomplete grade.
• IB credit.
• JST credit.
• Military credit.
• Repeated courses.
• USAFI/DANTES credit.
• Withdrawal.

## 29.2.5  AACOMAS Concluding Thoughts

Refer to the AACOMAS Applicant Guide at all times. *Carefully* read the sections on Course Entry, as they are liable to change since the time this book was written. Lastly, AACOMAS is very straightforward about the consequences of inaccurate transcript entry; check again to make sure you have avoided the following errors:

### Posting Delays

The following scenarios can cause delayed application posting/processing and should be avoided whenever possible:
• A transcript is not accompanied by a Transcript Request Form or is accompanied by the incorrect form.
• A transcript is not addressed specifically to "AACOMAS."
• A school you attended is missing from the Colleges Attended section. We cannot attach a transcript to your application unless the school is listed.
• An incorrect school name is listed in the Colleges Attended section. We cannot attach a transcript to your application until it is corrected.
• The name on a transcript cannot be found in the AACOMAS database, either because your name changed, was misspelled on the transcript, was misspelled on the application, or you have not yet created a AACOMAS account.

### Rejected Transcripts

The following scenarios can cause transcripts to be rejected and should be avoided whenever possible:
• A transcript is unofficial, marked as student-issued, or is addressed to someone other than AACOMAS.
• A transcript is missing pages or was severely damaged in the mail.
• A document received by AACOMAS is not a transcript.
• An incorrect transcript was received; this can occur when another student at your school has the same or similar name and you did not provide enough information to the registrar when you requested your transcript. Be sure to provide your schools with as much information as possible so they can properly identify your records.

## 29.3  TMDSAS

### 29.3.1  Transcript Requests to Yourself

Do this *before* the application service opens (~May 1) so that you can accurately enter your courses. You also need copies of transcripts from other colleges where you took courses, even if your undergraduate institution accepted the transfer credit. If you took college-level courses (*excluding AP or IB courses*) in high school, TMDSAS also requires official transcripts from those institutions (even if they did not count for credit at any college).

TMDSAS also distinguishes between types of study abroad experiences: if the study abroad took place through your undergraduate institution and appears on its transcript, you do not need a separate transcript from the abroad institution. For other study abroad programs, refer to TMDSAS instructions.

## 29.3.2 Transcript Requests to TMDSAS

After listing the schools where you *attempted* college courses on AACOMAS, you will be able to print a Transcript Request Form to send to your registrar(s). This form allows TMDSAS to easily file the mailed transcript(s) with your submitted application. Thus, you should request that the registrar include the Transcript Request Form with your mailed transcript. Throughout the application cycle, you will update your TMDSAS with grades for future courses; *you must also send updated official transcripts with these grades*. TMDSAS also allows for electronic transcript delivery. Refer to TMDSAS instructions and discuss with your school's registrar for additional information.

You should only send your transcript(s) to TMDSAS *after Spring grades are finalized*; otherwise, your application may have significant delays.[11]

You will be notified upon transcript receipt, but you should also regularly monitor the "Supporting Documents" section of the "Status" page on TMDSAS.

## 29.3.3 TMDSAS Transcript Entry Synopsis

Transcript entry is done in the "Transcripts" section. You must enter your courses in chronological order, exactly as written on the official transcripts. First, select how your institution classifies terms (e.g., quarter, semester). Next, specify the terms that you attended each institution listed in your "Colleges attended" section. Note that TMDSAS defines **Winter** terms by the year in which the coursework was completed, which may differ from how they are listed on your transcript. For example, "Winter 2018" on your official transcript that ended in January 2019 should be listed as "Winter 2019" on TMDSAS.

Next, enter the course name, number, credit hours, and grade exactly as they appear on your transcript; refer to the official instructions if you cannot fit the information exactly. TMDSAS also requests that you capitalize the first letter of all words for the course name, even if it appears in all caps on your transcript (e.g., "INTRODUCTION TO BIOLOGY" should be written as "Introduction To Biology")

Of note, if your institution uses "**credit units**," e.g., 1.0 or 0.50 formats, check whether your transcript has a *conversion ratio* to semester hours, e.g., "1 unit is equivalent to 4 semester hours." If not, contact your registrar's office to confirm. If there *is* a conversion ratio, you must *manually* convert the credit units to semester hours and enter the convert semester hours on TMDSAS. For example, 0.50 credit units may be converted to 2.0 credits; you would enter this as 2.0 credits on TMDSAS. Refer to the Applicant Guide for additional guidance.

You will also classify each course by the **subject matter** (e.g., biology, chemistry, arts, education, philosophy and religion, etc.); refer to "TMDSAS Course Listings" for an exhaustive list of recommended classifications.[12] You will also select whether the course included a lab component, as well as whether it was an honors course.

Refer to TMDSAS instructions for "Academic Status" (e.g., high school, freshman, sophomore, junior, senior), particularly if you did not complete a college degree in 4 years (e.g., 3 or 5 y), or if you participated in a combined program (e.g., BA/MS) or post-baccalaureate program.

If there is no grade on your transcript because the grade has not been finalized, simply leave "grade" empty. Designate "**Planned/In Progress**" courses without grades accordingly.[13]

---

[11] Spring grades are required to submit your TMDSAS application. Note that you can submit your application before sending your transcripts, but you *must* have Spring grades on the official transcripts when they are sent.

[12] Mathematics other than calculus and statistics are classified as "Other Science." However, they still count toward the Biology-Chemistry-Physics-Mathematics (BCMP) GPA.

[13] Again, note that you must have Spring grades to submit TMDSAS. "Planned/In progress" will refer to courses to be taken in summer, fall, and spring (of next year) after initially submitting your application in Spring.

Note that **AP credit** is only accepted if it is broken down on your transcript(s). Lump sum AP credit is *not* accepted by TMDSAS; if this is the case on your transcript, you should ask your registrar to send a letter detailing AP credit breakdown. Designate the AP credit as your first undergraduate term unless your transcript specifies a specific term for them, and designate your academic status as "pre-freshman."

If you attended multiple institutions (e.g., university during fall/spring and community college during the summer), you MUST list where the courses were taken, even if credit was transferred elsewhere. For example, a summer biology course at your community college should be listed as taken at the community college, even if your main university accepted credit for that course.

TMDSAS also asks to designate "Last Time Taken" for courses. This will be the case for all courses taken only once. However, you will also assign this to courses repeated for additional credit *only* (i.e., not a better grade): independent study, orchestra, etc.

Upon transcript(s) receipt, TMDSAS will generate its *own GPA* for your application to create a more standardized GPA across applicants receiving interviews.

## 29.3.4 TMDSAS Course Entry Special Cases

Refer to the TMDSAS Guide for specific instructions if the following circumstances apply to you:
• Audited courses.
• Canadian transcripts.
• Continuing Education Units (CEUs).
• CLEP credit.
• Courses with narrative evaluations.
• Courses with "suggested" credits and/or grades.
• Foreign coursework (with specific instructions for American colleges overseas).
• Distinguished from study abroad.
• Specific instructions for English vs. French-Canadian Canadian institutions.
• Graduate coursework taken as undergraduate (or vice versa).
• Incomplete grade.
• International transcripts.
• Study abroad, overseas US institutions.
• IB credit.
• JST credit.
• Military credit.
• Repeated courses.
• USAFI/DANTES credit.
• Withdrawal.
• Zero-hour courses.

## 29.3.5 TMDSAS Concluding Thoughts

Refer to the TMDSAS Applicant Guide at all times. *Carefully* read the sections on course entry, as they are liable to change since the time this book was written.

## 29.4 Summary

No matter which primary application(s) you are submitting your transcript to, focus on (1) getting all your official transcripts as early as possible, (2) requesting they be submitted to your application service ASAP, and (3) ensuring you submit the information accurately as delays will put your application at a significant disadvantage. Do not be afraid to consult the guide associated with your application service frequently.

# 30 Activities and Meaningful Experiences

*Joel Thomas*

Each primary application has an open-ended section for extracurricular activities. This section can be challenging for applicants because there is very little explicit instruction on what to write. For example, what is the right balance to strike between an austere, resume-style description and rich narrative? Moreover, this section can distinguish you from the thousands of applicants with similar academic credentials. The different primary applications also have subtle but important differences in their formatting. Lastly, AMCAS and TMDSAS ask you to expand on a number of your "most meaningful experiences," giving ADCOM members additional insight into your values and personal characteristics.

We will first discuss general recommendations for all three primary application services.

- *Show and tell.* The extracurricular section serves two purposes: to explain to ADCOM members *what you did* during your extracurricular activity (e.g., day-to-day duties, length of involvement, leadership roles, broader impact on the group) and *what you learned/demonstrated* by doing the activity. Here are examples from the author's own AMCAS application (▶ Fig. 30.1):
  - **Tell:** The first 20 to 33% of the entry should succinctly describe your personal involvement in the activity (*what you did—do **not** obfuscate with intentionally vague "resume-speak"*).
  - **Show:** The rest of the entry should describe what you learned, as well as the personal characteristics you actively developed. Refer to the AAMC's *Core Competencies for Entering Medical Students* when brainstorming your phrasing, and "show" with descriptive, specific examples.
    - This does *not* mean that you have to directly relate everything to medicine. The ADCOM will collectively roll their eyes when they read that you learned to snowboard to become an excellent surgeon. Instead, you should expand on the activity and speak about how it developed a useful, transferable skill in its own right (e.g., developing "resilience" through repeatedly getting back up on the board after wiping out).
- Draft your entries in a plain text word processor (e.g., Notepad) first, then copy and paste them in the primary application, and finally preview the finished product. The application services use plain text,

## Sample AMCAS Activity Entry

| Experience Type: | Community Service/Volunteer - Medical/Clinical | | Most Meaningful Experience: No | | |
|---|---|---|---|---|---|
| Experience Name: | Free Clinic Volunteering | | Dates: 03/2014 - 04/2014 | Total Hours: 15 | |
| | | | 09/2014 - 05/2015 | Total Hours: 59 | |
| Contact Name & Title: | | | | | |
| Contact Email: | | | Contact Phone: | | |
| Organization Name: | | | | | |
| City / State / Country: | | | | | |
| Experience Description: | For the past three semesters, my duties involved dispensing medications to patients, writing labels with dosage instructions, and maintaining the general cleanliness of the free clinic pharmacy. The clinic serves a diverse immigrant population, and I learned much about culturally competent care. Instructions to "take by mouth" on a pill bottle initially seemed redundant to me, but I came to realize that it's best to be as explicit as possible because many patients grow up with alternative, non-Western medicine. I also witnessed difficulties in obtaining information about income and insurance status from the patients and learned how to inspire the trust required to overcome these obstacles. | | | | |
| Experience Type: | Community Service/Volunteer - Not Medical/Clinical | | Most Meaningful Experience: Yes | | |
| Experience Name: | Lessons Coordinator: Science Program for Low-Income Students | | Dates: 09/2012 - 05/2015 | Total Hours: 500 | |
| Contact Name & Title: | | | | | |
| Contact Email: | | | Contact Phone: | | |
| Organization Name: | | | | | |
| City / State / Country: | | | | | |
| Experience Description: | I volunteered as a science educator for low-income elementary school students 1 hour a week and was elected to lessons coordinator. I created about 70 original 30-minute lessons for elementary school students and helped organize a science fair for fourth graders. Serving as a mentor to 6 science fair presentations, I helped students design experiments and understand the scientific method. I organized science enrichment events at a museum for the local community and created and gave two 20-minute lectures on general physics and rubber band dynamics to elementary school students. We wanted to show students that science can be fun and done with inexpensive materials at home. | | | | |
| Most Meaningful Experience Remarks: | This experience showed me the value of teamwork and the importance of tackling large projects by dividing them into small pieces. I largely attribute the success of this entirely student-run project to the synergy of the executive board; it was incredibly satisfying to work with a highly competent team towards a common goal of giving back to the community. Tasks were clearly delegated and the rare conflicts were amicably and quickly resolved. Taking on the position of lessons coordinator was initially daunting because I had to completely revise a year's curriculum for 4 grades. I first reviewed the literature on elementary science education and incorporated suggestions after talking to school teachers and other executive board members. After devising a general framework, I spent about 6 hours per week revising 4 lessons at a time. In my senior year, I was happy to hear from school teachers and returning volunteers that the new lessons were a great improvement.<br><br>The most rewarding part was cultivating a love of school and learning in young children. I had also mentored high school students from similar backgrounds who grew up hating school. Hearing from children that they tried the experiments at home and told their parents what they learned made me feel as though I made a real impact in the community. | | | | |

**Fig. 30.1** Sample AMCAS Activity Entry.

and you want to avoid missing formatting issues that may arise from copying and pasting from your word processor.

- Likewise, do *not* use bullet points to describe your activities. Instead, use succinct but full sentences.

- Resist the temptation to write just for the sake of writing—it's perfectly fine if you do not use up all of the available options for extracurricular entry. Similarly, we encourage grouping similar activities (e.g., multiple short-term shadowing experiences) whenever possible.

- Ideally, your extracurriculars will include some form of clinical experience (shadowing, volunteering), +/− research (especially if you are applying to research-oriented schools), +/− nonclinical volunteering, and ideally some unique activity that distinguishes you from other applicants (e.g., horseback rider, karate black belt, ocarina master).
  - When describing your research, use nontechnical language accessible to an educated lay reader.
  - Published abstracts that appear in a journal are acceptable to list as publications (unless explicitly stated otherwise).
  - Note that publications are *extremely* rare among applicants. Many successful MD/PhD applicants do not have any publications.

- Don't repeat information found elsewhere in your app. That said, you *can* mention the same experience in your personal statement or secondary applications as long as you introduce *additional, new* insights into your character and development.
  - For example, your "Work/Activities" section on your AMCAS may simply describe your involvement with the free clinic, as well as what you learned about immigrants' experiences with the healthcare system. You're free to expand on this experience in your personal statement by discussing how you *also* gained valuable insight into the intersection of public policy, economics, and medicine. You *should not* just rehash your insight into immigrants' experiences with the healthcare system in your personal statement.

- Generally speaking, you should only include extracurriculars from the beginning of college to immediately before matriculation. This includes future, anticipated activities; note that different application services have their own rules for including future activities, however.
  - You *may* include activities before college if they are substantial (e.g., research publication, significant experience abroad), longitudinal (starting before college but continuing into the time you were enrolled), or contribute to your narrative significantly (the story you are telling about yourself). This is more likely to be the case if you took time off between graduating high school and beginning college. However, you should refer to the specific application service as to whether they allow high school activities.

- It is extremely rare for the ADCOM to contact the listed "contact person." That said, you should list someone who would be able to verify your involvement. For solo activities, you may list yourself (depending on the application instructions). If, in doubt, discuss with your prehealth advisor.

- You will quickly realize how unforgiving the character limits are, and you will probably deliberate over every word in your entries. As such, you should start drafting early because you'll likely surprise yourself by your ability to eliminate fluff with repeated read-throughs and edits.
  - That said, you will probably not be able to include *everything* you'd want to in your entries. Fortunately, you will likely have ample opportunity to expand in your secondary applications and interviews.

We will now discuss nuances specific to each primary application.

## 30.1 AMCAS

AMCAS allows up to 15 entries for "Work/Activities." We believe that a competitive application should have at least 10 entries. Each entry allows 700 characters (including spaces) at maximum. You are allowed to pick up to three activities as "Most Meaningful" and expand on them with 1,325 additional characters (including spaces). You can list up to four separate date ranges for a recurring event.

Activities are broadly characterized as "honors/awards/recognitions," "military service," community service/volunteer ("medical/clinical" vs. "not medical/clinical"), paid employment ("medical/clinical" vs. "not medical/clinical"), research ("presentations/posters," "publications," "research/lab", "teaching/tutoring/teaching assistant"), "physician shadowing/clinical observation," and miscellaneous (i.e., "artistic endeavors," "conferences attended," "hobbies," "intercollegiate athletics," "leadership—not listed elsewhere," "other"). You can only use *one* of these 18 categories to describe each activity you list.

Your entries will be ordered chronologically based on the dates you enter. However, ADCOM's can re-order them in whatever way they desire.

- We recommend taking full advantage of this section by discussing three "Most Meaningful" activities, as these prompts give you ample opportunity to highlight your qualitative strengths in the context of experiences that will be memorable to the ADCOM.
- For the "Most Meaningful" activities, you can use the full 700 characters to vividly describe your role in the activity; use the additional 1,350 characters to discuss what you learned and appreciated. You do not necessarily need to explicitly relate the experience to medicine, but you *must* tie it to a core competency that a physician would exemplify.
  - *At least one "Most Meaningful" experience should be a clinical experience* (you *are* trying to convince the ADCOM that you're committed to becoming a physician, after all). If you're applying to research-heavy schools, another "Most Meaningful" experience should be research-related.
- For the activities that you did not pick as "Most Meaningful," spend the first 25 to 33% of the available space to describe your involvement, and use the remaining space to discuss what you learned and the competencies you used.
- Lump similar activities if you're pressed for entries (e.g., multiple physician shadowing experiences, multiple publications in the same field).
- "Zero" hours is appropriate for honors/awards/recognitions, publications, and presentations/posters.
- If you anticipate participating in an extracurricular during your application cycle, it is acceptable to include expected hours and to list the end date as graduation (or immediately before medical school matriculation, if applicable).
- You cannot add onto the "Work/Activities" section after submitting AMCAS, but you *can* expand further in secondary applications, interviews, and update letters.

## 30.2 AACOMAS

AACOMAS allows *unlimited* entries for "Experiences." We recommend including at least 10 and no more than 20 entries altogether. AACOMAS also has an "Achievements" section for "awards, honors, presentations, publications, and scholarships." In both the "Experiences" and "Achievements" sections, you are allowed 600 characters (including spaces) for each entry.

Activities may be categorized as "non-healthcare volunteering or community enrichment," "non-healthcare employment," "healthcare experience" (paid and unpaid), and "extracurricular activities" (i.e., unpaid).

- DO schools often emphasize community service and working with the underserved. You should highlight similar interests in your extracurricular descriptions.
- Lump similar activities if you're pressed for entries (e.g., multiple physician shadowing experiences, multiple publications in the same field).
- "Zero" hours is appropriate for honors/awards/recognitions, publications, and presentations/posters.
- If you anticipate participating in an extracurricular during your application cycle, it is acceptable to include expected hours and to list the end date as graduation (or immediately before medical school matriculation, if applicable).
- You cannot change your entries once you submit AACOMAS, but you can *add new ones.*

## 30.3 TMDSAS

TMDSAS uses a unique format for extracurricular entry. All applicants will be given the same categories with the option of submitting an entry for each category. **This means that an applicant may include the *same* activity under *multiple* categories to highlight different aspects of that activity** (e.g., president of a volunteering club may be listed under "leadership" and "community service"). There is also no limit to the number of entries; we recommend including at least 10 and no more than 20 entries altogether. The categories are "academic recognition," "non-academic recognition," "leadership," "employment" (including *before college*), "research activities," "healthcare activities," (non-healthcare) "community serv-ice," "extracurricular and leisure activities," and "planned activities."

TMDSAS has the strictest character limits at *300 characters* (including spaces). Applicants may choose up to 3 "Top Meaningful Activities," each of which has an additional 500 characters (including spaces) for discussion. Note that "Top Meaningful Activities" *must* be completed or ongoing experiences; they cannot be activities that you will start in the future.

- We recommend taking full advantage of this section by discussing three "Top Meaningful" activities, as these prompts give you ample opportunity to highlight your qualitative strengths in the context of experiences that will be memorable to the ADCOM.
- For the "Top Meaningful" activities, you can use the full 500 characters to vividly describe your role in the activity; use the additional 500 characters to discuss what you learned and appreciated. You do not necessarily need to explicitly relate the experience to medicine, but you *must* tie it to a core competency that a physician would exemplify.
  - *At least one "Most Meaningful" experience should be a clinical experience.* If you're applying to research-heavy schools, another "Top Meaningful" experience should be research-related.
- Pay close attention to the TMDSAS Application Handbook as to whether you may include entries before college (e.g., after high school graduation) for each category.
- For "Research Activities," do *not* separately list end products of the research (e.g., publications, posters, abstracts). Instead, each entry should list a research experience *along with* its final product.
- If you shadowed multiple physicians at the same location, create *one entry* for the location and list each doctor in the description. However, if each physician practiced a different specialty, then you may make separate entries for each specialty.
- Note that TMDSAS uses the first 50 characters (including spaces) of each activity description to populate the "Chronology of Activities" document. As such, be strategic with the first 50 characters, as you'll ideally want to convey the maximum amount of useful information in your Chronology of Activities (i.e., that you're a well-rounded applicant involved with a variety of extracurriculars).
  - It's perfectly acceptable if the first 50 characters in the Chronology of Activities cuts off midsentence. You are not expected to manipulate the formatting to make it appear perfect.
- You cannot edit this section after submission. If you must do so, TMDSAS recommends creating an addendum to your application to be taken to interviews.

## 30.4 Summary

Extracurricular activities may be categorized as "non-healthcare volunteering or community enrich-ment," "non-healthcare employment," "healthcare experience" (paid and unpaid), and "extracurricular activities" (i.e., unpaid). The extracurricular section serves two purposes: to explain to ADCOM members *what you did* during your extracurricular activity (e.g., day-to-day duties, length of involvement, leader-ship roles, broader impact on the group) and *what you learned/demonstrated* by doing the activity. This section is a great way to differentiate yourself from other applicants.

# 31 Personal Statement

*Landon Cluts and Joel Thomas*

The personal statement is one of the most dreaded parts of the medical school application. In 5,300 characters, you must paint a vivid picture of your personal journey to applying to medical school, with admirable but realistic expectations for the future to come. This is a rare opportunity to be creative. Up to this point in college, you have most likely been writing scientific papers or book reports that have a specific format. The personal statement is different. You determine the format, there can be dialogue, and there can be surprise twist endings because this piece is truly a short novel about you. All the while, you'll want to walk the fine line between sharing too much intimate detail and being overly guarded.

With all the options in shaping your personal statement, there is one goal that you must keep in mind. Every single experience you describe must be directly tied to why you chose medicine, why you would make an excellent physician, or why you deserve an interview with every admissions committee that will see your application.

As you fill out your application, you will painstakingly detail your awards, leadership opportunities, service activities, and so on. You will be able to write a snippet about most and more extensively about a few. The personal statement is not the place to simply rehash the rest of your application. It is the place to help a busy Admissions Committee (ADCOM) member get to know you so that he or she can advocate for you and sell you to the rest of the committee. Ideally, the ADCOM will learn new things about you that are not covered in the rest of your application. That said, you can reference the same activity as long as you significantly expand on why that specific thing has shaped your choosing to pursue medicine.

### Student Perspective
*I was a camp counselor the summer after my first year of college. In my application, I described my responsibilities as a counselor and what they taught me. In my personal statement, I described a specific event that truly affirmed in me my desire to be a physician and how my actions at that time displayed the values or skills that a committee may be looking for in potential colleagues. In my case I wrote about an injured camper and described how I handled it and how I felt after his mother thanked me (it was a simple scraped knee, nothing major).*

## 31.1 Timeline

You may be asking, "When should I start writing my personal statement?" The good news is that *you already have.* The experiences you have had since starting college all are fair game for inclusion in your personal statement as long as they are important enough and convincing enough for the admissions committee to want to meet you. You will want to make sure you give yourself enough time to have your personal statement proofread—*a lot*—by multiple people. Your university may even have a writing center that will be able to help you through the process. One of the authors, for example, began outlining his personal statement about 6 months out from application day, had a working draft about 2 weeks afterward that was taken to the writing center, and then had friends, family, the writing center, and advisors look at it over the next 4 months until it was as good as it was going to be.

## 31.2 Everyone's a Critic

Keep in mind that your personal statement will never be *perfect.* Read that last sentence 10 times and then refer back to it whenever you feel anxious about your personal statement. At some point your personal statement will need to be submitted and you will forever think of different ways to do it and that is perfectly okay. Also, keep in mind that everyone's a critic: the more people you ask for feedback, the more likely it is that you will get conflicting advice. If there's no clear majority or consensus among readers on a particular topic, it probably does not matter too much. Alternatively, different ADCOM members may react differently to it—you can either play it safe by omitting some of the more controversial content, or you can decide that it's out of your hands how people will perceive your writing (e.g., 50% may love it, 50% may think the writing is slightly awkward but not bad enough to affect the essay as a whole). These are judgment calls with no easy answers, but we generally advise playing it safe and omitting a section that continually invites polarizing feedback.

## 31.3 Pitfalls

We will first discuss common pitfalls to *avoid* in your journey to craft your imperfect personal statement that will absolutely get the job done.

- "I have always wanted to help people."
  - This is a cliché phrase that should be kept out of your personal statement.
  - Everyone goes into medicine (hopefully) because they have some underlying drive to help people. Your personal statement, instead, should demonstrate this trait without explicitly saying it and allow your experiences and actions to do the talking for you (show, don't tell).
- Not demonstrating empathy or compassion:
  - There are many legitimate reasons why someone may be motivated to go to medical school (e.g., love of research, desire to become a leader). However, possessing a genuine concern for the well-being of others and *demonstrating* this through specific examples is essentially necessary for admission.
- The excuse essay:
  - Some people have had legitimate obstacles in their lives. These are absolutely fair game to be part of your personal statement. This is *not* the same as trying to explain away a bad grade or a reprimand you received from your university.
  - Take full responsibility. Use your personal struggles and strife to demonstrate you are resilient or how you are able to overcome despite the circumstances or that you can be quick on your feet to come up with solutions to big problems.
- Psychiatric history:
  - This is controversial but an unfortunate reality of pursuing a medical career. Despite our society's enormous strides in fighting mental health stigma, many ADCOM members are apprehensive about selecting candidates with a history of mental illness—*even if it's well-controlled*.[1]
    - Presumably, this is because medical school often introduces students to unprecedented levels of stress that may cause controlled mental illness to become uncontrolled.
    - ADCOM members also have thousands of qualified applicants to choose from. Given the choice between two similarly qualified applicants with and without a history of mental illness, many would choose the one without—regardless of the ethics of the choice.
    - In addition, as described in Chapter 18, Self-Care and Wellness, several states have questions on their medical license applications about any history of mental illness.[2] States vary considerably in the intrusiveness of these questions, but there have been several high-profile instances of physicians facing significant obstacles for disclosing well-controlled mental illness.[3]
- The recap:
  - This is a personal statement that essentially rehashes what you have already listed in other sections of your application. The personal statement should offer up new information and really let the committee know who you are as a *person*, not just as a medical school applicant (you should definitely have a life outside of getting into medical school, as well as a plan to continue your personal interests once you matriculate).
- The cocky essay:
  - It is bad form to make your personal statement all about how awesome you are. Instead, it should show that you are able to work as part of a team (i.e., virtually every moment of a physician's working day) and that you are humble.
- The "Did you go to English Class?" essay:
  - Your essay will never be perfect, but it *will* be grammatically flawless. This is non-negotiable. Refresh yourself on the proper use of commas, semicolons, colons, verb-tense agreement, gerunds, hyperbole, similes, "there, their, and they're," etc.

---

[1] Medical Students with Disabilities: A Generation of Practice. Available at: https://store.aamc.org/downloadable/download/sample/sample_id/156/. Accessed July 8, 2022.
[2] Physician-Friendly States for Mental Health: A Review of Medical Boards. Available at: https://www.idealmedicalcare.org/physician-friendly-states-for-mental-health-a-review-of-medical-boards/. Accessed July 8, 2022.
[3] Samuel L. Doctors fear mental health disclosure could jeopardize their licenses. Available at: https://www.statnews.com/2017/10/16/doctors-mental-health-licenses/. Accessed July 8, 2022.

- There are no "objective" rules for writing well, but George Orwell's *6 Rules for Writing* will serve you well[4]:
    1. Never use a metaphor, simile, or other figure of speech which you are used to seeing in print.
    2. Never use a long word where a short one will do.
    3. If it is possible to cut a word out, always cut it out.
    4. Never use the passive where you can use the active.
    5. Never use a foreign phrase, a scientific word, or a jargon word if you can think of an everyday English equivalent.
    6. Break any of these rules sooner than say anything outright barbarous.
  - Multiple pairs of eyes and your university's writing center are invaluable resources here.
- The snoozer:
  - Most of what you have written for your application up to this point is boring. You've had to objectively describe experiences and their significance, but you had very little room to add flair. This is not the case for the personal statement. Your personal statement should be exciting and engaging, and it should captivate the reader from the beginning to the end.
  - *Don't do this*:
    - *I worked in a soup kitchen one time while I was in college. We served chicken noodle soup to homeless people. It made me happy to see them happy when they had a hot meal. That made me realize I wanted to be a doctor because I could help people every day.*
    - While this is an extraordinarily good thing this person did, the writing is horrendously dull and I almost fell asleep reading it.
  - Do something like this:
    - *I walked into the small kitchen and smelled the delicious aroma of chicken noodle soup being cooked by the busy volunteers on a cold winter's day. This was my first day volunteering at _____, and I could not wait to get to work. I took my place in the serving line and was shocked by the crowd standing there waiting for a warm meal. "I never realized how many people were homeless here in _____" I thought to myself, stunned by my ignorance… etc.*

## 31.4 How to Write the Personal Statement

Each primary application service has slight differences in the character limits and prompts for the personal statement (refer to Chapter 28, Primary Application: AMCAS, AACOMAS, and TMDSAS). Here, we will discuss how to answer the "Why do you want to become a doctor?" prompt common to all three primary applications.

- Understand the big picture view. Your personal statement supports the following thesis: Becoming a physician best integrates my personal and professional values and interests. I have explored and tested this interest through X, Y, and Z, and I have come to the conclusion that starting medical school now is the best next step.
  - You need to support this thesis with arguments that use *specific* examples from your life.
  - Our recommended outline is:
    - **Introductory paragraph**—Your *first sentence* should captivate the reader and immediately grab his or her attention. At the same time, *do not go overboard*. While we've emphasized that this is your chance to be creative and distinguish yourself from other applicants, you still need to show restraint. It's safer to veer toward a conservative, cautious essay—that runs the risk of being boring and unmemorable—than a bold, over-the-top essay that runs the risk of making you appear unprofessional and unhinged.
    - **Three or four supporting paragraphs** that each center around a major experience/theme that supports the thesis.
    - **Concluding paragraph** that ties everything together and essentially restates the thesis while leading the reader on a good note based on your attitude, optimism, and healthy amount of confidence.

---

[4] Trautner C. George Orwell's Six Rules for Writing. Available at: https://infusion.media/blog/george-orwells-six-rules-for-writing/. Accessed July 8, 2022.

- Each paragraph should center around an AAMC Core Competency, i.e., how you appreciated this competency in others and/or demonstrated it yourself.
  - *One of these supporting paragraphs should focus on empathy or compassion.* Other suggestions include intellectual curiosity (e.g., through scholarly work), leadership, teamwork, cultural competence, and being an advocate for the underserved.
- Each unit of the essay—individual characters, words, sentences, and paragraphs—should serve the overall purpose of supporting your thesis. Words should work together to form sentences that flow, creating a cohesive set of paragraphs that strengthen your argument.
- Whenever possible, you should introduce statements showing that you have thought carefully and honestly about the known challenges of being a physician, e.g., not being able to help everyone, working with uncertainty, the changing role of the physician in society. This demonstrates to the ADCOM that you've done your research and you *still* believe that medicine is the best career for you.
- Before you begin brainstorming, you should read examples of successful medical school essays that can be found online and in various books. This will familiarize you with the different essay styles, the type of experiences and themes people tend to focus on, and how to properly relate things to medicine. Try to understand how the writer uses their experiences to help bring the ADCOM onto their side and see them as a part of their medical school community.
  - Do not plagiarize any of this material. Be careful to avoid doing it inadvertently, too. It's extremely easy for ADCOMs to run your material through plagiarism checkers.
- Devote a week to serious introspection and brainstorming. *Who are you?* Seriously, what do you genuinely enjoy and value in life? Who are your heroes, and why do you look up to them? What has kept you motivated to aggressively work toward a high grade-point average (GPA) and Medical College Admission Test (MCAT) while sacrificing many things your peers have enjoyed?
  - What were the most formative experiences in your life up till this point? Ideally, this should include longitudinal extracurricular experiences, i.e., the "most meaningful" activities you discussed in your primary application. *At least one of these experiences should focus on compassion and/or empathy.*
  - Vividly picture a specific day or instance of that experience that would allow you to use descriptive language to share the experience with the ADCOM.
  - You're allowed to mention experiences before college (e.g., high school), as many applicants became interested in medicine in adolescence. That said, the bulk of your essay should expand on more *recent,* in-depth experiences.
  - During this brainstorming period, do the things that normally make you *happy.* Positive psychology research suggests that subjective well-being improves creativity, as well as the ability to stay committed to uninteresting tasks.[5] So take walks outside! Bake fancy desserts! Lift some serious weights! Hang out with your friends and have life-chats to encourage introspection!
- Not everyone was a combat medic in Iraq or had a blockbuster-worthy life event. The majority of applicants likely had comfortable middle- to upper-middle-class lives and gradually explored an interest in medicine through common activities like hospital volunteering, biomedical research, and physician shadowing.
  - The important thing is to expand on what **you**—*an individual with unique interests, values, and motivations—took from these experiences*. Was it seeing patients' gratitude when you were able to help them in seemingly insignificant ways as a volunteer? Was it the sense of excitement and optimism you experienced in the lab when you explored a novel hypothesis explaining the pathogenesis of a disease?
- If you're a career changer, do *not* be overly negative and outright disparage your former career. You do not want to give the impression that you're a complainer, as many parts of being a medical student and physician are—frankly—extremely boring and common to virtually all jobs (spending hours filling out redundant paperwork, sitting in meetings, regurgitating the same information to multiple people on the phone and being placed on hold).
  - Instead, speak about the unique aspects of being a physician that you feel are lacking in your job and why these aspects matter to you. Do you desire to meet people across all walks of life and work with them on specific problems and personally witness the impact of your interventions? Why?

---

5 Boniwell I. Happiness and subjective well-being. In: Positive psychology in a nutshell: the science of happiness. McGraw Hill, Open University Press; 2012: 38.

- You don't need to use the full character limit; quality is more important than quantity.
  - That said, if you find that your personal statement is < 75% the allotted character limit, consider expanding on an experience to more vividly support your thesis.
- Minimize quotes. Your space is limited, and the ADCOM wants to hear *your* voice.
- Don't be overly formal or excessive with thesaurus words. Imagine your reader as an educated colleague who is genuinely interested in learning about you.
- Draft your personal statement in a plain text word processor (e.g., Notepad) first, then manually retype it in the primary application, and finally preview the finished product. The primary application uses plain text, and you want to avoid formatting errors that may arise from copying and pasting from your word processor.

## 31.5 Example Personal Statement

The following is the author's AMCAS personal statement with commentary (▶ Fig. 31.1).

- **Introduction:** The first paragraph immediately draws the reader's attention with vivid sensory detail. That said, the author received some criticism that this detail was over-the-top and "childish". Ultimately, he decided to leave it in, as he also received praise from other readers that it was enjoyable to read. This example illustrates the point that everyone's a critic and that you will never be completely happy with your personal statement. Ultimately, you will have to make some judgment calls on what's worth keeping as is versus revising.

### PERSONAL COMMENTS

A fluffy, golden-brown English muffin. Warm, gooey peanut butter. Tart blackberry jam. I'm no Gordon Ramsay, but I will admit to shamelessly channeling my inner gourmet on Monday mornings at ███ Hospital. If I've learned anything from hospital volunteering over the past seven years, it's that simple gestures — be it an unexpected ketchup smiley-face or even a shared grin — can often make an enormous difference to patients caught in a web of uncertainty and sickness. Unfortunately, while I can currently offer patients my time and good intentions, these alone will not stop a metastatic tumor from tearing apart a family. From a young age, I have been aware of the devastating effects of disease. Witnessing my blind aunt struggle to attend to her son bedridden by cerebral palsy and my childhood friend's fatal brain cancer left me with a desire to enter medicine that has only grown over time.

I also learned as a child that a physician can inspire hope when all seems lost. That morning was like any other - so much so that I had to hear the screaming twice to realize that something was wrong. When I found my mother sprawled on the kitchen floor in a pool of blood after deeply cutting her hand, I began to panic. I immediately phoned my father, a primary care physician, who calmly asked me to describe the situation. Upon concluding that she did not face any serious harm, he taught me how to manage my mother's wound with ice until he was able to come home. My father's ability to take control of the situation and save my mother from what appeared to be imminent danger left a profound impact on my development. Over the past four years, I have tested my childhood interest and come to the conclusion that only a career in medicine would integrate the practices and beliefs I already value in my personal life in a professional context.

Throughout college, I mainly pursued knowledge to understand the world around me and to make evidence-based decisions rather than to fulfill pre-professional or major requirements. I focused on taking upper level classes in as many subjects as possible and questioned the methodological assumptions and limits of these different fields through philosophical analysis to arrive at a cohesive, interdisciplinary web of beliefs. Medicine exemplifies this ideal. The physicians I shadowed possessed not only an understanding of the natural sciences, but also human psychology, the social determinants of illness, and other structural forces and life circumstances that lead people to poor health. I look forward to a career of continually keeping up with advances across multiple fields and directly applying them to secure the health of my patients.

Moreover, a rigorous medical education would allow me to not only serve as an informed practitioner, but also to improve existing treatments through research. This motivation was the key to my success at ███ Rather than seeing my work as an endless series of aliquots and assays, I was motivated by the prospect of making an impact on human suffering by discovering therapeutic targets for fibrosis. I was particularly inspired by the physicians who actively sought better patient outcomes through clinical trials and cohort studies. Although there are many paths to research or patient care, only a medical career offers the possibility of blending the two. Becoming a doctor would allow me to identify and treat clinical problems among my patients that have yet to be addressed in the literature and to draw on an extensive science background to find better solutions in the laboratory.

Most important, however, is the privilege of bearing the ultimate responsibility for the health of my patients. While medical care requires the perspectives of nurses, pharmacists, and other professionals, only a physician has the technical expertise to make final and even unorthodox treatment recommendations. A plastic surgeon I shadowed illustrated this role through her care for a young child. The boy in question, who would eagerly tell anyone about his adventures in school, gave no suggestion of the severe cleft lip he had suffered since birth. His surgeon, however, had taken a calculated risk despite doubts from her colleagues by operating even though the boy was under the recommended age for surgery. Her risk clearly paid off, as the gratitude on the parents' faces was unmistakable. While it is true that the practice of medicine is not limited to doctors, no other health professional receives the autonomy afforded to physicians.

I understand that the road to becoming a physician is fraught with sacrifices and the frustration of not being able to cure all those we treat. I also recognize that the very role of the physician in the American health care system may change radically in the face of shifting health policy. Despite these realities, I am still dedicated to becoming a doctor because no other career would allow me to have such meaningful relationships with people in their most vulnerable moments. I am also immensely attracted to the opportunity to add to our arsenal of knowledge - be it scientific or philosophical - in the ongoing war against disease. Although the battles will undoubtedly be arduous, I can think of no better way to spend the rest of my life.

**Fig. 31.1** AMCAS personal comments, Joel Thomas.

- Specific examples—ketchup smiley-face, shared grin—communicate the more abstract realization that small gestures can make a big difference to patients.
- The author communicates that while his current healthcare experiences are gratifying, he would like to be able to do more for patients by going to medical school and becoming a physician.
- The author makes references to early childhood events in the context of his long-standing desire to become a physician. Notice how he doesn't elaborate on these experiences (son with cerebral palsy, brain cancer) because it would not be the best use of the character limit. Instead, he moves straight to the first body paragraph to redirect the essay to *his* journey to medical school.
- **Body Paragraph 1:** First sentence sets the theme for paragraph: "physician can inspire hope when all seems lost."
  - The author again captures the reader's attention with a vivid description of a traumatic event.
  - After describing the event, the author reflects on what he found admirable in the physician's actions and how they made a lasting impact.
- **Body Paragraph 2:** The first half of the paragraph reflects on the author's personal values and interests: developing a unified web of knowledge and exploring multiple academic disciplines.
  - He then ties these personal interests to the professional expectations and opportunities in medicine.
- **Body Paragraph 3:** First sentence sets the theme for the paragraph: the rigor of a doctoral-level medical education would allow the author to change medical practice. Implicit in this idea is that the breadth and depth of basic science education is a *distinguishing feature* of pursuing an MD vs. PA or NP degree.
  - The rest of the paragraph refers to a specific research experience and how the prospect of impacting patients' lives motivated him to excel in research.
  - Again, he references something *unique* to pursuing an MD: having both the educational background to perform high-level biomedical research *and* the clinical skills to treat patients directly.
- **Body Paragraph 4:** The use of "most important" adds to the rising action and flow of the overall essay. The first sentence again sets the theme for the paragraph as a whole.
  - The second sentence pays homage to the teamwork in day-to-day medical practice while also acknowledging the *unique* leadership role of physicians on the healthcare team.
  - He supports this claim with a specific example from shadowing while giving a sense of realism to the "boy in question, who would eagerly tell anyone about his adventures in school."
- **Conclusion:** The author sets a sense of contrast and opposition by beginning the paragraph with the complexities and honest challenges of being a physician. Nonetheless, he is still motivated to pursue medical school because of (1) *empathetic, compassionate* contexts found solely in medicine ("… meaningful relationships with people in their most vulnerable moments") and (2) the appeal to scholarly work.
  - The final sentence leaves the reader with a sense of confidence and optimism without naiveté, as the author candidly acknowledges the challenges to come.

## 31.6 Summary

The personal statement is one of the most important pieces of your medical school application, and it's perfectly normal to revise it over tens of times over the course of several months. Your personal statement should artfully convey your narrative to the ADCOM and reveal perspectives about your character and aspirations that are not immediately apparent from your application. The introduction and conclusion should be particularly strong, as they are most likely to be remembered by the reader (and therefore will likely disproportionately affect their evaluation). The body paragraphs should expand on specific, concrete experiences that exemplify your character. You should have as many people critique it as possible and incorporate suggestions appropriately, being mindful that your personal statement will never be "perfect" and that everyone will find *something* to critique. Eventually you'll get to a point where you are ok with submitting it. Until then, spend as much time as you need to polish the prose; you only get one chance to make a first impression.

# 32 Altus Suite: CASPer, Snapshot, and Duet

*Joel Thomas*

CASPer (Computer-Based Assessment for Sampling Personal Characteristics), Snapshot, and Duet are components of the Altus Suite, a series of online tests required by certain medical schools as part of the overall application as of 2022. CASPer is a "situational judgment test" (basically an online multiple mini-interview [MMI]; see Chapter 34, Interviews) that presents examinees with realistic hypothetical scenarios and asks them what they would do and why. These responses are assessed to evaluate the applicant's behavioral tendencies, values, and overall interpersonal skills. Snapshot is essentially a one-way video interview in which the applicant provides recorded responses to 3 open-ended prompts that explain their motivations for pursuing medicine, as well as aspects of their personal history (e.g., "Tell me about a time you identified and addressed injustice").

Duet is an online questionnaire in which applicants grade their preferences for various aspects of medical training (e.g., "I highly value research output" vs. "I highly value early, in-depth exposure to underserved communities"). These answers are then sent to participating medical schools, ideally allowing them to identify applicants who would be exceptionally great fits based on their personal preferences.

As of 2022, CASPer consists of 15 total stations divided into a typed response section and a video response section. The typed response section includes 3 written prompts and 6 video prompts. The video response section includes 2 written prompts and 4 video prompts. There is an optional 5-minute break in the middle of the typed response section, as well as an option 10-minute break before beginning the video response section. Examinees can take the test in the comfort of their own home. The videos are approximately 3 minutes, and examinees have approximately 30 seconds to read the text prompts. The scenarios *are not* clinical. Instead, you might be told that you are at a party with friends or at an office work environment. In addition, some of the text prompts may not be scenarios but instead behavioral questions, e.g., "Tell me about a time in your life when you've had to disagree with an authority."

After viewing or reading the prompt, examinees in the typed response section have 5 minutes (with a timer at the bottom of the screen) to *type* their responses to three questions that appear on the next page. Examinees in the video section have 1 minute to answer each question, for a total of 3 minutes of video-based response per prompt. Of note, *the examinee cannot return to the text or video prompt during the question phase of the station.* As such, it is critically important to memorize key details of the prompt before addressing the questions. Fortunately, you will not be penalized for spelling mistakes and typos. Altogether, the exam takes approximately 1.5 hours.

Your responses are graded by a panel of 12 independent human scorers from a diverse pool of professions and backgrounds. Frustratingly, you will never receive a detailed score beyond your quartile performance for CASPer; it is simply sent to the schools that request it. The exam takes $85 to take (this allows you to send your results to 8 programs at no additional cost) and $15 per program to send to additional programs beyond the first 8 program. You cannot retake the CASPer, and your score is only valid for a single application cycle. Thus, if you reapply in a future application cycle, you must retake CASPer. You will need a working webcam to take the test, as you will be watched during administration for adherence to testing rules.

As of 2022, Snapshot consists 3 sequential prompts that each require a video response. You have 30 seconds to read the prompt, followed by up to 2 minutes to respond to the prompt. *Your video responses are automatically saved and therefore you cannot re-record your answer.* Fortunately, you take a mandatory practice session before answering the questions that are actually sent to ADCOMs. Snapshot should be completed within 2 weeks of taking CASPer to allow timely transmission to programs that request it. Applicants applying to French-speaking medical schools (i.e., certain Canadian medical schools) will need to complete Snapshot in both English and French.

As of 2022, Duet consists of 21 pairwise comparisons between hypothetical aspects of medical training. You will score your preference (or lack thereof) for one aspect in each pair. For example, if you *had* to choose *between* research opportunities and team-based learning when comparing medical schools, then do you have a strong preference for research output, slight preference for research output, no preference, slight preference for team-based learning, or strong preference for team-based learning?

## 32.1 Which Schools Require It?

The list of schools that require CASPer changes fairly often; several schools that once required it dropped the requirement, and several schools have recently decided to demand it. As such, you *must* check whether your particular schools of interest require CASPer. That said, the following medical schools required CASPer for admission in 2021.

### 32.1.1 AMCAS

1. Albany Medical College (for the BS/MD program).
2. American University of The Caribbean School of Medicine (International).
3. Baylor College of Medicine.
4. Boston University School of Medicine.
5. Central Michigan University.
6. Drexel University.
7. East Tennessee State University Medicine.
8. Florida Atlantic University.
9. Hofstra University (for the BS/MD program).
10. Howard University.
11. Indiana University.
12. Marshall University Joan C. Edwards School of Medicine.
13. Medical College of Georgia at Augusta University.
14. Medical College of Wisconsin.
15. Meharry Medical College.
16. Mercer University.
17. Michigan State University.
18. New York Medical College.
19. Northeast Ohio Medical University.
20. Oregon Health and Science University.
21. Pacific Northwest University (for the BS/MD program).
22. Penn State College of Medicine.
23. Rosalind Franklin University.
24. Rutgers New Jersey Medical School.
25. Rutgers Robert Wood Johnson Medical School.
26. San Juan Bautista School of Medicine.
27. Stony Brook University.
28. SUNY Upstate.
29. Temple University.
30. Tulane University.
31. University of Colorado, Denver.
32. University of Illinois at Chicago.
33. University of Miami.
34. University of Michigan.
35. University of Nevada, Reno.
36. University of Vermont.
37. University of Washington.
38. Virginia Commonwealth University.
39. Virginia Tech Carilion School of Medicine.
40. Wake Forest School of Medicine.
41. West Virginia University.
42. Dalhousie University (Canadian).
43. McGill University (Canadian).
44. McMaster University (Canadian).
45. Memorial University (Canadian).
46. Queen's University (Canadian).

47. University of Ottawa (Canadian).
48. Université de Montréal (Canadian).
49. Université de Sherbrooke (Canadian).
50. Université Laval (Canadian).
51. University of Alberta (Canadian).
52. University of Manitoba (Canadian).
53. University of Saskatchewan (Canadian).

## 32.1.2 AACOMAS

1. Alabama College of Osteopathic Medicine.
2. Arkansas College of Health Education.
3. California Health Sciences University.
4. Idaho College of Osteopathic Medicine.
5. Michigan State University College of Osteopathic Medicine.
6. Oklahoma State University.
7. Touro College.
8. Western University of Health Sciences.
9. William Carey University.

## 32.1.3 TMDSAS

1. Texas A&M University.
2. Texas Tech University El Paso Paul L. Foster School of Medicine.
3. Texas Tech University Health Sciences Center (for the BS/MD program).
4. University of Texas Medical Branch Galveston.
5. Long School of Medicine, UT Health San Antonio.
6. Sam Houston State University (DO program).
7. University of Texas Houston, McGovern Medical School.
8. University of Texas Southwestern.

## 32.2 When Should I Take It?

It takes 3 to 4 weeks to send your score report to schools. As such, we recommend taking CASPer as early as possible, i.e., the first test date in May. Early July is the latest we recommend taking CASPer, as some schools begin to send out interview invitations in late July. Additionally, some schools may not require all parts of the Altus Suite. That said, Duet and Snapshot must be taken within 14 days of CASPer to be successfully submitted to requesting medical schools. There have been cases of schools later requiring additional components of the Altus Suite (i.e., during the application cycle) after initially only requiring CASPer. In these cases, applicants were not able to submit Duet and/or Snapshot because they were out of the window when they had recently taken CASPer. *Therefore, we recommend that everyone who takes CASPer should also take Snapshot and Duet within 14 days to safeguard against this possibility.*

## 32.3 How Do I Prepare?

Our approach to preparing for CASPer is twofold: how to *type* your response and how to *formulate* your response.

We specifically emphasize typing speed because many applicants have complained of not being able to answer the prompts in time. We specifically recommend https://www.keybr.com/ and https://10fastfingers.com/ for improving your typing speed to at least 40 to 50 words per minute (wpm). While the scorers are instructed to ignore typos and grammatical errors, you should still aim to be able to type quickly without major grammatical errors and typos, as it would not be unsurprising for scorers to be biased by poor diction and grammar.

You should answer the easiest question(s) first to give yourself enough time to brainstorm and answer the harder question(s).

*Formulating* your response to the scenarios requires a (1) basic working knowledge of professional and personal ethics, (2) the ability to identify multiple perspectives and sides in an interpersonal conflict, (3) the ability to articulate your values and responsibilities, and (4) the ability to *choose* one side and justify it.

For the video response sections of CASPer and Snapshot, we recommend creating a professional recording (i.e., clean background, good lighting, no distracting noise). You should be dressed professionally in your interview attire.

For Snapshot - as with MMI preparation, - you should practice responses to common interview questions (e.g., "Tell me about yourself" and "Why do you want to become a doctor?"). Additionally, you should be able to give abbreviated (<2 minute) versions of answers to meet the time limit for Snapshot.

To prepare for Duet, we recommend being as honest as possible with your motivations and preferences for medical training to ideally be matched with a school that's a great fit. That said, if there are certain schools that you really want to attend, then we recommend reviewing their mission statements and emphasizing those while completing Duet. This - of course - assumes that you're being reasonably honest; if you're seriously exaggerating your preferences and values for the sake of getting into a "dream school", then you should probably re-assess whether your dream school is actually your dream school.

## 32.3.1  Ethical Knowledge

- CASPer scenarios and behavioral questions aren't directly related to medicine. However, the same *ethical principles*—honesty, justice, nonmaleficence (avoiding doing harm), respecting others' autonomy—are highly relevant. In addition, developing a working understanding of these *general* ethical principles and knowing how to apply them to *specific* situations will prepare you for MMIs.
- As reference materials, we recommend skimming through the University of Washington's Bioethics Topics page[1] +/– *Doing Right* by Philip C. Hébert[2] to get a comprehensive overview of medical (and really professional) ethics as a whole. *This is probably overkill for CASPer*, but it will help you tremendously for MMI interviews.
- **Behavioral Questions**—We recommend searching online for "common interview behavioral questions" and having an answer for the following general questions that you can shape accordingly for specific prompts:
  - Tell me about a time you failed.
  - Tell me about a time you handled an interpersonal conflict.
  - Tell me about a time you disagreed with a superior.
  - Tell me about a time you worked with someone unlike yourself.

## 32.3.2  Identifying Multiple—Potentially Unspoken—Perspectives in an Interpersonal Conflict

- You may run into scenarios that have "obviously bad actors." For example, you might be the cashier at a fast food restaurant, and a customer may be needlessly rude and ask for a free meal. Here, you will want to avoid the *fundamental attribution error*,[3] the tendency to explain other people's bad behavior as products of their innate personalities, rather than as potentially arising from particular circumstances.
  - For example, consider that the customer is normally a very pleasant person but had just been laid off from her job that day. You may wish to respond with, "*Naming and reflecting the emotion - > open-ended question*", e.g., "You seem frustrated. What is bothering you?"
  - Essentially, your answer should demonstrate that you're willing to give people the benefit of the doubt and can explore other people's emotions and circumstances without being hastily accusatory.

---

[1] Bioethics Topics. Available at: https://depts.washington.edu/bhdept/ethics-medicine/bioethics-topics. Accessed July 8, 2022.
[2] Doing Right. Available at: https://global.oup.com/academic/product/doing-right-9780199031337?cc=us&lang=en&. Accessed July 8, 2022.
[3] The Fundamental Attribution Error: What it is and how to avoid it?. Available at: https://online.hbs.edu/blog/post/the-fundamental-attribution-error. Accessed July 8, 2022.

### 32.3.3 Articulating Your Values and Responsibilities

- At the same time, you should be aware of your specific responsibilities. For example, as the cashier, you have a duty to the company to ensure its function, and you would not be able to simply give the woman free food (as an example).
- Your response should specifically mention the variety of perspectives and how they clash in the scenario.

### 32.3.4 Choosing a Side and Justifying It

- Once you have considered the multiple perspectives and issues in the scenario, you must choose a plan of action and justify it. To do this, we recommend the course of action that maximizes utility ("What would do the most good for the most amount of people?" i.e., *utilitarian ethics*) while also avoiding actions that are straightforwardly "wrong" or "unethical" by most conventional ethical systems (e.g., avoiding murder or lying, i.e., *deontological ethics*—an ethical system that emphasizes avoiding actions that are "wrong" under a series of rules, e.g., societal norms for conduct).[4] Whenever possible, you should also try to invoke *principlist biomedical ethics* by explicitly making mention of your concerns for **autonomy** (the patient's right to control their body), **nonmaleficence** ("do no harm"), **beneficence** (doing whatever you can to help the patient), and **justice** (balancing respect for fairness, judicious allocation of scarce resources, and upholding the law[5]).
- We suggest using conditional "if/then statements," e.g., "If I discovered that the woman was seriously ill, then I would find out more and be prepared to ask someone else to call 911. On the other hand, if the woman did not have any serious extenuating circumstances and simply wanted a free meal, then I would uphold my responsibility to the restaurant and politely refuse."
- When justifying your answer, you should state the anticipated *consequences* of your decision.

Realistically, you only need 2 to 7 days to prepare for CASPer if you're crunched for time. However, we highly recommend taking the time to read through at least one of the reference books on ethics, as you'll also knock out much of your MMI prep by doing so.

### 32.4 Is There Any Practice Material?

The CASPer website has practice material at the "CASPer System Requirements Check." You can also take a free CASPer practice test at https://www.caspertest.com/casper-sample-questions/.[6]

### 32.5 Summary

CASPer is an online situational judgment test required by an increasing number of medical schools. You will be presented with hypothetical scenarios, and will have to formulate a response based on (1) basic working knowledge of professional and personal ethics, (2) the ability to identify multiple perspectives and sides in an interpersonal conflict, (3) the ability to articulate your values and responsibilities, and (4) the ability to *choose* one side and justify it. We recommend skimming the above resources if you feel shaky on professional and medical ethics, and improving your typing speed and significant practice if you find you have trouble finishing the prompts.

---

[4] Mandal J, Ponnambath DK, Parija SC. Utilitarian and deontological ethics in medicine. Trop Parasitol. 2016 Jan-Jun; 6(1): 5–7. Available at: https://www.ncbi.nlm.nih.gov/pmc/articles/PMC4778182/. Accessed July 8, 2022.
[5] Of course, the history of medical ethics abounds with examples of providers choosing to go against unjust laws.
[6] We have no affiliation with this website and cannot vouch for how well their practice test mimics the actual exam.

# 33 Secondary Application

*Joel Thomas*

Pat yourself on the back. After much soul-searching and several personal statement revisions, you've finally finished your American Medical College Application Service (AMCAS) application—the digital representation of your lifetime of sweat and tears in the pursuit of medicine.

Unfortunately, virtually all schools will require *even more* writing (and payment) through a "secondary application," a series of prompts specific to each school. While some programs screen applications and only send secondaries to a subset of applicants, these are in the small minority. As such, you should expect to complete a secondary for each medical school you've applied to. Because these secondaries are the only school-specific piece of your application at this point, they are closely scrutinized by admissions committees to gauge applicants' specific interest in their program.

Because applications are generally evaluated on a rolling basis, it's in your best interest to submit your secondaries within a few days of receiving them. Unfortunately, many schools send their secondary applications at around the same time in the application cycle. Thus, you will be expected to produce high-quality writing for multiple schools at a moment's notice to be submitted almost immediately.

Yes, this does sound daunting, but it's not actually as bad as it could be. First, the 150 + medical schools in the United States mostly ask about the same themes, albeit at different word limits; your recollection of "your greatest challenge" may range from 1,000 words for one school to 2 sentences for another. In total, you will realistically only have to introspect and respond to unique 10 to 15 essay prompts.

Second, almost all schools use the same prompts each year, and these prompts are neatly catalogued on studentdoctor.net. *Thus, we strongly recommend prewriting your secondary application essays using the previous year's prompts.* This way, you won't be overwhelmed with having to submit multiple essays to different schools on a short notice. You may have to add or remove detail depending on whether character limits have changed. At worst, you might spend a day or two on intensive writing if a school completely changes its prompt; some schools (e.g., Duke School of Medicine) are famous for doing this, and such information is publicly available on studentdoctor.net.

We have reviewed the secondary prompts from all 155 MD and 37 DO programs in the United States for the 2021 to 2022 application cycle. Fortunately, we were able to distill them into 20 unique themes that will allow you to comfortably brainstorm material for whatever secondary prompts you encounter. While reflecting on these questions, think about what material is essential to your narrative versus additional detail that can be added or removed to fit character limits. We also encourage you to practice speaking out loud your responses to these questions, as they are also frequent topics of conversation during interviews.

## 33.1 The Prompts

### 33.1.1 Diversity

How will you contribute to the diversity of our class/what makes you special/why is diversity important to the medical profession? This is arguably the most common secondary theme. Recognize that it **is** possible to give a fantastic answer to this without being an under-represented minority. In fact, the majority of accepted students are not under-represented minorities (by definition).

To answer this well, really reflect on what makes you unique compared to other pre-medical students that you know. Did you study or do research on some unusual topic in college? Are you a serious athlete who cultivated excellent time management skills through competing while being a full-time student?

Medical schools value diversity in two ways. First, they want a diverse class (remember what we said earlier about being a "pointy applicant") because physicians are expected to be leaders in whatever niche they carve in medicine. There are many different ways to specialize and make a difference in medicine. Presumably, a class of students with a wide variety of perspectives and experiences will branch out to become leaders approaching patient care from different angles. The second way is recruiting students who have personally worked with people from many different backgrounds, which brings us to…

## 33.1.2 Breadth of Perspectives

Tell us about a time you've worked with people unlike yourself/how have you advocated for people unlike yourself? Tell us about a time when you were in the minority and what did you learn from this experience? Physicians must be able to reliably make good impressions with people from all walks of life. They're expected to do this very quickly, often in the most harrowing moments of people's lives. Understanding the lived experiences of people unlike yourself helps you empathize with them on a deeper level, appreciating what they value over what you might find important[1] (source?).

## 33.1.3 Why Us?

Why are you applying to this school? How will you contribute to the mission of the school? At minimum, you'll want to know all of the information on Medical School Admission Requirements (MSAR) and the school's website. We also recommend reading the school-specific threads on studentdoctor.net, as current students and other applicants frequently discuss unique aspects of the program.

You should also invoke your *narrative* (as discussed in Chapter 5, Building Your Narrative). How does the school's mission align with your application's strengths? For example, if you have significant experience working with underserved populations, you may want to highlight X program's area of concentration for working with underserved populations.

## 33.1.4 Explain Yourself

Explain any shortcomings/inconsistencies in your applications (e.g., gaps in employment or education, poor performance, prior failed application cycle, disciplinary action, or criminal history). If you have previously applied, how have you strengthened your application to make sure you get in this time? The biggest mistake you can make with this prompt is making excuses (or appearing like you're doing so). Explain in neutral terms exactly what happened and provide evidence to suggest that it was an atypical, one-off occurrence. You should also provide details showing how you have worked to make sure that this event won't occur again.

## 33.1.5 Challenge

Tell us about the biggest challenge you've faced. What have you learned from it?
• What challenges do you anticipate in medical school (and beyond) and how will you address them?
• Tell us about a time you failed. What did you learn from it?
• What are your coping mechanisms for stress?
• Give us an example of feedback/criticism you received that was surprising/difficult to receive. How did you respond, etc.?
• Tell us about a time you faced a challenge working in a group and how you overcame it.

*Try not to write about academics.* Throughout your medical career, you will face significant interpersonal and emotional trials. In this context, academic competency is expected as a bare minimum while facing these other challenges. You want to share an event that demonstrates your resiliency and ability to adapt to emotional or interpersonal challenges.

Keep in mind that schools are not looking for epic war stories—unless you have them; most applicants have had a fairly comfortable middle- to upper-middle-class upbringing. What's most important here is demonstrating your ability to cope with adversity.

---

[1] Cao Y, Contreras-Huerta LS, McFadyen J, Cunnington R. Racial bias in neural response to others' pain is reduced with other-race contact. Cortex 2015;70:68–78. https://doi.org/10.1016/j.cortex.2015.02.010

### 33.1.6 Most Rewarding Experience

Tell us about your most rewarding experience. Invoke your narrative. Show (don't tell) that you exemplify the virtues and core competencies that medical schools value.

### 33.1.7 Academic Interests

Why did you go to X for undergrad? This is less common of a secondary prompt but a somewhat common interview question. Again, invoke your narrative.

### 33.1.8 Back-up

What would you do if you didn't get into medical school this cycle? Very straightforward—you will identify your weaknesses this cycle and apply again next year, having patched those weaknesses. You should explain your specific back-up plans to strengthen your application (e.g., research year, working in a clinical setting, etc.).

### 33.1.9 Alternate Universe

What would you do if you couldn't become a physician? This is a very different question from the previous one.. You could pick a career that also incorporates the professional values you appreciate in medicine, e.g., physician assistant, clinical researcher who spends much time volunteering on their own time, etc. Picking careers outside of medicine is obviously also acceptable. Most of us had career opportunity costs for picking medicine, and it's OK to say you wanted to be an economist, writer, etc.

### 33.1.10 Continuity

What are your plans for this year while you're applying to medical schools? Just demonstrate that you're committed to keeping up the things you've been doing throughout college (again, keep your narrative consistent).

### 33.1.11 What Else?

Tell us something that isn't already on your primary (e.g., significant aspect of your personal background or identity, e.g., religion/cultural upbringing/gender identity; significant passion/hobby/interest).
• What do you do for fun? Any recent travel?
• Anything new since you've submitted your primary?

You can invoke your narrative here. However, some schools are genuinely just curious about your hobbies and interests outside of medicine. As such, consider this question in the context of the secondary as a whole—if there's an extremely small character limit or if other questions already ask you serious introspective questions, then you're probably free to mention your interests in surfing or pie making.

### 33.1.12 Looking Ahead

How do you ideally see your medical career (e.g., 20 years from now?) Do any particular areas of medicine interest you? Why do you think you're a good fit for this interest? Invoke your narrative. Refer to specific experiences or accomplishments to substantiate your stated interests.

### 33.1.13 Values

What qualities ("which five"—on Geisinger's secondary) are essential to success in medicine? Tell us about how you demonstrate those qualities and/or continue to work on them. Refer to the AAMC

Core Competencies.[2] Of note—the University of Massachusetts secondary has prompts based on "competencies that are important for a physician to possess": leadership, teamwork, empathy/compassion, communication, inquiry, persistence/grit, advocacy/cultural competence. You probably can't go wrong with discussing any of these.

## 33.1.14 Looking Ahead

What challenges/changes do you anticipate for the medical profession in the future? You should have a passing knowledge of current events, especially related to healthcare economics. Wikipedia articles are a reasonable and efficient place to start, at least in terms of getting a basic overview and a list of other sources to check.

## 33.1.15 Narrative

Tell us about your community/family (and how they've shaped you).
• Tell us about what you have learned from your clinical (and/or nonclinical) volunteering experiences.
• Tell us about a leadership experience.
• Tell us about your role model.

Invoke your narrative.

## 33.1.16 Community

What is the role of the physician in the community? One possible way to address this question is discussing the role of advocacy. As a physician, your professional opinion holds significant weight in convincing public figures to effect change that improves the health of the underserved. A letter to a representative or even an Instagram post by a physician can make a large difference in convincing the right people to change the laws.

## 33.1.17 Ethics

How can a physician balance being empathetic/openly caring with being efficient/having enough emotional distance? This is difficult to answer without having the experience of working as a physician. We recommend approaching this question by first acknowledging that there *is*—indeed—a tricky sweet spot of emotional closeness that physicians should offer. This sweet spot is likely context dependent, as well. A physician could probably discuss his or her specific difficulties with more experienced physicians to gain a better perspective on how to balance the two extremes.

## 33.1.18 Regional Ties

Do you have any ties to the region? If you have immediate family or a significant other in the region, mention so. This will likely increase your chances of acceptance (schools prefer to admit applicants they think are likely to matriculate).

## 33.1.19 Miscellaneous

Schools with specific focuses (e.g., primary care, Spanish-speaking school, historically black, religious affiliated, military, research) will have a question related to that aspect of the school, why that appeals to you, and why you think you'd be a good fit. Refer to specific experiences/accomplishments in your life to substantiate your stated interests.

Some schools have very "out-of-the-box" secondaries (e.g., USC Keck—"Write a sentence that is not true, then tell us why you wish it were."). Just demonstrate that you can think creatively while also showing the competencies and characteristics that a physician should exhibit.

---

[2] Core Competencies for Entering Medical Students. Available at: https://www.aamc.org/services/admissions-lifecycle/competencies-entering-medical-students. Accessed July 8, 2022.

## 33.2 Summary

Virtually all schools will require *even more* writing (and payment) through a "secondary application," a series of prompts specific to each school. Because applications are generally evaluated on a rolling basis, it's in your best interest to submit your secondaries within a few days of receiving them. Second, almost all schools use the same prompts each year, and these prompts are neatly catalogued on studentdoctor.-net. *Thus, we strongly recommend prewriting your secondary application essays using the previous year's prompts.* In total, you will realistically only have to respond to unique 10 to 15 essay prompts due to the overlap and redundancy of prompts between different schools.

# 34 Interviews

*Joel Thomas*

Congrats! You got an interview invite! The interview is the last major step in your medical school journey. It's understandable to be nervous at this point. It's absolutely possible to torpedo your efforts over the past few years in a single day. That said, our experience with Admissions Committees (ADCOMs) has shown us that most applicants don't dramatically strengthen or weaken their overall application on interview day. So *relax*. You've already done most of the legwork over the past few years by forging yourself into a competitive applicant. At this point, there isn't much that's in *your control* for you to worry about. While you definitely need to prepare for interview day, you should also remember that it's just as much an opportunity for the schools to try to sell themselves to you.

In this chapter, we will discuss the role of the interview in your overall application, as well as strategies for succeeding on interview day. In the next chapter, we will share strategies for making your months of travel and interviewing as painless as possible.

## 34.1 How Important Are Interviews?

Interviews are counterintuitive in terms of their effect on the overall application. ADCOMs rank them as the most important variable for acceptance.[1] At the same time, from our own experience on ADCOMs, interviews generally don't help or hurt most applicants. This is because your application is still judged holistically after interview day. It is *not* the case that all applicants are on an equal footing come interview day, with the interview being the deciding factor afterward. Instead, ADCOMs meet periodically throughout the interview season to discuss applications *as a whole*, incorporating interview impressions with the rest of the application.

To illustrate this point, imagine that applicants to a medical school are on various levels of a ladder (▶ Fig. 34.1) based on their overall application's competitiveness (e.g., grade-point average [GPA], Medical College Admission Test [MCAT], extracurriculars). Applicants above a certain level will get invited to interview. The interview can raise or lower the applicant even further, and applicants that hit the "acceptance" level get accepted. Some applicants will already be above this level before they interview. For these applicants, the interview is essentially a formality, and they will get admitted unless they do exceptionally poorly on the interview. Likewise, some applicants are barely above the "interview" level, and they will need to perform exceptionally well on interview day to gain admission.

So it's true that an excellent interview has the opportunity to dramatically improve an applicant's chances. Likewise, a brutally poor interview will destroy an otherwise outstanding application. Most applicants, however, have "decent" interviews that don't move them much on the ladder. The rest of their application will do most of the leg work for admissions. What this means for *you* is that you should prepare as hard as you can for interviews, but you should also realistically expect that it won't make or break your application because virtually everyone else at the interview stage will have also prepared extensively. Instead, you should use interview day to *meet your future colleagues*[2] and learn as much as you can about each school, *especially from current medical students.* The medical students will give you the most unfiltered, honest take on what daily life is actually like at that school because they don't have the same pressures and incentives as the ADCOM to dazzle you with rosy PowerPoint presentations. That said, they may not necessarily be completely forthcoming about the less-than-ideal aspects of their experiences because they may feel uncomfortable about painting the school in a potentially negative light. Therefore, you will need to learn how to ask the right questions and how to read between the lines when discussing difficult topics.

---

[1] Medical School Admissions: More than Grades and Test Scores. Available at: https://www.aamc.org/media/5916/download. Accessed July 8, 2022.

[2] Seriously! You will meet some incredibly interesting people on the interview trail who will end up as your classmates and colleagues down the line. These are the people you will meet on the medicine wards, the operating room, etc. As exhausting as the interview trail can be, you should try to become energized by these people. Make the effort to meet at least one person each interview day who you genuinely enjoy hanging out with!

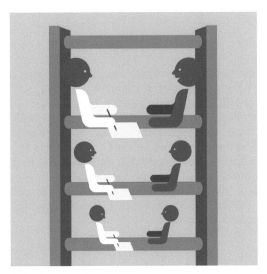

**Fig. 34.1** Ladder model for medical school interviews.

## 34.2 So How Do I Maximize My Face Time with Current Medical Students?

Be extremely enthusiastic, positive, and charming. Medical students are very busy, and they're taking time out of their schedule to talk to you. They know that you're probably nervous, as they were in your shoes just a few years ago.

- Begin the interactions with easy questions about positive things: "What do you like the most about being here?" "Why did you pick this program?" "What kind of medicine do you want to do, and what sorts of opportunities do you have to explore that?" "What are some of the more unique features of this program that really appeal to you?".
- If you're at a lull in conversation, ask "What do you do for fun?" "What's a typical day like for you?"
- Try to understand what a typical, boring Wednesday would be like! Ask them where people get groceries, how easy it is to work out, etc.
- What is the advising like? Are there big class-wide events that many people attend? *Do you anticipate any curriculum changes in the next few years? (i.e., something that would affect **you** if you matriculate).* Do students feel prepared for board exams—how similar are in-house exams to NBME material? How receptive is the administration to proposed changes by the students? Is there much interaction—if any—with other schools (e.g., undergrad, law, pharmacy, etc.) How do you like the city/town? How is parking for clinical rotations, and how far do people have to go? What are the study spaces like?
- On a typical week, how much mandatory material is there? (e.g., workshops).
- (If pass/fail)—is it true pass/fail, or are there internal rankings? If so, do they affect placement in AOA? (Tread carefully with these questions—you want to avoid appearing like a cutthroat gunner).

Once you've established some rapport, dip your toes into the harder-hitting territory that is critical to explore. "What would you change about the program if you could?" "Is there anything in the program that hasn't lived up to your expectations so far?" In addition, *read between the lines*. If the applicant is struggling to come up with compelling answers to "What do you like the most about this program" or "Would you choose this program again?", then take note of that. Of course, the student simply may just be having a "meh" day, and you should not totally discount the program on this basis alone. At the same time, you will recognize throughout the interview trail that students who love their schools and would wholeheartedly recommend it interact *very* differently with applicants compared to more disheartened students.

# 34.3 Interview Day Preparation

You need to strike the right balance between "rehearsed presentation," "feel-good conversation between two good friends," and "impromptu introspection out loud" in your interviews. You will have to balance "being yourself" and "leading with the aspects of your personality that click best with your interviewer." This is both an art and science. We recommend the following:

- Know your application in and out, and be prepared to speak at length about any little detail. Literally down to the last word; we've been in interviews where we've been asked to expand in great detail about a half-sentence tucked away in our extracurriculars or biographical information.
  - Be prepared to address any weakness—real or perceived—in your application. I literally had an interviewer probe me about a "C" in gym class on my *high school* transcript[3] because the grade for that class was entirely my grade on a physical fitness exam. The grade did not even count toward my GPA.
  - Take time before your first actual interview to do deep introspection about everything on your application. At every experience—what motivated you to do it? What were your expectations heading in? How was it different? What did you learn? What are the insights you gained? How did it affect you as a person, your perspective, your beliefs, and the role of what medical training could play? The role of what you could play in the future? What is the theme and common thread that connects your experiences, or why you pursued them, or what insight you took away from them? How does this tie into your motivation to pursue medicine and reinforce your best qualities?
- Be able to speak intelligently about current events in medicine and—to a lesser degree—the news in general.
- **There's only a limited amount of time in each interview,** and therefore only parts of your application will receive attention. That said, there are certain things we *strongly advise* you to bring up—even if not already done so by the interviewer—*at every interview*: evidence of your commitment to hard work, demonstration that you're empathetic and genuinely care about patients' well-being, and that you're a multidimensional, interesting person who's a delight to work with under stressful conditions, capable of being a team player, *and* a leader depending on the situation.
- **Continue your hobbies and interests throughout the interview season.** Interviewers want to admit applicants who can demonstrate that they are multidimensional and continue to pursue interests outside of medicine.
  - This includes reading for leisure. Be able to intelligently discuss a book for, "What was the last book you read/what are you currently reading?"
- **The "interview" isn't just the interview.** Treat the whole day as the interview. *Everything you do the entire day is under scrutiny.* We have heard too many horror stories about applicants who were (inadvertently?) standoffish to the administrative assistant or security guard—perhaps because they were running late or nervous—only to have it communicated to the ADCOM. Treat everyone with the same enthusiasm and warmth you would give to your interviewer.
- **Introverts—take heed.** If you are introverted at baseline, you should make an effort to appear sociable. Medicine, for better or worse, tends to reward extraversion,[4] and introversion may be mistaken for asociality. Unfortunately, this is something you will need to carry forward into your clinical rotations, as well. Fortunately, there tends to be less of an expectation to appear outwardly extroverted the farther you advance in your career (presumably because your reputation and evaluations will begin to speak for themselves).
- **Don't lie.** If you genuinely don't know the answer to a question, then say so. If you need to speculate/ offer a reasonable guess, but *qualify* your answer as such.
- **PRACTICE PRACTICE PRACTICE.** Do at least three to four full-length practice interviews under real conditions (i.e., wearing your interview attire, at the same time of day). Your prehealth advising office will usually offer these, but it is much better to get them from people in medicine. Try to find medical students, residents, and—ideally—attending physicians who can interview you and give you honest

---

[3] This was for an "early assurance" program that required high school transcripts.
[4] Lievens F, Ones DS, Dilchert S. Personality scale validities increase throughout medical school. J Appl Psychol 2009;94(6):1514–35. Available at: https://pubmed.ncbi.nlm.nih.gov/19916659/. Accessed July 8, 2022.

feedback. Also, *record* your interviews. Yes, it will be painful to watch, but the throes of embarrassment are your best teachers for avoiding the same mistakes on interview day.

- If you can't find anyone in healthcare to interview you, we recommend Googling "medical school interview prep" to find medical students and doctors willing to interview you. If you're trying to save money, we recommend posting on reddit.com/r/premed, reddit.com/r/medicalschool, reddit.com/r/residency, reddit.com/r/medicine, and SDN to find people willing to help you for free.

- **Body language is crucial.** The moment you meet your interviewer, sport a warm, resting smile at all times, introduce yourself confidently, and *meet the handshake* if you are offered one (conventions have changed during the COVID-19 pandemic).

  - If your interviewer is meeting you in a public space and walking you to his/her office, make small talk en route (e.g., where you are traveling from, what you've done already in the day, etc.).
  - Maintain strong but not overpowering eye contact throughout the interview (it helps to look at the bridge of the nose between the eyes if direct eye contact is too intimidating for you).
  - Speak slowly and deliberately while minimizing the use of filler words, e.g., "um" and "like."
  - Maintain a fine balance between formal and casual. You don't want to appear robotic, but you don't want to be overly casual with your interview. You want to appear incredibly warm and caring.
    1. Try to emulate how popular politicians speak to their electorate. Give your interviewer the same feeling that you get when you finally meet up with your best friend in a warm coffee shop on a bracing winter night.
  - Get into the habit of *thinking several steps ahead* before you speak. For every question that the interviewer asks you, delay answering the question for a second or so, and use this time to quickly think of the general theme of the answer you will give and how you will elaborate on it. As you begin your answer in a general format, mentally fill in the gaps on the details. If you're truly at a loss, stall for time and gather your thoughts with, "That's a really interesting/great question. Let me gather my thoughts for a second" < Take up to 15 seconds >.
  - Strike the fine balance between appearing prepared and extemporaneous. You will need to have general answers to the most common questions *cold*, but be flexible in how you present them, depending on the disposition of the interviewer and the specific format of the question you are asked, e.g., "When did you first decide to go into medicine?" vs. "Why do you want to become a doctor?"
  - For virtual interviews, invest in an HD webcam and ring light setup. Have a clean background, but you may get bonus points if you have a conversation starter in plain view (e.g., musical instrument, interesting book). Wear the usual interview attire. Have interruption-free internet connection. Minimize distracting background noise (e.g., dog, baby, other people in your house or apartment, notifications from your computer or phone).

## 34.3.1 Know Your Answers to the Following Questions Cold

- *"Tell me about yourself."* This will likely be the first question you are asked, and it's very easy to stumble aimlessly and frustrate your interviewer. This is your opportunity to speak about your life in a broad sense (e.g., upbringing, nonmedical interests), but you also need to keep it relevant. We recommend where you were born/grew up, where you went to college and what you majored in, major extracurriculars you did in college (particularly research if applicable), what you did in your gap year (if applicable), your personal hobbies/interests, and what you hope to achieve in medicine.

  - "So my name is Kevin James. I'm from Long Island, New York, and I went to SUNY Stony Brook for college. I majored in psychology, and I was on the track team and speech and debate team. I volunteered weekly in the ED at Winthrop Hospital for 4 years, and worked in a lab doing bench research on fruit flies. During that experience, I became interested in the translational aspects of bench research as it could apply to clinical practice. After medical school, I'd like to go into academic medicine and eventually conduct translational research."

- *"Why medicine?"* Don't completely rehash your personal statement; the interviewer has likely already read this. Instead, *hit the major themes again*, but restate the major themes and *show* (through your body language, tone of voice) that you were genuinely moved by the major points you spoke about in your application. This is the time to give life to your application and to clarify any questions the interviewer may have.

- *"What excites you the most about medical school?"* Tie it back to your narrative. Leave the interviewer with a lasting impression about your core values and what genuinely excites you. Speak to your extracurriculars thus far and how you hope to additionally pursue similar opportunities at a higher level in medical school.
- *"Why this school?"* This is your opportunity to show that you have done extensive research about the school. If you stayed with a student host, then hopefully you picked their brain about features of the school that aren't immediately apparent on the website or admissions brochures. To knock this question out of the park, you will need to tie overarching themes (e.g., working with special patient populations) or unique opportunities at the school to your personal narrative.
  - "I got the impression that the school really values clinical acumen—both in specialized academic medicine *and* primary care—while also empowering students to be community leaders. This really appeals to me, and I pursued this interest throughout college by… I really think I'd be able to continue my professional development in that regard by…."
- *"What areas of medicine interest you the most?"* or *"Where do you see yourself in 10 years?"* You need to demonstrate that although you've done much research about medicine and sought clinical experience, you still have an open mind and are willing to explore other areas of medicine. If you have some particular interest, then talk about it! Just also make it clear that you're open to falling in love with other specialties.
- *"What questions do you have for me?"* This may literally be the first and only question in the interview. You *need* to have thoughtful questions that cannot be answered by a quick Google search. Don't leave the interviewer hanging!
  - "Why did you choose to work here, and what keeps you excited to come to work?"
  - "I get the impression that many different types of students could thrive here. I'm curious—what type of student would *not* do well here?"
  - "What would you say is an underappreciated feature of this school?"
- *"What is your biggest weakness?"* This is an incredibly difficult question. Frankly, we don't even know if interviewers expect an *honest* answer to this and instead simply ask it to see if applicants can come up with convincing, "on-paper appropriate" answers on-the-fly (versus genuinely gauging applicants' capacity for self-reflection). This is because you run the risk of having your entire application tossed out if you give a weakness that is sufficiently worrisome to the interviewer—even if you provide strong evidence that you're actively working on the weakness and that it's unlikely to affect your ability to practice medicine. Unfortunately, "sufficiently worrisome" is highly subjective and likely to be fraught by bias on the part of the interviewer.
  - We recommend reading this excellent article on Savvy Premed about this question: https://www.savvypremed.com/blog/5-rhetorical-tricks-for-answering-whats-your-greatest-weakness-in-medical-school-interviews
- *"What do you anticipate struggling the most with in medical school?"* or *"What worries you the most about medical school?"* Again, don't reveal anything that would make the interviewer seriously question your ability to handle medical school. We recommend more "reasonable" fears that most students struggle with and overcome, e.g., adjusting to the workload, maintaining social relationships with people outside of medical school, etc.
- *"Is there anything else about you we should know about?"* YES. This is the interview version of the "optional essay." Re-emphasize something about you that makes you unique. Alternatively, mention a major update since submitting your application that hasn't been brought to light. Echo a major theme in your narrative and how this particular medical school would be a perfect fit with that theme. Don't leave the interviewer hanging!
- **Hypothetical ethical scenario:** Demonstrate that you can hold multiple opposing views at once and understand that the issue is complex and multifactorial.
  - "This is a difficult scenario. On the one hand, you could argue for X. On the other hand, you could make a convincing point that… Ultimately, I would do Y for reasons 1, 2, and 3."
  - When in doubt, refer to the principles of medical ethics: autonomy, nonmaleficence, beneficence, justice (including issues of social justice): https://depts.washington.edu/bhdept/ethics-medicine
  - Pick the more conservative sounding answer if in doubt.
  - As discussed in Chapter 32, Altus Suite: CASPer, Snapshot, and Duet, *Doing Right* by Philip C. Hébert is a fantastic resource for ethical questions.

- **Your thoughts on current events:** Similar approach as above for ethical scenarios. Current events also suffer from having polarized and sensational coverage on the media cycle. You'll shine if you can distill a controversial topic into its most neutral, objective account and approach it from multiple perspectives before ultimately offering your perspective—while also stating that you can understand why it's a controversial topic.
  - "As a future healthcare professional who has done reviews of the scientific literature, I am strongly in favor of wearing masks in public during the COVID-19 pandemic. At the same time, I can understand why many libertarian-leaning individuals—as well as those skeptical of government recommendations—are against the idea, particularly in light of clarion calls for public health interventions in the past that were not duly evidence-based. For this particular case, I am convinced by the body of evidence, but I can understand why people could be skeptical"
- **Stressful question:** Generally speaking, interviewers don't *want* to stress applicants. If they do, it's intentional, and they're *gauging your ability to handle unexpected stressful situations on the fly* (like you will have to do regularly as a physician). As such, handling stressful questions requires a level of emotional awareness.
  - We're going to recommend mindfulness meditation *yet again* to improve this skill. When you feel your sympathetic nervous system acting up (increased heart rate, sweating, vague abdominal pain from decreased gastric perfusion), take a second to be mindful and *recognize your internal state of mind*. Then, take a deep breath, gather your thoughts, and follow with a measured, strategic response.
- **Group interview:** This is rare, but some schools may have interviews in which more than one applicant is interviewed at a time.
  - *Do not appear overly competitive or cut-throat.* Do not interrupt or overpower the other applicant(s). Instead, *bolster* them and present yourself as a team player who can support colleagues. In doing so, you will actually gain the upper hand in this setting because medicine is a team sport. For example, if the other applicant(s) makes a good point, *explicitly acknowledge it as such* (e.g., "Matthew makes an excellent point"), and then *elaborate on it* ("…and I would also add…").
- **Behavioral questions**: These are questions that take the form of "Tell me about a time you…" to understand examples of your *past behavior*. These are frustrating for many applicants because they require pouring through the memory bank on-the-fly for applicable examples. They do, however, appear to be more evidence-based than standard open-form questions in terms of standardizing interview performance among applicants.[5] In general, we recommend using the **STAR Format** (situation, task, action, result). Describe the background situation, the specific task you faced, your action (elaborating on *other possible actions* and *why you picked your specific action based on your values*), and the result (including what you learned).
  - "Tell me about an ethical dilemma you navigated"—Describe the tension you faced between multiple possible choices you could have made but why you ultimately made the choice that you did (based on your individual values) and what you learned for future situations/what you might do differently in the future (if applicable).
  - "Tell me about a time you managed interpersonal conflict."
  - "Tell me about a time you served as a leader."
  - "Tell me about a time you worked with someone unlike yourself."
  - "Tell me about a time you failed."

## 34.4 Multiple Mini-Interview (MMI)

This is an interview format started at McMaster University in 2002. Instead of a few traditional open-form interviews of 20 to 40 minutes, all applicants rotate through the same 6 to 10 stations that each have a standardized set of questions or objectives. This format was developed because it presumably minimizes the effects of bias that may disproportionately color applicants' outcomes if they only have 1 to 2 interviews (e.g., with interviewers of similar vs. radically different backgrounds). With 6 to 10 stations, positive and negative outliers would be less influential, and applicants' performance would regress to the mean.

5  Easdown LJ, Castro PL, Shinkle EP, Small L, Algren J. The Behavioral Interview, A meThod to Evaluate Acgme Competencies in Resident Selection: A Pilot Project. J Educ Perioper Med. 2005 Jan-Jun; 7(1): E032. Available at: https://www.ncbi.nlm.nih.gov/pmc/articles/PMC4803420/. Accessed July 8, 2022.

- Most schools do not use this interview, but many do—including many top 20 schools (e.g., NYU, Stanford).
- The stations include ethical dilemmas, patient actor scenarios, teamwork exercises, writing prompts, and even short traditional interviews.
- *Learn how to interact with patient actors. This was a major blind spot for the author, and he failed miserably on his first patient actor station because he literally had no idea how to act like a healthcare professional interacting with a patient.*
  - YouTube "standardized patient history taking" for suggestions on how to introduce yourself and interact with the patient actor.
  - As awkward as it can be, you'll get points for being a good actor and playing along with the scenario. Don't make it more painful than it needs to be for the patient actor.
- Written prompts are essentially the same as any other interview question. As with CASPer, just make sure your typing speed is reasonable (see Chapter 32, Altus Suite: CASPer, Snapshot, and Duet for tips on improving typing speed).

**Thank You Notes/Emails**

Thank you correspondence has become a major source of frustration on the interview trail. Ideally, every applicant is sincerely thankful to the interviewers and sends them thank you correspondence out of genuine good will. The reality is that many applicants feel compelled to send them because other applicants send them, and they don't want to hurt their application by not sending them. At the same time, ADCOMs can't reliably distinguish between sincere and insincere "thank you" notes. Moreover, different schools have different policies about postinterview correspondence.

To simplify things, we recommend the following:

1. You *should* be appreciative to the ADCOM, particularly medical students. They typically don't stand to gain much from volunteering their time, and most do so out of genuine concern for selecting the best new class for their medical school. At the same time, we understand wanting to refuse to participate in the thank you note pageantry, especially considering how it has essentially evolved into a calculated gesture by many applicants.
2. Nonetheless, because you stand to gain from writing a thank you note (or you stand to look worse than other applicants by not writing one), **we recommend writing thank you notes/emails *unless explicitly told not to*** by the school.
   - Get the contact information of the people who interviewed you and send them an email expressing your gratitude *on the same day of the interview*—ideally immediately afterward, as their impression of you is still fresh.
   - Use the following format: "Hi Dr. X (or medical student's first name, if applicable), Thank you so much for taking the time to interview me for admission at XXX. I particularly enjoyed our discussion about YYY (elaborate in 1–2 sentences). I really enjoyed my time on campus, and I look forward to a final admissions decision."

## 34.5 Summary

While an interview can obviously tank your chances of admission, most applicants probably don't dramatically strengthen or weaken their overall application on interview day. The day is an opportunity for you to present a polished version of yourself and advocate for your chance to be admitted. Likewise, it is the best time to get to know the school, the people, and their environment. You aren't just there to sell yourself, but to experience what you might be walking into if you decide to matriculate there. If you are fortunate to be offered admission at multiple schools, this is an excellent time to gather information on factors that might help you decide between them. You should know, and practice (but never memorize) your rough answers to the most common interview questions. Going on mock interviews can be helpful in picking up on and mitigating red flags you may not be aware of, and polishing your presentation; we recommend this for every applicant. Be sure to practice some MMI questions and formatting as well. After your interview, be sure to write thank you emails to those that took the time to be with you on interview day.

# 35 Interview Trail Travel and Attire

*Joel Thomas*

The interview trail is a unique feature to medical school admissions, and you likely haven't experienced anything like it thus far. Here, we will discuss travel strategies and interview attire. Note that this chapter describes in-person interviews. Since the COVID-19 pandemic, the logistics of medical school interviews have been in flux, with multiple admissions cycles switching to 100% online interviews. As of 2022, it's still unclear when/if programs will return to in-person interviews, but we hope this chapter proves useful at that time.

## 35.1 Interview Trail Travel

Barring exceptional circumstances (e.g., global pandemic), you will need to physically show up to every medical school you interview at. This will be extremely expensive: $3,000 to $8,000 as described in Chapter 20, The Big Picture. Nonetheless, there are certain strategies you can employ to save hundreds, if not thousands of dollars.

- If you plan on having multiple flights, apply for **TSA Precheck**. This is a service that allows you to get expedited security checks for domestic and certain international flights. You can do this several months before interview season. Not having to stand in long lines at airports is a game changer.
- Get a **credit card with travel rewards.** As described in Chapter 22, Before You Begin: Application Cycle Prophylaxis, specific credit cards (i.e., Chase Sapphire Reserve, Chase Sapphire Preferred, Southwest Airlines Rapid Rewards Card, etc.) offer generous travel parks that can save you hundreds to thousands of dollars with flights, as well as generous flight perks (e.g., lounge access). The specifics of choosing among cards are beyond the scope of this chapter; we recommend reading multiple articles on Google on this very topic. That said, you should consider getting a card with an annual fee for the interview season, as these tend to offer better rewards that are ultimately worth it from a cost/benefit perspective. You can always "downgrade" to a card without an annual fee next year with the same institution.
  - You can gain even more flight rewards by exclusively flying with the same airline and using points judiciously.
- If possible, avoid checking bags. Many applicants successfully bring everything they need in carry-on luggage. The last thing you want to add to interview stress is lost luggage.
- Whenever possible, **cluster interview dates in the same geographic region**. Do not be shy about contacting programs you've already scheduled interview dates at to see if you can change the original interview date after getting another interview at a program nearby. Programs understand that applicants are trying to be economical.
- All things considered, **it's ok to spend more money for more opportunities**. That means you *should* pay the extra $500 for the opportunity to interview at another "reach" school on your list. Yes, the trail is expensive, but these expenses are ultimately a drop in the bucket in the grand scheme of your medical career. The difference of a few thousand dollars on the trail is nothing compared to the tens of thousands' dollars difference in cost of attendance between different schools that may admit you.
- Bring toiletries, casual clothes, over-the-counter as needed medications (e.g., ibuprofen, sleep aid, decongestant, etc.), a reusable water bottle (empty it before the security check at airports—it's extremely expensive to buy water at airports, and we recommend refilling your reusable bottle instead), lint roller, +/− a travel steamer to minimize wrinkles in clothes.
- **Lodging:** Whenever possible, stay with a student host. You'll gain invaluable insider information about the medical school experience that you can use when choosing among schools. This can also be excellent fodder for the interviews the next day. *Just make sure to be exceptionally courteous to the student: leave everything as clean as you found it, minimize noise/distraction at night, etc. Do NOT say or do anything that would present you in a negative light (e.g., being inappropriately casual—even if the student emphasizes that he/she is not associated with admissions).*
  - If no student host is available, ask friends and family across the country for overnight accommodations. Make good use of your network!

- Carefully vetted Airbnb's are a great economical option—the author exclusively used them for residency interviews. Otherwise, you can consider commercial hotels if you're concerned about the quality and safety of your lodgings.
- If you plan to do heavy driving, make sure you are up-to-date on **vehicle maintenance**. You should also **check the traffic laws** of whatever states you anticipate driving through. For example, it is a misdemeanor to drive > 10 mph beyond the speed limit in Virginia. This may not be immediately obvious to someone in a nearby state who plans to drive to a medical school interview in Virginia. If you're facing a misdemeanor, you will have to update all your medical schools with this!
  - Otherwise, we recommend audiobooks and podcasts to feed your brain (and provide interview fodder for the trail).

## 35.2 Interview Day Attire

Despite an increasing emphasis on open mindedness for an increasingly diverse patient population, the medical profession still expects specific professional norms for its practitioners. Unfortunately, what constitutes "professional" may be heavily biased by problematic historical attitudes. For example, a paper originally published in the *Journal of Vascular Surgery* identified female surgeons wearing bikinis on personal social media pages while off-hours as "potentially unprofessional," and the Editors ultimately retracted the paper in view of the fact that "professionalism has historically been defined by and for white, heterosexual men and does not always speak to the diversity of our workforce or our patients."[1]

What this means for you as an applicant is that there's a non-negligible likelihood that you will be judged harshly for violations of "professionalism," some of which may be archaic. As such, you are *strongly* encouraged to present yourself in a way that is least likely to offend, even though that may mean obliging outdated, potentially problematic norms. This means making fashion and grooming choices to avoid ill judgment that may not be immediately obvious. Some of these deliberations will be different for female-presenting applicants and male-presenting applicants. Therefore, we *strongly* encourage female-presenting applicants to read the recommendations on "Women's Interview Attire"[2] from Student Doctor Network (SDN) by female ADCOM members, and we encourage male-presenting applicants to be aware of avoidable strikes against their application on interview day by reading the "Men's Interview Clothing" thread by ADCOM members.[3]

Specific considerations aside, what follows are some general recommendations for "safe" interview attire. There are many deviations from these that are more than acceptable. This section is designed not for those who are experienced in professional attire (who can probably skip this section), but for people who feel they need a heavy amount of guidance, who just want something that will work in all interview situations.

- **Suits**: Get a two-piece suit of reasonable quality. This includes dress suits, skirt suits, pant suits, etc.
  - The suit should be fitted, but not too tight. Get a more traditional style—this is not the time to experiment with the cutting edge of fashion.
  - Appropriate colors for the suit are navy blue, charcoal, dark gray, dark brown. Avoid black or other colors. Avoid shiny fabrics.
  - Get a solid white or solid light-blue dress shirt.
  - If wearing a tie, make sure it matches the rest of your outfit, and make sure you know how to tie it.
  - Wear conservative solid black socks or something similar.
  - Avoid large, visible logos.
  - Dry clean the suit every few interviews and make sure that your clothes are not wrinkled.
- **Undergarments**: Avoid visible undergarments and showing a lot of skin.

[1] Hardouin S, Cheng TW, Mitchell EL, Raulli SJ, Jones DW, Siracuse JJ, Farber A. Retracted: Prevalence of unprofessional social media content among young vascular surgeons. Available at: https://www.jvascsurg.org/article/S0741–5214(19)32587-X/fulltext. Accessed July 8, 2022.
[2] Women's Interview Attire #4. Available at: https://forums.studentdoctor.net/threads/womens-interview-attire-4.1220512/. Accessed July 8, 2022.
[3] Men's Interview Clothing #4! (2017). Available at: https://forums.studentdoctor.net/threads/mens-interview-clothing-4-2017.1269021/. Accessed July 8, 2022.

- **Shoes:** Your shoes should match your belt color. The focus should be on professional, comfortable walking shoes. Oxfords or Derbys are generally your safest bets for traditional formal menswear. Closed-toed shoes are recommended. For shoes having heels, make sure you are comfortable walking several miles in them; flats are often the way to go.
- **Facial Hair/Beards: Corporate conventional wisdom, even recently, cautions that people should be clean shaven for professional interviews.** Given that many interviews are still conducted by older, likely more culturally conservative physicians, we recommend this as a defensive move. This is not to say that facial hair can't be professional, but it's better to play it safe than to risk having an unprofessional-appearing beard. Of course, you should use your judgment. If you simply feel more comfortable and confident with facial hair, then keep your *neatly groomed* facial hair.
- **Watch:** A smartwatch is perfectly fine, and we actually recommend it so you can respond to urgent emails during the trail (e.g., new interview invites).
- **Accessories**: Ear piercings, bracelets, and necklaces are fine, but avoid overly distracting accessories.
- **Hair:** Have a professional haircut close to the interview. Like all the other categories, just play it safe.
- **Luggage:** Consider investing in a carry-on bag with a suit compartment to keep the attire as wrinkle-free as possible.
- **Organization:** Consider bringing a professional portfolio binder. You can have copies of your CV in there (but you can also assume your interviewers will have this information) as well as a notepad to jot down questions for later, thoughts, etc.

## 35.3 Summary

For interview travel: get TSA precheck and a credit card with travel rewards. Try to group interviews in the same geographic region together so you can go from one to the next without returning home first. If you don't yet have an acceptance, you should be interviewing at every school that offers you one. If this means spending an extra thousand dollars, do it—that's cheaper than may be having to apply again in the future. Stay with medical students when interviewing if you can, both for cost and perspective on the program.

For interview attire: We realize we recommend a defensive, conservative approach—similar to what we recommended for your social media and online presence. This can be restrictive for those that like to express themselves online or in fashion. Our only point of emphasis is that the margins between applicants are very thin, and most people on your interview day have similar application statistics, and taking a risk without much upside doesn't make a lot of sense when the downside is so significant (even when that downside is present for unfair reasons—i.e., stodgy old doctor that has opinions on what constitutes "professional" attire).

# 36 Wait-List and Update Letters

*Phillip Wagner and Joel Thomas*

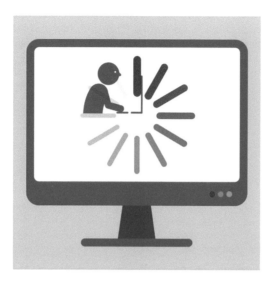

Medical schools interview a small fraction of those that apply, and an even smaller fraction is accepted. There are, however, a similarly small fraction of people who apply, are interviewed, but not accepted or rejected outright. They are instead alternates, and they are placed on a wait-list. The school likes you and would be happy for you to matriculate there, but you aren't among their first choices.

Each school sends out acceptances to a small proportion of those that interview (generally slightly more than their class size). If an accepted applicant is accepted to another school that they prefer, they reject their acceptance. At that point, the school turns to the wait-list to fill empty seats of accepted students who have decided to go elsewhere. Candidates on the wait-list are ranked, and your place on that list greatly affects your chances of admission.

Your position on the wait-list matters in three distinct scenarios: (1) The school at which you have been wait-listed is preferable to one you have already been accepted to, (2) the school at which you have been wait-listed is your number 1 school, and (3) the school at which you have been wait-listed is the only school (so far) that has not rejected you. If you aren't in one of those situations, you should skip the rest of this chapter.

If you fall into one of the above groups, then you need to get accepted by a school that has wait-listed you. You have only a few options at your disposal. They are as follows:
- Update letter.
- Letter of intent.

## 36.1 Update Letter

Your application will have been received roughly 1 year before you would matriculate. For many of you, your life doesn't stand still for that year. Events relevant to your application strength nearly always take place in that year. If you are still in school, you'll accumulate a year's worth of grades. If you are working, you'll gain one further year of experience. If you are doing research, you might produce one or more papers. Maybe you got a promotion, a newly defined role, joined a new club, participated in a new volunteer experience, or took on a novel leadership role. The point is that a lot of interesting stuff can happen in a year.

An update letter is sent to schools that have yet to finalize a decision on your application (i.e., wait-list or decision unknown so far). It shares significant updates, including (a) new grades, (b) new employment, (c) new clinical or nonclinical experiences (e.g., publication), and anything else that you think would aid in that school looking more favorably upon you as an applicant. These letters should be sent to every school that has wait-listed you, as well as to every school that has yet to communicate their decision to you *after admissions decisions have already been sent to other applicants.* These are often low-yield interventions. Virtually every applicant sends them, and they are likely never as important as anything in your primary application. That said, they have the benefit of being almost exclusively high reward/low risk. If your updates moved you up a couple spots on the wait-list, it may not matter, but it could also be the difference between you being accepted or not. In addition, the only cost is a small amount of time. Here is an example of an update letter the author used during his application cycle:

"Dear Office of Admissions:
   before "I am…"
   I am writing to add an update to my application since interviewing for the MD Program.
   I am currently participating in the NIH Academy Fellows Program, a selective yearlong program on health disparities sponsored by the NIH Office of Intramural Training and Education. This program meets every week and includes coursework on health disparities, regular talks from renowned experts in public health and policy, and a month-long workshop on promoting diversity and overcoming bias in professional settings.
   A major component of this program is a long-term community outreach project. For this project, I am working with a team of four other postbaccalaureate researchers to create new lesson plans for the Health Education Outreach Program, an organization that provides education on healthy living and integrating into society for the local homeless population in Bethesda, Maryland. Although the current lessons include a wealth of well researched information about healthy living, they lack tangible, realistic suggestions for health improvement that an average homeless person could use. Therefore, I am currently trying to incorporate practical solutions such as learning how to pick cheap and reasonably healthy fast food options as well as understanding how to qualify for affordable health insurance through the Patient Protection and Affordable Care Act. My group plans to test these new lessons in early May, and we are also working to expand the education program to other shelters in the area.
   I would also like to make it known that I am still very interested in attending XXX School of Medicine. Thank you again for giving me the opportunity to interview. I look forward to receiving a final decision from the Office of Admissions. Sincerely,

XXXXXXXX

There's no hard and clear answer when to send these letters. It will depend on when you hear (or when you don't hear, i.e., prolonged silence) from a school, as well as when you have something important to tell them. In general, they should be sent out sometime between September (if you even have any significant updates that early, which is unlikely) and December. They can obviously be sent out later if you go on some late interviews stretching into January and February, so it's obviously determined on a case-by-case basis. You should also send them if you've been wait-listed and your schools of interest are periodically sending acceptances off the wait-list.

And remember—you can send more than one update letter, especially if you are really having trouble deciding when to send one, and something significant happens early on that you want to share with schools. Many schools' application websites even have dedicated sections for updates officially versus sending them by mail/email.

If you know a school is your number 1 choice, then it is important to communicate this. This is because the admissions process for medical school is very different compared to undergraduate institutions. In fact, it appears counterintuitive if you do not understand the incentives at play. Whereas at undergraduate institutions, schools would accept you if they wanted you to go there (simple, right?), this is not the case for medical schools. They will likely offer you acceptance if they would like you to attend and *they think you have a high chance of not rejecting their offer and going somewhere else.* You may find if you are a competitive applicant, some of the schools that turn you down first will be schools at the bottom of your preference list. While that sounds fairly ridiculous, schools don't want to extend offers that will be turned down. This is known as **yield protection.**[1] So, sometimes if you are wait-listed, it may mean you are a second-tier choice for them, but it may also mean they think you will end up at a more competitive institution.

---

[1] Where to Apply When You're Applying: How to Pick? Available at: https://medicalschoolhq.net/opm-188-where-to-apply-when-youre-applying-how-to-pick/. Accessed July 8, 2022.

In short, schools want people who want to be there. Many schools even train their interviewers to score you on how much they perceive you to want to go there—it actually affects your chances! It's hard to say exactly how much, but many competitive applicants are really similar in grade-point average (GPA), Medical College Admission Test (MCAT) scores, and research experience. In general, writing a generic update letter takes very little time and energy. It may be the difference between an interview offer or not.

So, if a school is your number one, they need to know. So, in addition to sending them an update letter, as described above, you need to emphatically state that it's one of your top choices and give specific reasons why you would be a great fit and would love to attend.

## 36.2 Letter of Intent

So what does a letter of intent look like? There is no standard format, but it should unequivocally express that if accepted, regardless of who else offers you a spot, regardless of incoming financial aid packages (information you almost certainly won't have by the time) or any other factors, you will choose to matriculate there.

That said, as discussed in Chapter 20, The Big Picture, we advise caution with sending a letter of intent. There's no convincing data that they affect admissions decisions, and our educated guess is that they're unlikely to turn a blatant "no" into a "yes." In addition, a letter of intent is sent before an acceptance—as well as a financial package. Locking yourself to a particular school may force you into attending a school with a much heftier price tag compared to other schools that may admit you. Of course, if you anticipate that you will not be getting significant need- or merit-based aid, then this may not be as significant a consideration for you.

## 36.3 Summary

Many applicants will find themselves not outright rejected or accepted, but on a wait-list. There are certain things you can do in this state of limbo that may tip you toward an admission. These include an update letter with significant additions to your application that may distinguish you from other applicants on the wait-list. Alternatively, you can send a letter of intent that demonstrates your interest in and commitment to attending one specific school. The decision to send a letter of intent should be carefully considered, however, as you make the decision without financial aid information, which may vary greatly among schools that ultimately accept you.

# 37 Financial Aid

*Phillip Wagner and Joel Thomas*

Financial aid is a complicated subject for those with an interest in going to medical school. The loans that students typically have to take out are infamous and a major point of anxiety among applicants. There are some simple misconceptions that surround the medical school financial aid process, but not a lot of ways to make it much cheaper. How much you consider financial aid in your decision-making depends on where you are in the application process.

## 37.1 A Snapshot of Current Debt, Income, and Wealth

As of 2021, the average medical student graduates with $241,600 in *total* student loan debt, of which the average medical school debt is $215,900.[1] Barring major changes in student loan policy, that number will likely continue to increase as it has done every year for which we have data. In addition, the range of debt that students possess is not normally distributed: *30% of medical school graduates in 2020 had absolutely no debt*[2] while others—those without aid, scholarships, or family assistance who are enrolled at certain schools—can easily possess well over $300,000 in debt by graduation.

These debt numbers can be daunting, and **your choice of which school to attend should absolutely incorporate cost** (more in Chapter 38, Acceptance and Decisions: What Really Matters When Choosing the One School). However, applicants should be encouraged by what is known about physician income. Lists of annual income organized and stratified by physician specialty are abundant, and indicate that even the least lucrative specialties—pediatrics, urgent care, and family medicine—currently average between $200,000–300,000 in yearly salary, slightly over the total average expected medical school debt.[3] Physicians in these specialties may not earn this much the moment they graduate from residency and begin practicing, however. In addition, one must consider the *take-home* pay after taxes for these salaries—which may only be 50 to 60%—compared to the debt *burden* that evolves over time with interest. You generally cannot anticipate paying back $200,000 in loans taken out at graduation in 2 years with a $170,000 salary. In addition, you will likely have new, major expenses by this point (childcare, mortgage, life insurance, etc.) that limit how much of your take-home pay you can funnel toward loans.

That said, studies about physician **net worth** (i.e., accounting for taxes, expenses, and loans) paint an encouraging picture. According to Medscape's 2019 Physician Wealth and Debt Report, roughly 50% of practicing doctors at the age of 45 have a net worth exceeding 1 million dollars. As the age approaches 60, that number increases to 75%, with roughly one-fifth of that 75% having a net worth of greater than 5 million dollars.[4] Even at the lowest end of yearly salary, 60% of family medicine doctors have a net worth of over $500,000. That latter number may not seem like very much, but keep in mind that the median net worth for those of 60 years of age in the United States is between $150,000 and $200,000.[5] So while debt is a long-term burden for roughly three-quarters of doctors, it is by no means insurmountable for most doctors, and a significant proportion go on to have lucrative careers. Factoring in the annual unemployment rate for physicians, which is always less than 1%—compared to 4 to 10% for the US economy as a whole[6]—finding rapid employment is rarely a concern for a doctor.[7]

[1] Hanson M. Average Medical School Debt. Available at: https://educationdata.org/average-medical-school-debt. Accessed July 8, 2022.

[2] Medical School Graduation Questionnaire. Available at: https://www.aamc.org/media/46851/download (2020 AAMC GQ) . Accessed July 8, 2022.

[3] Physician Starting Salaries by Specialty: 2018 vs. 2017. Available at: https://www.merritthawkins.com/news-and-insights/blog/job-search-advice/physician-starting-salaries-by-specialty-2018-vs-2017/. Accessed July 8, 2022.

[4] https://www.medscape.com/slideshow/2019-compensation-wealth-debt-6011524#1

[5] Average Net Worth By Age: How Do You Compare? Available at: https://turbo.intuit.com/blog/real-money-talk/net-worth-by-age-704/. Accessed July 8, 2022.

[6] The Employment Situation – June 2022. Available at: https://www.bls.gov/news.release/pdf/empsit.pdf. Accessed July 8, 2022.

[7] Hargreaves S. Jobs with the lowest (and highest) unemployment. Available at: https://money.cnn.com/2013/01/04/news/economy/jobs-lowest-unemployment/index.html. Accessed July 8, 2022.

None of this changes the fact that the debt burden is significant. Many doctors take all 25 allowed years to repay their debt, and that initial average student debt of over $200,000 does not reflect what you will have paid once 25 years of compound interest is included. To illustrate the point, $170,000 of loan amounts to ~$360,000 paid back over 18 years when interest is included.[8] In addition, the cost of medical school has skyrocketed since the responders of those surveys had trained. Debt should certainly be a factor in your decisions, as its presence can obviously dampen your earning potential, but it can also pressure young doctors into working in geographic locations they would rather not, or working in more lucrative fields rather than in ones that they may enjoy more but are less lucrative. It is, and should be—for most applicants—an important factor in your decision making, but likely not the primary one.

Of course, finances more broadly are beyond the scope of this book. We recommend the following books as the best "bang for your buck" in terms of time invested to learn as much as possible about personal finances in medicine: *The White Coat Investor* (and its accompanying website)[9] and *The Bogleheads' Guide to Investing* (and its accompanying website).[10]

## 37.2 Financial Aid Doesn't Matter Early in the Process

The cost of medical school can seem burdensome at the outset, but you shouldn't concern yourself with it right away. When selecting which schools to apply to—a topic covered more thoroughly in Chapter 27, Making Your List: What Schools Do I Apply To?—it is important to make sure to apply to all of your state schools and apply broadly to many schools throughout each tier of competitiveness. Beyond that, financial aid should not affect your early considerations.

*The exception to this rule is if you are uncertain you want to go onto clinical medicine, i.e., residency training and beyond. Leaving after 2 years of medical school does not provide you with much increase in earning potential, but will provide you with a large increase in personal debt. Doctor-level debt is generally only OK if you are going to make doctor-level wages. While there are exceptions to this—some applicants transition successfully to medical or pharmacologic consulting or equally lucrative alternative careers every year (an MD degree can itself be lucrative without residency training)—several hundred thousand dollars in debt is something not everyone will be able to overcome without a medical degree or substantial family assistance.*

What this means is that you should apply while ignoring the "sticker price" of the listed tuition. If you have spent any time browsing any medical school guide, you have probably checked the annual tuition of each medical school. The listed price in whatever guide you have should more accurately be known as the "sticker price." What is a sticker price? If you have ever been shopping for cars, the sticker price is the price listed on the car when it is in the lot. However, this is not the price that everyone pays, and the real price depends upon many other factors.

Much like the sticker price on cars, you don't have any idea what you will end up paying in the end. You also have no idea what other people will end up paying. Unlike the sticker price on cars, however, much of the difference—or lack thereof—between the sticker price and what you pay will probably not be up to you and your negotiating ability. It is largely out of most applicants' control. You will not know the actual cost of your attendance at a particular school until your acceptance. At that point, you will receive a personalized Financial Aid Award letter from the school, and a much clearer view of your financial outlook. But while you are applying, ignore the prices.

## 37.3 Financial Aid: When You Are Applying

Application cost: Most application sources—this one included—recommend that you apply to between 12 and 25 schools. Say you apply to 18 schools—somewhere in the middle of that range. That will cost, at minimum, about $2,500, just for the primary and secondary applications. In addition, you should expect to spend quite a bit of money travelling for interviews, depending on how many offers you receive. Based on travel expenses, as discussed in Chapter 20, The Big Picture—the application process can easily cost $3,000 to $8,000.

[8] Hargreaves S. Jobs with the lowest (and highest) unemployment. Available at: https://apps.aamc.org/first-gloc-web/#/calculator/details. Accessed July 8, 2022.

[9] A Doctor's Guide to Personal Finance—Book Overview. Available at: https://www.whitecoatinvestor.com/the-book/. Accessed July 8, 2022.

[10] Getting started. Available at: https://www.bogleheads.org/wiki/Getting_started. Accessed July 8, 2022.

If you or your family cannot provide that money, consider using student loans—if you are a student currently—or applying to the AAMC's Fee Assistance Program,[11] which allows you to apply up to a certain number of schools at a reduced rate based on a sliding scale of family income. It will not eliminate your costs, but can mitigate your common and secondary application costs substantially. Your travel costs are, however, not covered by any widely available financial aid.

## 37.4 Financial Aid: After You Have Applied (Submitted Your Primary and Secondary Applications)

Do nothing! All you have so far is the sticker prices. Wait until you're accepted and get aid packages.

## 37.5 Financial Aid: After Acceptance

If you receive an acceptance from a medical school, you will be asked to submit personal information regarding yours and your parents' financial status. Eventually you will receive a Personalized Award Letter, showing you what kind of aid you are eligible for if you choose to attend this institution. This letter can be confusing, as can navigating the other types of available aid. Below you will find a brief description of the various types of aid that are available.

## 37.6 Understanding Your Personalized Award Letter; What Types of Aid Are Available?

If accepted by a medical school, you will receive a personalized aid package. In this aid package, you may receive several types of aid. Among them are:
- Government-backed loans (available to everyone).
- Institution-based loans (from the medical school, institution dependent).
- Need-based aid (from the medical school, available to some students).
- Merit scholarships (available to *almost no one*).

Outside those sources of aid listed in your award letters, you may receive aid from:
- Outside scholarships.
- Private loans.
- Special admissions/combined degree programs (MD/PhD and others).
- Mandatory service clauses (primary care, underserved communities, military-based).

So what are these different options?

### 37.6.1 Government-Backed Loans

Sadly, this type of "aid" is loans given to you by the federal government. These types of loans start accruing interest immediately, and will have the interest capitalized and compounded over time. You have to pay these back at a rate of interest which is generally higher than that charged for government-backed undergraduate loans.

The only way to have these paid back for you is to go into medical service in some sector of the nonprofit or government sector for a certain period of time (aka **Public Service Loan Forgiveness [PSLF]**, in which case your loans will be forgiven—more in Chapter 41, Real Talk on a Medical Career], or to enter into some incentivized service contract (i.e., **National Health Service Corps [NHSC]**—agreeing to work in a medically underserved area for some variable amount of years during your career[12]). Several branches of the United States Military offer a similar incentivized contract, as well (i.e., the **Health Professions**

---

[11] Fee Assistance Program (FAP). Available at: https://students-residents.aamc.org/applying-medical-school/applying-medical-school-process/fee-assistance-program/. Accessed July 8, 2022.

[12] NHSC: Scholarship and Loan Repayment Programs. Available at: https://students-residents.aamc.org/financial-aid/article/nhsc-scholarship-and-loan-repayment-programs/. Accessed July 8, 2022.

Scholarship Program [HPSP]).[13] However, this should all be beyond your scope of interest at this point; worry about getting into medical school first, then work out the mechanics of how you want to pay back your loans. The government, special foundations, and the United States Military will not consider entering into one of these contracts with you *until you are accepted to at least one school*. The good news regarding some of these loan mitigation strategies is that they can be entered into during medical school or residency, and you do not need to figure these out during the application process.

For an *extremely* thorough, user-friendly, and **free** explanation on how to best approach medical student loans, we refer you to Dr. Ben White's book, *Medical Student Loans: A Comprehensive Guide:* https://www.benwhite.com/studentloans/

## 37.6.2  Institution-Based Loans

These are loans given to you by your institution to aid with your tuition and living expenses. These loans can be some of the most generous loan packages out there, and are normally superior to both government-backed loans and loans from other private lenders. What makes these loans better is a much lower static interest rate, a significant period of time before interest starts to accumulate, or a prolonged deferment period—this is, of course, institution specific.

For institution-based loans, keep these potential limitations in mind:
- Not all medical schools have them.
- They vary widely in quality between different institutions.
- They generally have an upper limit to how much you can borrow, which is far less than what you will need to pay tuition.
- They often cannot be consolidated after graduation (which is the way most people like to simplify their loan repayment strategy after graduating medical school).
- They generally are not eligible for the special repayment or forgiveness strategies available to federal loans (e.g., public service loan forgiveness).

## 37.6.3  Need-Based Aid

This aid, much like the name suggests, is awarded to accepted students based on demonstrated financial need. The institution generally came to possess this money by way of donations from alumni, foundations, or other sources.

What is good about this type of aid?
- You don't have to pay it back.
- The award is almost always good for the entire 4 years of school.
- You don't have to do anything to receive it other than make sure you, your parents, and your spouse have filed your taxes and FAFSA, and you may have to write a yearly thank you letter.

What is bad about this type of aid?
- There is a finite amount of it per school.
- You can't do much to increase your chances of it being awarded to you; it is based almost entirely on your previous income, your accumulated wealth, your spouse's income, and—for most people—**your parents income**. This last clause is what disqualifies so many medical students from need-based awards; rightly or wrongly, **most medical schools consider you financially tied to your parents, even if you are married or 48 years old.** They expect your parents will be contributing. If you think this is shocking, remember that 25% of medical school graduates leave medical school with no debt in a setting where almost no one gets merit money. This means that parents' fronting the bill is not unusual.
- Many people—in most places, even a majority—do not receive any or much. The assumption is that almost all doctors will make enough money to live comfortably, regardless of loan burden.

---

[13] Health Professions Scholarship Program (HPSP). Available at: https://www.medicineandthemilitary.com/joining-and-eligibility/medical-school-scholarships. Accessed July 8, 2022.

### 37.6.4 Merit-Based Institution Scholarships

This type of aid was more common in undergraduate institutions. When it comes to medical school, most applicants have displayed an incredible amount of merit already, and even people that do not get accepted can have impressive applications. It is very hard to determine who would receive a merit scholarship and who would not. Furthermore, there is a preponderance of people qualified to attend medical school who apply, and less than half of those people will succeed in matriculating. When the demand far outpaces the supply, and when there's no worry about doctors being able to pay off their debts, a medical school does not need to throw money at applicants to attract them; their entering class will be full regardless. For that reason and others, many medical schools do not offer any or few awards of this nature, and these should not be expected or counted on.

Indeed, applicants who receive merit-based scholarships tend to have truly exceptional applications (e.g., near-perfect GPA and MCAT scores, multiple publications, underrepresented minority status, or combination thereof) and are frequently offered scholarships by lower-ranked schools to entice them to attend over higher-ranked schools.

### 37.6.5 Outside Scholarships

These need little explaining. Much like the outside scholarships offered at undergraduate institutions, these generally require some type of application consisting of an essay, a transcript, a letter of recommendation, and some particular quality about yourself. These qualities can be based on ethnicity, gender, career interest, specific merit requirements, geographic origin, or other variables specific to the type of scholarship. These, much like merit scholarships, are small, infrequent, hard to obtain, and should therefore not be counted on to provide more than a small fraction of your expenses. For those that are interested, drug companies (e.g., Tylenol FutureCare scholarship) have a collection of options that may be a good place to start.

**Note:** Try to stick to reputable, well-known, or local scholarship applications. Scholarship scams are common, and you should be wary of any scholarship application that requires a fee.

We also recommend reaching out to your college's pre-med advising office for additional local resources, as well as whatever may be available in your county's medical society. Your Dean's List and other honor societies through your university may also offer scholarships for general academic excellence. In addition, scholarships may be offered for specific ethnic subgroups or from certain geographic areas (e.g., https://www.aaip.org/programs/student-programs/scholarships-internships-fellowships/scholarships/—Society for American Indian Physicians).

### 37.6.6 Private Loans

Available to everyone, these loans can be used to supplement the government-backed loans if you need additional funds. They should generally be used to supplement your needs as their interest rates are often higher than the government-backed loans. In addition, they tend to lack the loan forgiveness and special repayment plans available to federal loans.

### 37.6.7 Special Service Contracts

In general, these should not be considered when applying. While some schools have these implicit in the applications process—Tufts, for example, has a Maine-Track program you apply to semi-separately—most schools do not. The reason these special service contracts should not consume much of your time when you are applying is that (1) these programs will not consider you until you are accepted, and (2) these programs can be applied to once enrolled in and attending medical school. Some, such as programs incentivizing practicing in an underserved medical community or certain other geographical areas, can even be joined later in medical school, residency, or beyond. You should have more important things (e.g., getting accepted) on your mind instead. Once you are accepted at multiple (hopefully!) schools, you can begin to consider these programs.

## 37.6.8 MD/PhD, and Other Combined Degree Programs

Although we have another section (Chapter 25, Dual-Degree Programs: MD/PhD, MPH, MBA, JD, and Others) dedicated to combined degree programs, we again discuss the financial situation of MD/PhDs.

MD/PhD programs must be applied to separately from the standard MD track. From a financial standpoint, being an MD/PhD student allows you a tremendous amount of aid. Not only is your tuition covered for the entire time you are earning your MD and your PhD (about 8 years), but you receive a stipend the entire time as well—somewhere between 20 and 35 thousand dollars per year currently. While this seems very enticing to those that are very debt averse, the financial benefits should not be what draws an applicant to a path as arduous and research-driven as the MD/PhD track.

That said, we will again emphasize that the financial benefits of attending an MD/PhD program may wash out over time. Assuming the same age of retirement for an MD vs. MD/PhD physician, you will be losing 3 to 4 years of attending physician salary ($600,000–$2,800,000). In addition, most MD/PhD graduates enter academia, where compensation is typically much lower.

## 37.7 So What Does the Debt Data Tell Us?

Medical school applicants typically learn as much as they can about the schools to which they are interested in applying. To this end, many new resources have popped up, and many existing ones have been modified, to address this demand.

There is a wealth of seemingly helpful data out there to indicate which schools give the most financial aid, and whose graduates have the most debt. There are a number of sources that publish data relating to variables such as these below:
• Average debt per graduate.
• Number of students receiving aid.
• Number of students receiving scholarships, etc.

If you are someone who is hungry for data and convinced that with the right analysis and algorithm, you can find the "perfect" medical school for you, you may fall into the trap of using this information. While there is generally nothing bad about the data itself—except that it is self-reported by the schools and unverifiable—it just isn't the right kind of data to complete the analysis you want to do.

For instance, you may want to know what everyone else wants to know: "When all is said and done, after factoring in aid and cost of living and everything else I will need, how much does each school cost, relatively?" This data cannot tell you that. What you will end up spending on medical school is a highly personalized question, and the averages shouldn't mean much to you. These numbers do not factor in which students were helped by parents, supported by spouses, or engaged in the aforementioned post-school service agreements. A medical school where many people are from wealthy families often will have a preponderance of students who will graduate with very little debt, skewing the average toward the lower end, making the school look very generous with its aid money. However, you have no way of telling if this is the generosity of the parents, the school, or if these numbers can even apply to you. There are similar problems with every statistic reported in the financial aid criteria section of these sources. Just don't use them.

## 37.8 Financial Aid: After You Are Accepted

Now that you have been accepted, congratulations! Now is the time to start thinking about financial aid packages and compare them. This section will focus on common questions and problems regarding financial aid after you are accepted. These don't really show up in many application resources, so make sure to pay attention!

### 37.8.1 I Was Accepted, Where Are My Financial Aid Packages?

Schools release financial aid packages at different times, generally loosely correlated with when you were accepted. Most importantly, to receive an aid letter, you need to turn in a large amount of documentation, often consisting of, but not limited to:
• Your tax returns.

- Your W2 s and 1099s.
- Your parents' and spouse's tax returns.
- An aid application.
- A completed FAFSA.

If you want to know what your award will consist of—and receive your award letter ASAP—you need to have these forms ready to be sent ASAP after acceptance to the school's financial aid office. If you are not in typical contact with your parents, then you may experience significant delays in receiving your aid package.

### 37.8.2 We Are Quickly Approaching the April 30th Deadline, and I Haven't Received All My Award Letters Yet. What Should I Do?

This is a very common issue. For those of you that don't know, by April 30th, applicants that hold multiple acceptances are forced to give up all but one of them. Problems arise when you have not received a financial aid award letter from all of the schools to which you have been accepted.

So what do you do? In simplest terms, you politely hassle the school's financial aid office. This is done all the time. Just make sure to be polite, professional, and informative. Insist that you are very excited about being offered acceptance into their institution, but that you cannot make an informed decision about the offer when your financial aid situation is uncertain. Most applicants feel uncomfortable about politely pressuring medical school administrators, and prefer to do this over email. By all means, send an email to the financial aid office. However, your email should be immediately followed up with a phone call within the next day or so. There is no need to overexplain; this type of thing happens all the time. They know the drill.

Above everything, ask for an estimate of when you will receive the letter. If the letter does not arrive on that day, you should call the next business day to politely remind the office that you **need** the letter ASAP. Call every day after to ask for an update until you receive what you want. While this may seem pushy, where you will go to medical school is an incredibly big decision—too big to be decided for you by administrative backlog.

*Side Note: You may still get accepted to other schools after this date, and you are allowed to attend that school rather than the one you chose by the April 30th deadline.*

### 37.8.3 The School I Want to Attend Gave Me Much Less Aid than Another School. Is There Any Way to Appeal My Aid Award?

Short answer: negotiate. This is more common than you think. While you may feel uncomfortable with trying to assume a position of power—something incredibly common after the generally humbling process of applying to medical school—don't worry. Like all correspondence with those at the medical school, you should be polite and professional. However, you shouldn't be afraid to try to increase your aid.

How should you approach this? You should call the financial aid office to talk to the director. State why you would like to appeal your aid award. Whatever you decide to say, it should focus on this theme: *I want to attend this school more than I want to attend the other school(s) to which I was accepted. The only thing holding back that option is I received a much more generous offer from another school. Is there anything you can do for me?*

Nothing bad can come of this, so you shouldn't be worried. The worst thing that can happen is that they do not increase your aid amount. However, you potentially have a lot to gain.

### 37.8.4 The School I Most Want to Attend Gave Me Much Less Aid than Another School and Will Not Negotiate with Me. What Should I Do?

There is no easy answer to this one, and there is no "right decision" that applies to everyone.

There are a lot of factors to weigh when deciding between schools, and financial factors are just one of them, and only you can answer how important the difference in aid packages is to you, and how important the difference is in regard to the other factors you prioritize. In general, we strongly recommend attending the cheaper school if they're both roughly similar in terms of reputation (and other factors) and there's a dramatic price difference. This will be a highly personal decision, as different applicants ascribe different weight to price differences. Should you pay an extra $100,000 to attend a school ranked #25 vs. #50 (If you care about rankings, that is)? It depends. If you're strongly interested in a competitive specialty, and your gut feeling about the more prestigious, expensive school was so much better than the other school, then it *may* be worth it for you.

Most people accepted to medical school are only accepted to 0 or 1 school, so this will be a decision (sadly) that most accepted applicants will not have to make.

## 37.8.5 How Much Should the Cost of Medical School Matter?

Like the amount of aid available to you specifically, this is a highly personalized answer that we cannot answer. Cost should be one of many factors affecting your final choice, and we urge you to carefully consider the variables described in Chapter 38, Acceptance and Decisions: What Really Matters When Choosing the One School.

## 37.9 Summary

Medical school debt increases every year, and for applicants that bear it, it currently sits in the several hundred thousand dollar range. Given the employability of doctors and current salaries, almost all doctors *who continue to practice* have no trouble dealing with this debt over the span of their careers. You can review statistics on debt-dollar per student that schools and third-party organizations publish, and analyze them in the context of the tuition "sticker price" of the school, but these numbers should be interpreted with caution when applying them to your situation. When considering tuition, we favor considering instead the total cost of attending a school (tuition + living expenses in that area-financial aid).

When deciding between schools, your anticipated debt burden and total cost of attendance should generally factor in, and all other things being roughly equal, we favor a much cheaper school over a slightly more prestigious one for most applicants. However, only you know your financial situation, your anticipated specialty (well, some of you think you know it), and the things that matter to you—geography, weather, family, etc. Before deciding where to attend, you should wait for your financial aid letter, crunch some numbers, weigh your values, dollars, and your options, consult others if you want to—and then make the decision you feel is best for your future.

# 38 Acceptance and Decisions: What Really Matters When Choosing the One School

*Phillip Wagner and Joel Thomas*

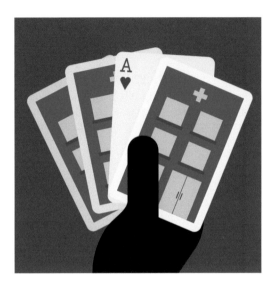

Congratulations on your acceptance to medical school! You did it!

Many applicants accepted to medical school are only accepted to one school, so this chapter is not for everyone. If you were accepted to more than one school, congratulations! You have a decision to make. This is a complicated decision with a lot of factors, and the decision will ultimately be a decision about what matters to you.

Here are just some of the typical factors on which to compare schools, in no particular order of importance.

## 38.1 Cost

- Discussed more in Chapter 37, Financial Aid.
- Cost is a tricky subject. The bottom line is that you will be able to pay back your loans—no matter how high—through *some* mechanism as an attending physician. This will definitely take more creative foresight if you are graduating with over $500,000 in debt vs. $200,000. You might have to do the public service loan forgiveness program (PSLF) (described in Chapter 41, Real Talk on a Medical Career), for example. More worryingly, you might be less inclined to pursue lower-paying specialties (e.g., pediatrics) because of your loan burden.[1] You might feel pressured to find jobs within your specialty that pay extremely well at the cost of demanding soul-crushing hours and call burden that limits time with your family (or to find jobs in rural, or "less desirable" areas). That said, we generally recommend choosing the cheapest medical school you get into if there are no significant compelling reasons otherwise. Compare the total "cost of attendance" between two schools—rather than just the tuition difference—because cost of living can be significantly different even if tuition is similar.
- Compelling reasons to pick the more expensive school include:
  - You get into a US MD school and a cheaper DO school. Unless you are certain that you're not interested in competitive specialties (dermatology, plastic surgery, neurosurgery, orthopedic surgery)—and this is

---

[1] Hsu AL, Caverzagie K. Educational Debt and Specialty Choice. Available at: https://journalofethics.ama-assn.org/article/educational-debt-and-specialty-choice/2013-07. Accessed July 8, 2022.

virtually impossible to conclude before you start medical school—we recommend choosing the MD program to leave as many educational opportunities open as possible.

- You get into two schools of the same type (US MD, DO school) that have *significant* differences in rank/prestige. If you're considering a competitive specialty, then it may be worth it to go to Duke Medical School vs. SUNY Upstate. That said, people match into competitive specialties every year from lower ranked schools, but it is much harder. It will ultimately be an individual, personal decision regarding how much the peace of mind of going to a more prestigious school matters to your career aspirations.
- Noticeable quality-of-life differences. Paying a bit more money (e.g., $10,000–$50,000 more over 4 years) to live in a more desirable location or closer to family may be reasonable depending on who you are and what matters to you. If you have significant personal ties to a region, then that may simply be priceless to you. Wanting to be close to a sick family member may be worth the financial difference. Picking a lower ranked medical school with better weather and climate if you have serious seasonal affective disorder may lead to a massive difference in quality of life and performance while you are at school. There is no point going to a high-ranked rural medical school if you know you need to be in a city to be happy.

## 38.2 Rank/Prestige

There is a full chapter here (Chapter 26, Medical School Rankings) dedicated to ranking systems and their strengths and flaws. While they are an imperfect standardized system, they are most useful at the ends of the spectrum. That is, you generally should **not** use the rankings to choose between school 45 and school 60, or school 21 and 30. This is because there will almost certainly be *some* more important difference between the schools (e.g., cost of attendance, geography, curriculum, etc.). That said, if you got into schools ranked 3 and 80, it would not be unreasonable to use rank as a significant factor in this decision, although certainly not the only factor. The prestige of your school absolutely factors into what specialties you will match into and how competitive your residency application is. The fact is that if you want to be a neurosurgeon and need every advantage you can get to be sure you match, then rank/prestige matters more. If you know you are going to be a primary care doctor, it matters far less, maybe even not at all.

## 38.3 Culture

While medical schools are universally full of hardworking, ambitious, and caring people, cultures can vary considerably. Are the students more cut-throat or laid-back? Does the incentive structure created by the administration create this kind of environment (e.g., true pass/fail vs. "fake" pass/fail in which there's an internal ranking of grades that determines AOA status and goes on your Dean's Letter)? If you are struggling, will the administration support you? Is administration more forgiving/accommodating of genuine life circumstances (e.g., being late to a mandatory session because your car broke down), or will it be quick to label you as "unprofessional"? How does the administration deal with unprofessional behavior by superiors? Is student feedback valued? Do students generally all hang out with each other, or is it more cliquish? Culture is complex, and talking to as many students as possible during your interview day is the best way to assess it. Online anonymous reports of the school's red flags and green flags can be useful, but remember to read these with healthy skepticism.

### Student Perspective
One of the authors of this section was once in a program when a close friend passed away. In order to attend a funeral, a copy of the deceased's obituary had to be submitted to the school to allow for a day off without penalty. In stark contrast, other programs—upon hearing that a family member is sick—will support you without question, letting you have time off and make up activities without even prying into the exact nature of the issue. These events can be unexpected, and a school that gives you the benefit of the doubt when supporting you is invaluable.

## 38.4 Research

It's not for everyone, but if you want a career in research, then you should critically evaluate the school's research output. Certain schools have an established research infrastructure (i.e., funding, well-known faculty) *and* a curriculum that allows and incentivizes it. They make it easy to get involved. Funding, choice of project, and access to mentors and training are ample. This is not the case at all schools. If you want to do a more competitive specialty, and your school has no one in that specialty doing research, it will be much more difficult to get involved. You can still make it work, but you will have to travel and find opportunities elsewhere at other institutions. Find out if the school uses a comprehensive electronic health record that makes it easy to perform data gathering and analysis for clinical research. Are there ample funded research opportunities for medical students (e.g., research gap years, paid summers)? Is there collaboration with neighboring institutions (e.g., Carnegie Mellon and the University of Pittsburgh, Harvard and MIT)?

## 38.5 Match Success

Match success can tell you about the strength of reputation at a particular school. It is imperfect, however, and can only really be used—always with a significant grain of salt—for those programs with reasonably large sample sizes—pediatrics, internal medicine, general surgery—specialties into which 5 to 30 people generally try to match per year. Now, if you want to be a dermatologist, it's hard to glean much for 4 people one year, and 0 people the next year, as the sample size is just too small. Even at the most competitive medical schools, sometimes entire years come and go without anyone who wants to apply into a small specialty like dermatology. Likewise, many competitive applicants will choose to go into "less competitive" programs for a variety of personal, subjective reasons. For the bigger subspecialties, are people matching into places you want to go or well thought of programs? Are they matching to locations in which you want to eventually settle, indicating a good relationship between programs? Where is the "middle of the pack" for match outcomes in the most popular specialties? This one is a lot harder to use, but it is still something to be considered.

## 38.6 Personal

To some people, the best school is the one that will help advance their careers at all costs. And that's ok. Other people have other factors at play that only they can know. While the reasons are too numerous to go into, some people are very family-oriented or have a sick family member to which they would like to remain close. If you have a local medical school and a distant more prestigious school to which you have been accepted, there is no shame in wanting to stay close to your family if that is what is important to you.

## 38.7 Location

While this may seem flippant, to some people this really matters. You won't necessarily have a lot of free time in medical school, regardless of where you go, so why should this matter? Questions you should be asking yourself should be: can I do the things I normally enjoy? Can I do the things I normally do to de-stress? If you are an avid hiker, you may not like medical school in a big city. Will you need a car for medical school vs. public transportation? If you are used to a bigger city, you may have trouble adjusting to a rural area with none of the things you generally like to do. Weather is important too—if you find that you have seasonal affective disorder, it might be worth going to a less prestigious school in warmer weather and shorter winters. If you are single and actively looking for a partner, then a school in a large city might be more appealing to you.

## 38.8 Work-Life Integration

- **Grading**: Some schools will have a Pass/Fail grading (the best system). This means as long as you pass the class exam, everything is fine. There are many different variants of the pass/fail system. The best is a "true" pass/fail system in which you simply need to pass the preclinical material and there is no internal ranking of grades that's shared with residency programs in any way (e.g., not-so-subtle comments on the Dean's Letter) or used for AOA Medical Honor Society selection. We encourage you to (tactfully) follow up on a school's claim of "pass/fail" grading with questions of how AOA status is chosen and whether there's internal ranking or whether the preclinical grades are used for Dean's

Letter comments. True pass/fail can make for a *dramatically* less stressful and more collaborative study culture between medical students. It gives you freedom to learn what you need to without obsessing over low-yield minutiae or class rank—you can spend that time doing anything else, either improving your resume or enjoying hobbies. We actively recommend avoiding schools with graded preclinical years if possible.

- **PBL/TBL**: Problem-based learning (PBL) and team-based learning (TBL) are newer educational styles in which groups of medical students collaborate on cases. These are mandatory educational sessions throughout the week. Some students really enjoy this, whereas others abhor it. It can also be very hit-or-miss. If you generally hate group work, then you might want to veer toward schools with less PBL and TBL (although it's worth noting these teaching tools are very trendy, and may be foisted upon you eventually regardless of where you decide to go). At the same time, the group work experience in medical school is typically very different from undergrad because medical students tend to be much more Type A and eager to participate in groups. In addition, if the PBL/TBL sessions are structured around challenging clinical cases and have faculty providing appropriate assistance, then this may be a valuable learning experience that simulates actual team-based care.

## 38.9 Resources and Support

- **Mental Health Counseling**: Med school is difficult, and some schools support you during this time with free and available counseling services. Some of you may not struggle with mental health until medical school, as it's an environment that can put you through more stress than you have ever experienced. Even if you don't think this will be an issue for you, make sure to ask on interview day what sorts of resources are available to promote mental health and wellness. That said, as described in Chapter 18, Self-Care and Wellness, be careful in how you ask about this (i.e., not disclosing any personal history of mental health issues), and be very scrupulous in evaluating the quality of wellness resources (e.g., truly confidential counseling that will not get reported to the administration).

- **Academic Counseling**: While no one anticipates academic struggle, a percentage of medical students at *every* school will perform below average. This is just a statistical fact. How a school supports you when you are struggling academically says a lot. While the range of resources is vast, make sure you ask how a school deals with failing a test, needing help, etc. Do they pay for a tutor for you? Do they make you repeat a year? Will the school allow you to delay taking board exams if you feel that you are not adequately prepared?

- **Test Performance**: This used to matter more when Step 1 was graded. Our theory is that Step 2 CK grades will still matter for residency, and we encourage you to be wary of schools where students underperform on board exams. Ask whether the in-house exam questions are modeled off of NBME questions. Is there co-curricular education that prepares students for board exams? How often do students take NBME shelf exams?

## 38.10 Curriculum

- Many curriculums are very similar, especially with respect to the most important aspect: the clinical years. That said, there are still important differences with respect to clinical years that you can suss out on interview day.
  - Is there ample interaction with *attending physicians* on the clerkships. That is, are there active opportunities for attendings to evaluate you performing histories and physical exams on patients? Will you be encouraged to scrub into and assist with surgeries? Will you be writing clinical notes and presenting patients to showcase your reasoning to your supervisors? The unfortunate reality is that attending physicians are extremely busy, and working with medical students is often low priority for them. Many medical students end up working mostly with residents and mid-level providers.
  - How far will you have to travel for clinical rotations? If you have to travel far, are there accommodations such as lodging and reimbursement for travel and parking? Are there any meals provided on rotations?
- The preclinical years, however, are increasingly being used to demonstrate innovation, and some schools are trending away from the traditional "2 years of basic science preclinical (i.e., biochemistry,

anatomy, histology, immunology, etc.), 2 years clinical experience." If a school is condensing the first 2 years, and then turns the second year into a research year (e.g., Duke[2]), that may appeal to someone who wants more research experience and training. Other aspects that may matter are mandatory classes. If you are someone that does better studying on their own schedule, mandatory class attendance may be very annoying and unhelpful. If you are, however, someone that excels in that type of structure, you may not do as well learning remotely as some schools are trying out now. Some schools podcast the lectures so that if you miss it, you can watch it at a later time. Don't get caught up in the specifics and the educational jargon, but ask yourself, big picture—does this curriculum support my learning style and further my career?

- Don't ask "how many students are assigned to each cadaver?" For some reason, this question *always* gets asked during tours of anatomy labs, and it is absolutely meaningless in the grand scheme of things.

## 38.11 Summary

Choosing a medical school is a very personal decision. Cost, culture, prestige, match success, location, as well as other factors play a big part in that final decision for most applicants. Like any important life decision, choosing what medical school you attend has massive implications, and has multiple factors that should come to bear. There is no objectively right decision, but you should be weighing all these factors in terms of what matters to you.

At the same time, aim to be flexible and adaptable to a variety of learning environments. Remember that all US medical schools will give you an excellent education if you work hard, and your final decision will ultimately be very personal.

---

[2] Curriculum. Available at: https://medschool.duke.edu/education/student-services/office-curricular-affairs/about-duke-curriculum. Accessed July 8, 2022.

# 39 Before and After Matriculation

*Ray Funahashi*

You are set on where you will be attending school. Get excited! Soon an avalanche of onboarding materials to sign and process will be sent your way, so keep an eye out. We have a few tips for what to do in the months leading up before school begins.

## 39.1 Relax and Enjoy

Soon you will be studying all day, every day. Resist the urge to do any heavy studying ahead of time to prepare for the medical school curriculum.

We recommend that you relax and recharge your batteries. **Visit friends and family.** You should generally enjoy your life now while you can because med school will get very busy very quickly, and your opportunities to see them will greatly decrease, especially if you need to travel to see them. Don't feel guilty about slacking off or "not doing enough." Between the options of doing too much and doing too little, we recommend erring on the side of "doing too little."[1]

Taking the time to relax now will help you to avoid early burnout at school. Starting med school fresh, rested, and inspired will pay big dividends as the year progresses.

## 39.2 Finding a Place to Live

*Should I prioritize living... close to the medical school, in a cheaper location, or a more "fun" location?*

Ideally, you could live in a location that satisfies all criteria, but these are all definitely up to personal preference.

Here are the pros and cons for each situation.

### 39.2.1 Close to School

#### Pros

- Depending on your school, you will likely spend a lot of time at the medical school during the first 2 years. Being able to roll out of bed and roll into classes quickly and arrive home quickly is a plus in stress reduction.
- If you can walk (or use public transportation), then you can get by without a car.
- You can bet that a significant portion of your classmates will be living near the school, and this makes social hangouts and building your inner circle much easier.
- If your hospital is also near the medical school, the proximity benefits extend into your clinical rotation years. This is a lifesaver for rotations with intense hours and overnights.
- You could always move to a more fun, cheaper, or farther location after the first year of medical school. You may even find potential roommates to move with once you establish a good social circle.

#### Cons

- Locations close to the school are usually high in demand and more expensive.
- Depending on your school, locations close to your school may not be "fun" (aka limited food options, grocery, bars, gym, activities, etc.).

#### Note

Some students have family who live near the medical school and so they may live there and commute to medical school. Obviously, this saves on cost and it could be worth it based on this alone despite social drawbacks.

---

[1] Within reason, of course. This doesn't suddenly give you free reign to start devouring candy and gain 50 lb before medical school.

## 39.2.2 Cheaper Location

### Pros

- Saving costs and minimizing your loans is a very smart thing to do in general.
- Areas may be more "quiet" which could help you focus on your studies and/or relax.

### Cons

- The location may be far from school, food options, groceries, and activities.
- Depending on the distance and your ability to drive/travel, this makes socializing a little more difficult.
- Public transportation options may be more limited.
  - If you need to rely on public transportation very frequently to go back and forth to the school/hospital, this can get very exhausting over time.
- All things considered, differences in housing costs are drops in the bucket in the overall budget for medical training. Reassess paying more during medical school across the scope of your *entire* lifetime earnings. $500 more per month to live in a dramatically nicer apartment is an extra $6000 a year, which translates to around $12,000 more paid over the course of your career (accounting for interest that accumulates on loans). On an attending salary, this might take about an extra *month* to pay back, which is a reasonable cost for an extra *year's* worth of happiness in medical school.[2]
  - As such, it may be reasonable to pay up for comfort and convenience, although this won't be for everyone. Not everyone succeeds in medical school (although the vast majority do), and burdening yourself with doctor-level debt when you may not end up making doctor-level money could be a decision you regret down the line. You will have to make your own decisions after weighing your values and preferences and budgetary constraints. The good news is that these decisions are often made 1 year at a time; if you aren't pleased living cheaply but commuting further, you can change it next year, and vice versa.

## 39.2.3 Fun Location

If your school is located in a city, there is often a tradeoff of living in a cheap location versus in a more "fun" location which is often more expensive. "Fun" here refers to areas with better food and bar options, grocery convenience, events, activities, and attraction. Often there is better public transportation also. Consider the things that you do for stress relief and happiness.

### Pros

- More food and socialization options.
- Easier to unwind when you are not studying.
- Dating/Easier to meet people outside of medicine/medical school.

### Cons

- Often more expensive in rent but also from the eating out and activities you end up doing.
  - Can drive up your loan debt.
- Depending on your work habits, it can be too much of a distraction from studying.
- Commuting can limit your leisure time.

## 39.3 Should I Live with a Roommate or Alone?

This is a highly personal choice of course, but here are some factors to consider.

---

[2] In addition, the price difference may be a moot point if you're doing PSLF (public service loan forgiveness), in which there's no cap on debt forgiven—thereby incentivizing you to take out more loans. More discussion in Chapter 41, Real Talk on a Medical Career.

### 39.3.1 Living with Roommates

Medical school is very intense and stressful. Having people you can talk to and destress with can be very helpful. On the other hand—depending on your study habits—this can also be distracting to your studies.

### 39.3.2 Classmates as Roomies

- You get to be very close because you go through the ups and downs of the medical experience together.
  - You can vent with people who understand the struggles of the med school experience.
- You can easily ask or confirm with your roommates about schedules, assignments, and other things in case you miss them—especially in the preclinical years because you share the same schedules.
- During the clinical years, you can share intel with each other about how to do well in clerkships that one of you already had.
- You can share rides to/from school.
- It can be more fun. If you share a house with several people, it can be a natural place to host social gatherings for your friend group or classmates.

### 39.3.3 Strangers as Roomies

- You can "get away" from studying and medical school easier.
- You have a higher chance of rooming with someone who doesn't understand the demands of medical training and therefore may not be as accommodating.

### 39.3.4 Living Alone

- All of the typical advantages of living alone in college.
- If you like studying in your house, it may be easier to stay focused without roommates.
- Can get lonely at times (especially during clerkships when you're on different schedules compared to your friends).

## 39.4 Preparing Your Study Space

Try to set up a nice space for you to study before school begins. If you like studying in your room, make sure you have all your office supplies, computer setup, lights, coffee/tea, and whatever else you need set up. If you like studying in public spaces like coffee shops or libraries, try to scope out a few places during the week and weekends to see which places you like.

**Interesting Option: Coworking Spaces**

There is a psychological shift when you physically move to a dedicated location to study. This can help you stay focused and be more productive, especially if you tend to get distracted at home.

Coworking spaces are office and meeting spaces that can be rented or shared with a membership fee. It is often used by remote workers and small businesses.

But it's also a great study location option for students. And many cities have at least a few. Chances are, there is a coworking space near your school.

You might be thinking, why would I pay to rent a space to study when I could go to a cafe or library?

The biggest advantage is psychological—you will be among mostly strangers who are also working (and less students) so you don't get as distracted as you would otherwise.

Unlike a cafe, it is typically quiet, with 24/7 access and often private rooms available. Because you are paying, you get the "going to work" feeling, like a gym membership.

Unlike the school library, you probably won't see any other students there, and you may have access to a fridge and unlimited coffee/tea so you can stay in place and stay focused.

And, of course, the internet will be fast and reliable, though, this is a given anywhere these days.

The downside, of course, is that this can be expensive, and depending on your own discipline, you could theoretically be just as productive at the library. Also, traveling to the coworking location could be inconvenient.

## 39.5  Orientation and Start to the Semester

When you first begin med school, depending on your school, you may get a week or two of orientation before classes (and studying) officially begin. Here are some general tips for this time:

### 39.5.1  Socialize Now

Med school is like college in that people tend to form tight friend groups/cliques. During orientation, since everyone is a stranger, people are looking to make new connections and friends. Take advantage of class-wide activities and meet as many people as possible. Now is the time to make the effort to step outside of your comfort zone. The friendships you make in med school can become life-long. And as medical school progresses, as everyone starts settling into their own study routines you will see less and less of your classmates unless you build friendships. Especially in the clerkship years, you may go even an entire year or two without seeing someone in your class because you never get to share a clerkship rotation.

If you can, get involved in organizing class events. Your classmates will appreciate the effort, and it builds great class comradery.

### 39.5.2  Explore the Area

Self-care and maintaining a sense of happiness, though it is a challenge, is essential in med school (and life in general). As school begins, explore your surrounding areas and try to find your "go-to" areas. For example, parks, running/hiking trails, study areas, hangout areas, cafes, restaurants, grocery stores, etc.

### 39.5.3  Seek Mentors and Tutors

We mention the importance of finding mentors many times in this book, but you can never start too early in finding upper-class and faculty mentors! If you know tutoring is something that helps you, seek this help early also. Don't be ashamed! You will never regret this decision.

### 39.5.4  Get Involved in Projects

The first year and—to a lesser extent—second year of med school are when you will have the most time for research projects. Explore interests early, meet with faculty and see what interests you. It is okay to switch projects and interests as med school goes on (almost everyone does). But if you are remotely interested in a uber-competitive specialty (e.g., dermatology, orthopaedic surgery, ENT, neurosurgery, urology, plastic surgery), starting early on authoring publications is going to help tremendously.

## 39.6  Summary

There are a few things to keep in mind in the time between acceptance and matriculation. First and foremost—*live it up*. Don't prestudy for medical school. Celebrate the culmination of years of effort and a stressful application cycle. Visit friends and family because it will be much harder to do so again once medical school has started. You should also think about a place to live once classes start, keeping in mind the pros/cons of different options.

# 40 Plan B and Reapplication

*Phillip Wagner and Joel Thomas*

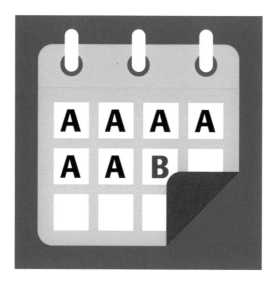

Every spring and summer, some applicants will be happy and holding acceptances. Most applicants (~60%), however, will be crestfallen with all rejections or will be nervously awaiting wait-list movement. Given the highly competitive admissions process and limited number of seats for acceptance, it's inevitable that some people will have to reapply the following year or rethink their aspirations altogether.

What should you do if it's now March or April and you have no interview invitations or acceptances? Unfortunately, it's time to start thinking about Plan B. In fact, if you have applied early in June or July and have no interview invitations in January, you should begin to *decide* on your Plan B and take active steps toward executing it at the end of the application cycle. That said, some applicants have been accepted off of the wait-list *the day before the start of classes at medical school.* As such, if you are still on a wait-list, you will need to let your Plan B supervisor (e.g., employer) know that there is an extremely small but nonzero chance that you will need to drop your Plan B and matriculate at medical school.

Plan B does not have to mean you are giving up on medical school. However, the first decision you must make at this juncture has to be whether you want to reapply to medical school. Are you willing to make more sacrifices and do whatever it takes to improve your application drastically? Do you have the financial resources to do so? Medical school applications are on a competitive uptrend, meaning you should not expect a different result by applying the following year with a similar application. Also, many medical schools do not look favorably on reapplicants (it ranges from irrelevant to hurting you to disqualifying you altogether, all depending on the school).

## 40.1 First Find Out What Went Wrong

Nearly anything could be a—or *the*—problem. It's possible you missed one of the deal breakers: GPA, MCAT score, or lack of research or volunteering (depending on the school). This also includes criminal records and professional/ethical red flags in your application. Not applying early enough—as we've repeatedly emphasized—is an easy way to tank your chances. Not applying to enough schools, or more likely, misjudging your competitiveness and applying to almost all reach schools, are common reasons to not be offered an acceptance.

Letters of recommendation are also silent killers. Even a slightly negative letter (e.g., a single sentence questioning or qualifying your ability) may universally invoke doubt by ADCOM. The worst part is that you wouldn't even be able to find out unless an ADCOM member explicitly told you because you waive your right to see letters of recommendation. This is why we emphasize asking for a "**strong, positive**" letter in Chapter 23, Letters of Recommendation and to carefully gauge your writer's reaction to this request. If you have any doubt about getting a strong, positive letter, then you should ask someone else because you will likely be anxious about what the letter says and its effects on admission.

Poor interviewing skills may be the explanation, as well. Every year, strong "on-paper" applicants get many interviews, yet fall short when they have to impress people in person. Either they are unprofessional, don't interact well with others, or unfortunately don't leave much of an impression. If you received three to four interviews but no acceptances, then we strongly recommend improving your interview skills. We recommend mock interviews (ideally recorded with feedback afterward) with people with actual ADCOM and interviewing experience.

You can obviously also have problems regarding other aspects of your application (a range that is so broad it encompasses every chapter title in this book and more).

On the other hand, you may have been one of many applicants who "fall through the cracks." That is, your stats and extracurriculars were good enough to get an interview, but nothing on your application was exciting enough to "wow" the ADCOM into an outright acceptance across all your schools. You didn't do anything *wrong*, per se. You just weren't good enough to stand out from the tens of thousands of other applicants.

If your deficiencies aren't immediately clear to you, then it's time to reach out. Call or email schools and politely ask for specific deficiencies or areas which could be strengthened. If you live nearby the school, you can also ask to make an appointment to speak to someone in person as well. Keep in mind some schools will not give you any feedback at all. In that case, you should have a professional medical school advisor, medical school student friend, or admissions consultant (if you're willing to pay) take a look at your application.

Here is an example of an email the author sent to the ADCOM after receiving a rejection:

*"Thank you for the prompt admissions decision. Is there any way I can find out how to improve my application to stand a better shot for regular[1] admissions? Thank you."*

He received the following response,

*"I re-reviewed your application and here is what I would recommend.*
*Keep doing what you're doing. Your GPA is obviously strong and should remain strong. Continue your research, clinical and service work experiences. Ideally these should be ongoing and current when you reapply. Take the MCATs in May, June or July if you can so that you will be able to complete your applications early.*
*If I could point to one weakness/specific area to focus on, while you did ok, I would encourage you to do some mock interviewing. Overall, your interviews went ok but they could have been stronger.*
*I hope this helps."*

If you are certain that what hurt your chances is applying very late in the application cycle, applying to too few schools (< 10), or applying to only "reach" (aka dream) schools, then you might apply the following year and be fine. Still, you will need to have adequate answers to the "reapplicant" questions you will be asked throughout the application cycle. These will still require some introspection. You cannot simply say, "I didn't apply early enough" or "I thought my application was more competitive." Instead, you will need to discuss how you failed to accurately assess an important metric—your application's competitiveness—and how you are actively working toward better calibrating your predictions for important decisions down the line. You will need to convince the ADCOM that you will not make a similar mistake for residency admissions. Likewise, if you simply applied too late, you will need to convince the ADCOM that you do not have a tendency for habitual lateness and have consciously implemented systems (e.g., multiple electronic reminders) to be more punctual.

---

[1] The author had applied via an early assurance program in his sophomore year of college. Hence, he is asking for guidance for regular MD admissions down the line.

## 40.2 Execute Your Plan B

If you had some easily overcomable obstacles (e.g., lateness, poor school selection), then we recommend simply applying again in the following year. You will still be expected to keep busy with productive work during this year. You cannot simply veg out at home and play video games all year while applying to medical school. Employment will also help cover the costs of reapplying, as you will again incur the same costs as applying the first time (i.e., thousands of dollars). Additionally, some applicants in this category might still be on wait-lists from the prior application cycle by the time June rolls around. **Do not hesitate to submit your primary application as early as possible, even if you are still hanging onto wait-lists from the previous year.**

If application lateness or some technicality wasn't your problem, we generally recommend that you work on improving your candidacy over the next year, and then apply the *following* year. That means a new two-year commitment, minimum. Full-time employment that addresses your weakness is the gold standard. If you didn't have enough clinical experience, then working as an EMT or ER scribe would greatly bolster your application. If you lacked research experience and only applied to research-heavy schools, then working as a post-bac researcher would be the best move. We recommend reviewing the other chapters in this book (e.g., Chapter 11, Extracurriculars; Chapter 12, Clinical Experiences; Chapter 13, Shadowing; Chapter 14, Volunteering; Chapter 15, Research; Chapter 17, Crushing the MCAT; Chapter 18, Self-Care and Wellness; and Chapter 19, Finding Mentors) to learn how to best improve the identified weaknesses in your application. We also recommend reading Chapter 16, Gap Years, Employment, Graduate degrees, and Post-baccalaureate Fellowships to better understand the range of possible "Plan B" opportunities.

In addition, you should check whether your MCAT score hasn't "expired," as many schools will not accept scores older than 3 years. If it will expire by your reapplication cycle, then you will need to retake the MCAT.

## 40.3 Reapply

Reapplication is a tremendously time-consuming and expensive ordeal. You should make your decision carefully. Before making your decision, you need to identify the weaknesses in your applications, mistakes you made in the application processes, and any red flags you may have inadvertently indicated. You will need to have a compelling story explaining how you identified your weaknesses and are actively working toward improving them during this application cycle. You will need to convince schools that they are not taking a risk by admitting you.

Be aware of the following:

- Almost all medical schools will only accept your application up to three times, many accept applications only twice.
- Schools will compare your new application to the previous application to see what improvements have been made. If there aren't many, they won't see you any differently than when they first reviewed your application and decided not to accept you or extend an interview invitation.
- You can strengthen relationships with your letter writers and get new, stronger letters.
- You can potentially become a much stronger candidate and open doors to schools that would not have originally considered you.
- You absolutely need to rewrite your personal statement and secondary essay responses (as well as virtually every free response in your applications, e.g., "Work and Activities" section).
  - While it may be tempting to talk about your application rejection as a hardship, avoid mentioning your rejection unless it is explicitly asked about. Instead, you should focus on strengthening your narrative with new evidence since you last applied.
- Apply very broadly—we would recommend applying entirely to schools within your range, and applying to at least 20 to 30, especially schools that value reapplicants and "reinvention."
- Consider applying to DO schools (more in Chapter 24, DO, MD, and International Schools). Many applicants who were close to getting into MD schools but fell short have no problem getting into DO schools, as they are overall less competitive. In addition, while you will definitely be at a disadvantage for competitive residency programs, great candidates from DO schools still match to very good programs. It may not be your dream title (DO) but it might still be your dream job.

- We generally recommend against applying to international medical schools. The only circumstances in which we would questionably recommend doing this is after multiple failed reapplication cycles with significant attempts at improving your application each time. At that point, however, we would question whether you have the core competencies necessary to thrive as a physician; you may simply be better off pursuing a different career altogether.

## 40.4  Summary

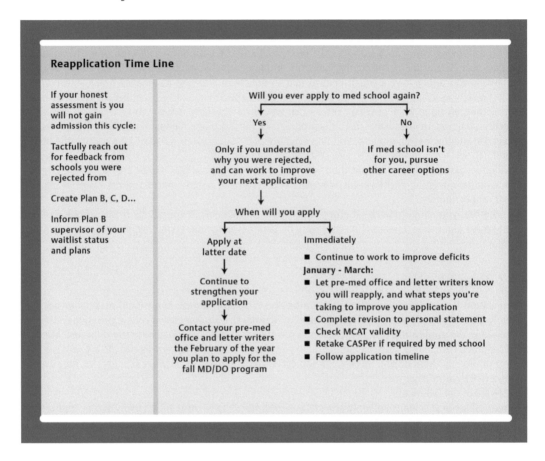

# Section IV

## Medical School and Career Insights

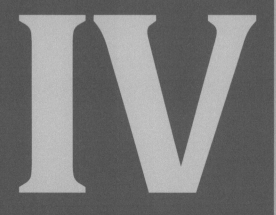

# 41 Real Talk on a Medical Career

*Joel Thomas*

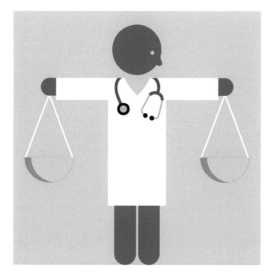

There is a strange conundrum in medicine. A significant portion of physicians—*up to 60–70% in some surveys*[1]—would not recommend their career. Burnout rates are continuing to rise,[2] take-home pay is generally stagnating or decreasing[3] as the cost of medical school attendance balloons,[4] and physicians increasingly find themselves fighting increased scope of practice from mid-level providers.[5] All the while, applications to medical school have increased to an *all-time high* at the time of writing this chapter.[6]

What explains this disconnect? Did the current generation of burnt-out, jaded physicians simply go into medicine for the wrong reasons? Did they fail to spend enough time shadowing and volunteering to truly understand what they were getting into? Did the landscape of medicine shift dramatically during their careers, pulling out the rug on their expectations? Were many of their current grievances too esoteric and insidious to understand back when they first applied to medical school? Does the current generation of pre-meds simply value different things, safeguarding it against many of these concerns? The answers are unclear, but they likely relate to all these factors.

In this chapter, we will explore common motivations for becoming a physician. We will evaluate the evidence behind these motivations, and we will vividly describe several harsh but often neglected realities of becoming a physician in the United States.

1   The Future of Healthcare: A National Survey of Physicians. Available at: https://www.thedoctors.com/about-the-doctors-company/newsroom/the-future-of-healthcare-survey. Accessed July 8, 2022.
2   Physician burnout: a global crisis. The Lancet 2019;394(10193):93. Available at: https://www.thelancet.com/article/S0140-6736(19)31573-9/fulltext. Accessed July 8, 2022.
3   Coffron MR, Zlatos C. Medicare physician payment on the decline: It's not your imagination. Available at: https://bulletin.facs.org/2019/09/medicare-physician-payment-on-the-decline-its-not-your-imagination. Accessed July 8, 2022 and Morris SS, Lusby H. The Physician Compensation Bubble Is Looming. Available at: https://www.physicianleaders.org/news/physician-compensation-bubble-looming. Accessed July 8, 2022.
4   The High Price of a Dream Job. Available at: https://www.aamc.org/media/24836/download. Accessed July 8, 2022.
5   AMA successfully fights scope of practice expansions that threaten patient safety. Available at: https://www.ama-assn.org/practice-management/payment-delivery-models/ama-successfully-fights-scope-practice-expansions. Accessed July 8, 2022.
6   Murphy B. Medical school applications up–what that means for premeds. Available at: https://www.ama-assn.org/residents-students/preparing-medical-school/medical-school-applications-what-means-premeds. Accessed July 8, 2022. Applications to medical school are at an all-time high. What does this mean for applicants and schools? Available at: https://www.aamc.org/news-insights/applications-medical-school-are-all-time-high-what-does-mean-applicants-and-schools. Accessed July 8, 2022.

We are choosing to focus on the negatives because they are difficult to conceptualize until you've experienced them first-hand. They are mostly things that we all heard ourselves from practicing physicians when we were initially contemplating medical careers. Like you, we had endured tremendous stress and delayed immediate gratification in college while fueling ourselves with distant dreams of professional fulfillment. We are very aware that it's easy to think of yourself as the exception to the rule: that although so many physicians before you had become disillusioned, *you—personally—*will not be phased by these challenges to come.

We can now emphatically say that this is the wrong attitude. We implore you to be kind to your future self as you read this chapter by imagining yourself facing these tribulations. We ask this because medicine has the sinister feature of essentially *forcing you to stay on the ride once you're on it.* Once you're over $200,000 in debt from loans, you have little choice but to grit your teeth and endure whatever suffering you may encounter, e.g., relatively inflexible working conditions in medical school and residency. This is because staying the course and eventually earning an attending physician's salary is—by far—the most reliable path to financial independence. At the same time, medical training is a Catch 22, in that *many of these grievances don't even become apparent until you're deep in debt*; you don't realize that you should have quit until it's too late to do so. As such, we encourage you to really push your imagination into overdrive and to imagine the worst-case future scenarios to test your commitment to becoming a physician.

Without further ado—let's separate fact from fiction about life in medicine. What follows are some of the most common reasons for wanting to become a physician and our commentary on these reasons.

## 41.1 "Becoming a Physician Allows Me to be a Lifelong Learner and Appeals to My Desire for Constant Intellectual Stimulation" (aka "I Like Science")

This is extremely accurate. The pace of discovery in medicine is staggering, and it's only getting faster in light of paradigm-shifting advances in genetics and computer science.[7] As a result, the ability to rapidly analyze and integrate scientific findings into day-to-day clinical decisions has become non-negotiable. Even the most "bread and butter" patient presentations and diseases can be more optimally managed (or mismanaged) with new, cutting-edge recommendations hot from the medical press. As the provider with the greatest breadth and depth of scientific training, you can truly rise to the occasion and find intellectual depth in even the most mundane encounters by critically evaluating the latest research to separate hype from reality. At the same time, if you don't feel like particularly taxing yourself on any given day, you can simply defer to the standard evidence-based treatment pathways. Essentially, once you have accumulated enough clinical experience through training, the basement for a "routine" medical career can be fairly thoughtless and algorithmic. On the other hand, the ceiling for patient care is essentially limitless, with the extreme end being conducting your own research to build on existing interventions.

That said, much of medicine can feel like rote memorization and mindless adherence to treatment algorithms. This is particularly frustrating early in training, when you spend most of your time on memorizing enormous volumes of information and honing your pattern recognition skills for common conditions. In addition, you will forget much—if not most—of the information you spend time learning throughout training (e.g., virtually all of organic chemistry and calculus). This is partially because the board exams place a significant emphasis on random minutiae about rare diseases that physicians should be *aware of* in the off chance that they encounter them in their career. Medical trainees—who ultimately end up specializing in some field—also learn an enormous amount of material pertaining to other specialties so that they can have intelligent conversations with consultants. Even if they no longer remember the specifics of that field, they still have to have the mental scaffolding necessary to quickly and efficiently relearn the relevant information.

---

[7] Gottlieb S. The Quickening Pace Of Medical Progress And Its Discontents. Available at: https://www.forbes.com/sites/scottgottlieb/2015/06/17/the-quickening-pace-of-medical-progress-and-its-discontents/. Accessed July 8, 2022. Krumholz HM. Big Data And New Knowledge In Medicine: The Thinking, Training, And Tools Needed For A Learning Health System. Health Aff (Millwood) 2014;33(7):1163–1170. Available at: https://www.ncbi.nlm.nih.gov/pmc/articles/PMC5459394/. Accessed July 8, 2022.

This foundational knowledge is essential, however. Imagine that you were trying to become a world expert in Ancient Greek philosophy. You would have to spend years putting in the rote memorization and intellectual effort to master ancient Greek *before* you spend any time engaging with serious philosophical arguments in the language. Medicine essentially has its own language, as well, and you need to brute-force learn the basics before you focus on complex reasoning.

In that vein, as you advance in your training, the emphasis shifts toward identifying subtleties in the "bread and butter," as well as the complex interaction between various medical conditions. One feature of medicine that is difficult to appreciate—especially if you're healthy—is that *many* hospitalized patients have 15 to 20 + comorbid conditions and are taking 20 + medications. Following the treatment algorithms (e.g., "If chest pain, get an EKG and troponins + /− chest X ray") for one to two diseases at a time is extremely straightforward—especially when you have a smartphone available. On the other hand, identifying (1) *why* a patient with 20 + medical conditions is coming in with abdominal pain, (2) *treating* that cause, (3) identifying and changing modifiable risk factors to prevent it from happening again, and (4) ensuring proper follow-up and referrals to other medical providers is exceedingly more complicated and requires significant thought and attention to fine detail—especially when the scientific literature for all of those 20 + diseases is rapidly evolving.

In addition, there is an expanding role of mid-level providers (more to follow) who typically see more routine, uncomplicated patients. As such, physicians of the future may have to see a greater proportion of these highly complex patients. This is even more so the case at highly academic medical centers, where patients with the most complex, rarest diseases are referred from other regional hospitals. If the idea of being Dr. House and treating patients with extremely complex illnesses appeals to you, then a career in academic medicine at a referral center is right up your alley.

That said, much of the day-to-day practice of medicine can be extremely mindless. Many physicians spend hours entering redundant information into electronic health records for billing and medicolegal purposes. Many physicians spend hours pouring through hundreds of pages of (mostly useless) outside healthcare records[8] because patients are often transferred between facilities, and the *medical record was originally designed to facilitate billing, NOT optimize patient care.*[9] Many physicians spend large chunks of their workday parroting the same insipid recommendations for diet and exercise to patients with overwhelming external barriers to health (e.g., poor health literacy, significant psychosocial stress encouraging poor health behaviors, severe poverty, etc.) because the current medical system essentially forces them to see massive volumes of patients in 15-minute time slots.[10] This can be incredibly demoralizing if you'd prefer to focus on big, systems-level problems versus focusing on the individual patient—whose problems are more likely to be affected by big-picture issues, anyway.

These issues tend to be most prominent early in training as a resident. Fortunately, there is tremendous flexibility in the work available to attending physicians. Working at an academic center with residents, for example, relieves much of your burden to chart in the health record because residents will write the notes. That said, physicians across all specialties rate the growing number of administrative tasks that feel like a waste of their training and expertise as a salient source of burnout.[11]

As such, *we advise you to temper your hopes of constant intellectual stimulation with more realistic expectations—especially when it seems that this expectation may directly lead to burn out because of the harsh contrast of the realities of day-to-day practice.* Most practicing physicians likely wrote vividly about the idealized aspects of medicine when they applied to medical school. Those hopes and dreams—again—likely kept them going through the more grueling aspects of training. As such, it can be deeply destabilizing to come to the conclusion that day-to-day clinical practice contains much fewer opportunities for those moments than they had originally anticipated.

---

[8] Physical copies, too. So forget that "Control + F" feature.

[9] Death By 1,000 Clicks: Where Electronic Health Records Went Wrong. Available at: https://khn.org/news/death-by-a-thousand-clicks/. Accessed July 8, 2022.

[10] This is a complex and changing topic, but essentially the overhead costs to practicing medicine tend to be high, and reimbursement plans for physicians have traditionally favored seeing large volumes of patients to be able to bill for more encounters, schedule more surgeries, etc.

[11] https://www.medscape.com/slideshow/2020-lifestyle-burnout-6012460

## 41.2 "Becoming a Physician Would Allow Me to Regularly Make a Deep, Personal, Positive Impact in People's Lives"

This is generally true, and it's a major distinguishing feature of medicine. There are many other jobs that allow for constant intellectual stimulation and on-the-job application of cutting-edge science (e.g., engineer, epidemiologist, high level management/finance, etc.). Many people in these jobs, however, eventually experience a deep lack of meaning behind what they do. For example, many of the highest-paying jobs in tech capitalize on your ability to design algorithms that get consumers to share personal information to advertisers or click on mindless ads for products of questionable utility.[12] Accordingly, many people in tech feel that their talents—while being handsomely compensated—are squandered for work that ultimately does not benefit society. People in corporate finance and law also frequently complain of similar woes. Most physicians, however, feel that they're doing work that's considered "objectively good" by most ethical theories. As a result, they tend to experience some of the highest rates of individual meaning related to their work compared to other careers—a feature of life that's strongly linked to overall wellbeing.[13] Specifically, 90% of physicians as a whole (and 96% of surgeons) surveyed reported "high meaning" at work, compared to 42% for lawyers, 39% of financial analysts, and 29% of computer and software engineers.[14] In addition, "gratitude/relationship with patients" and "knowing that I'm making the world a better place" are cited among the most rewarding aspects of being a doctor across all specialties.[15]

That said, there are many other jobs that are probably "objectively good for society"[16] and allow you to "help people." In fact, virtually all jobs benefit society in *some* way; after all, no one would want to spend money on paying you if you didn't provide some value. What distinguishes medicine is that it allows you to directly see the impact of your intellectual efforts on a personal level. Even in my last year of medical school, I was routinely serving as the first person to give my patients a new cancer diagnosis and to counsel them on the spot. On average, I was personally involved in serious conversations about life-changing medical decisions *at least once every 1 to 2 weeks*—ranging from delicate discussions about a new lifelong diagnosis of schizophrenia, severe intraoperative complications, harrowing death in the ICU, Munchausen syndrome by proxy, a new diagnosis of metastatic breast cancer, and progression of (an unknown diagnosis of) heart failure to name a few examples. Each time, I have taken care to be as conscientious as possible and to be 100% mindful of the patient and family's suffering. It has truly been a tremendous honor and one of the most gratifying and humbling aspects of this career.

The trade off, however, is that the overall impact of a physician on society *as a whole* is relatively low compared to other jobs with similar barriers to entry.[17] Physicians generally only treat a limited number of patients at a time when on-the-job, and it's difficult for an individual physician's efforts to scale as is the case with projects like public health and advocacy.[18] In addition, a disheartening conclusion in epidemiology is that *health care only accounts for ~10% of the contribution to premature death. Genetic and social determinants are far more important in determining a patient's health outcomes than that of any physician.*[19] Doctors also tend to train and practice in areas with the least need for physicians (urban and suburban areas with high healthcare density—versus rural areas that need providers),[20]

---

[12] Vance A. This Tech Bubble Is Different. Available at: https://www.bloomberg.com/news/articles/2011-04-14/this-tech-bubble-is-different. Accessed July 8, 2022.

[13] Having a sense of meaning in life is good for you-so how do you get one? Available at: https://theconversation.com/having-a-sense-of-meaning-in-life-is-good-for-you-so-how-do-you-get-one-110361. Accessed July 8, 2022.

[14] Most and Least Meaningful Jobs. Available at: https://www.payscale.com/data-packages/most-and-least-meaningful-jobs/full-list. Accessed July 8, 2022.

[15] https://www.medscape.com/slideshow/2020-compensation-overview-6012684

[16] Air-quoted because the notion of objective morality is still very controversial in ethical theory.

[17] Lewis G. Medical Careers. Available at: https://80000hours.org/career-reviews/medical-careers/. Accessed July 8, 2022.

[18] For example, you can't really expect to operate on 10 different people at the same time. The bulk of most physicians' contributions tends to be in skilled labor. Although, you might find someone trying from time to time: https://www.medpagetoday.com/special-reports/exclusives/94402

[19] McGinnis JM, Williams-Russo P, Knickman JR. The Case For More Active Policy Attention To Health Promotion. Health Affairs 2002;21(2). Available at: https://www.healthaffairs.org/doi/full/10.1377/hlthaff.21.2.78. Accessed July 8, 2022.

[20] Aka the "inverse care law"—https://www.thelancet.com/journals/lancet/article/PIIS0140–6736(71)92410-X/fulltext

further diminishing the marginal impact that a physician has on the world as a whole. In addition, because so many people want to go to medical school and residency—which are essentially bottlenecks to the physician supply—attending medical school does not make a significant impact on the aggregate physician work-force because the counterfactual is that if *you* didn't attend, someone else would be just as likely to take your spot in the medical school and ultimately in the workforce. Based on all of these factors and others, one career consultant and analyst has estimated (controversially) that *adding an additional doctor to the world health force is only expected to add 4 health years for every year of work—dramatically less than even modest donations to health charities.*[21] If you *only* wanted to do the best for the world, then it could be argued—per the effective altruist philosophy—your best bet would be going into finance (or really any high-paying job) and donating your money.

We highlight this point because it can be easy to fall into a deep state of existential angst and nihilism when you recognize that you're spending an inordinate number of hours on a job that has relatively low impact on the world as a whole—especially when you're dealing with disrespectful patients, administration, or poor life circumstances altogether. Imagine going to work 6 days a week as a vascular surgery resident—regularly pushing 80 hours a week—to continually operate on patients with serious diseases that would be largely preventable by avoiding smoking. In the right circumstances, it would be easy to feel that your herculean efforts at revascularizing around clogged vessels are largely hopeless because the patient continues to smoke and develop new blockages. On a deep level, you have to be at peace with the fact that the patient's behaviors and life circumstances will have a far greater impact on their health than your interventions.

At the same time, we believe that *because* healthcare in the United States is so deeply dysfunctional, those who are genuinely motivated toward systems improvement could find many opportunities to provide a lot of good for many patients by identifying and improving systems-based problems in healthcare delivery. Having the firsthand experience of being a physician provides invaluable insight to healthcare quality improvement projects, and we encourage those already in medicine who feel frustrated by their relatively low impact to consider this pathway.

## 41.3 "I Want to Become a Physician to Do the Best, Evidence-Based Medicine for My Patients. I Want the Most Breadth and Depth of Knowledge, and This Is Why I'm Not Content with Becoming a Physician Assistant or Nurse Practitioner—Even Though I Understand that These Providers Make Crucial Contributions to the Healthcare Team"

As described earlier, this is largely true. Physicians can use their clinical judgment to deviate from the usual textbook recommendations—especially if they cite cutting-edge research or their own professional experience to justify their decisions. This is why virtually every clinical algorithm includes a disclaimer that the algorithm is not meant to replace a physician's judgment. The healthcare profession recognizes that the years of grueling education and experience acquired over medical school and residency provides physicians with an entirely different level of expertise managing patients compared to "mid-level providers," i.e., nurse practitioners (NPs) and physician assistants (PAs).

Or so it did. One increasing source of frustration for physicians—one that is likely to get worse over time, given the current political attitudes around healthcare expenses in the United States—is the expanding scope of practice by NPs and PAs. As of 2020, NPs can practice independently in the majority of states.[22]

---

[21] Lewis G. How many lives does a doctor save?- Part 3- Replacement. Available at: https://80000hours.org/2012/09/how-many-lives-does-a-doctor-save-part-3-replacement-84/. Accessed July 8, 2022.

[22] Rappleye E. 28 states with full practice authority for NPs. Available at: https://www.beckershospitalreview.com/hospital-physician-relationships/28-states-with-full-practice-authority-for-nps.html. Accessed July 8, 2022.

Psychologists,[23] optometrists,[24] nurse anesthetists,[25] pharmacists,[26] *naturopaths,*[27] and radiology extenders[28] are also pushing for a similar expanded scope of practice.

The reasons for this are complex, but they are cogently explained in *Patients at Risk—The Rise of the Nurse Practitioner and Physician Assistant in Healthcare.* In a nutshell, it all began when the professional nursing organizations aggressively lobbied politicians to expand scope of practice for nurses, citing the physician shortage, healthcare costs, and the fact that multiple studies had suggested that advanced practice nurses provided noninferior outcomes to physicians. Allowing NP's expanded scope of practice (i.e., diagnosing and treating illnesses without physician oversight) seemed to be a cost-effective strategy to filling in gaps in healthcare access. Politicians were convinced by this argument and passed legislation allowing NPs to be billed directly for their services without supervision.[29] Many states now allow NPs to practice with minimal supervision by physicians. In response to this increased demand—as well as increased government funding—there was a proliferation of NP programs, *many of which have 100% acceptance rates.*[30] PAs and other mid-level providers followed suit in lobbying for expanded scope of practice for similar reasons.

At face value, the arguments for expanded mid-level scope of practice seem convincing. First, it's clear that mid-levels provide enormous value to the healthcare system when they work synergistically with physicians. In fact, the PA and NP roles were created by physicians in the 1970s to work with physicians under supervision.

In addition, the "physician shortage" is a misnomer, as it's really a physician maldistribution. Urban and suburban areas tend to be oversaturated with physicians because educated professionals tend to want to live with other educated professionals, who tend to move to urban and suburban areas. There is also no evidence that mid-levels tend to practice more in underserved rural areas. In fact, the data suggests the opposite: they go to the same urban and suburban areas where physicians practice.[31]

Lastly, the studies about mid-level safety and efficacy are misleading. As of 2020—there are *no* high-quality studies demonstrating that mid-levels provide equally safe and efficacious care to attending physicians without supervision; a careful reading of every single study will show that they had physician supervision.[32] Indeed, the most comprehensive systematic review analyzed all available literature up to 2017 to assess whether nurses could substitute for physicians in primary care. Only 18 studies ultimately were deemed to be of appropriate methodological quality, and the nurses in all of these studies were under physician supervision or following physician-created protocols.[33]

[23] Daly R. Psychiatrists proactive in scope-of-practice battles. Available at: https://psychnews.psychiatryonline.org/doi/full/10.1176/pn.41.5.0017. Accessed July 8, 2022.

[24] Expanding Scope of Practice: Lessons and Leverage. Available at: https://www.reviewofoptometry.com/article/expanding-scope-of-practice-lessons-and-leverage. Accessed July 8, 2022.

[25] Brusie C. The VA Granted Nurse Practitioners Full-Practice Authority & Doctors Are Outraged. Available at: https://nurse.org/articles/doctor-vs-np-va-grants-full-practice-authority/. Accessed July 8, 2022.

[26] Sachdev G, Kliethermes MA, Vernon V, Leal S, Crabtree G. Current status of prescriptive authority by pharmacists in the United States. jaccp 2020;3(4). Available at: https://accpjournals.onlinelibrary.wiley.com/doi/full/10.1002/jac5.1245. Accessed July 8, 2022.

[27] Licensing and Scope of Practice: How it affects your career as a naturopathic physician. Available at: https://nunm.edu/2019/05/nd-licensing-and-scope/. Accessed July 8, 2022.

[28] 10 Things Radiologists Need to Know About Radiology Extenders. Available at: https://www.radiologybusiness.com/topics/practice-management/10-things-radiologists-need-know-about-radiology-extenders. Accessed July 8, 2022.

[29] Sharp N. American College of Nurse Practitioners: experiment in democracy. Nurs Manage 1995;26(1):22-3. Available at: https://pubmed.ncbi.nlm.nih.gov/7898804/. Accessed July 8, 2022.

[30] Kerr E. Nursing Master's Programs With 100% Admit Rates. Available at: https://www.usnews.com/education/best-graduate-schools/the-short-list-grad-school/articles/nursing-masters-programs-with-the-highest-acceptance-rates. Accessed July 8, 2022.

[31] Shryock T. Replacing doctors. Medical Economics Journal 2019;96(3). Available at: https://www.medicaleconomics.com/view/replacing-doctors. Accessed July 8, 2022.

[32] Al-Agba & Bernard "Patients at Risk: The Rise of the Nurse Practitioner and Physician Assistant in Healthcare" 2020.

[33] Laurant M, van der Biezen M, Wijers N, Watananirun K, Kontopantelis E, van Vught AJAH. Nurses as substitutes for doctors in primary care (Review). Available at: https://www.cochranelibrary.com/cdsr/doi/10.1002/14651858.CD001271.pub3/epdf/full. Accessed July 8, 2022.

So what does all of this mean for a future physician?

- **You will likely be seeing a higher proportion of medically complex patients because mid-levels are more likely to see less complex patients when they can[34] and are more likely to make unnecessary referrals to specialists.**[35] While this might be appealing to those who crave a constant intellectual challenge, it can become extremely draining over time. Imagine—for example—that you are a professional sprinter. Even if you love the exhilaration of racing at a high level, you will get absolutely exhausted if you had to sprint at maximal capacity day-in and day-out for your entire career. Less complex patients allow you to mentally recharge in between challenging encounters, and physicians are already beginning to report increasing burnout from the increasing complexity of patient panels.[36] This trend will likely only get worse, as the population becomes increasingly medically complex due to rising proportion of obese[37] and elderly[38] patients.
  - In addition, the breadth and depth of medical training grants a sense of diagnostic humility and cautiousness that isn't as emphasized in mid-level training. That is, *physicians—by virtue of learning deeply about virtually every disease and understanding just how deep the rabbit hole goes—are better at knowing what they don't know.* Many deceptively simple patient presentations often end up being atypical presentations of deadly diseases, and the high-profile examples of patients' experiencing serious harm from mid-levels highlights this fact.[39]
- **You will likely experience a devaluation of your achievements.** There is now an intentional blurring of professional distinctions in healthcare settings. Mid-levels vehemently fight against the term "mid-level,"[40] PAs have campaigns in which they literally claim that they are not the physician's assistant,[41] and nonphysicians campaign to be called "doctor" in the hospital under the argument that doctor is no more than an academic title.[42] The white coat has largely lost its historic meaning; go to any hospital, and you'll find that virtually every employee will be wearing a doctor's length white coat nowadays.[43] This might sound like petty posturing, but the sense of pride and accomplishment behind surviving medical training used to provide psychological defense against its grueling stresses. The undertone behind these public campaigns is that the respect granted toward physicians is exaggerated—that the differences in training are not so great. In reality, an attending physician will have finished at least 11 years of schooling after high school and 15,000 to 16,000 hours of training after graduating residency, compared to 500 to 1,500 supervised patient care hours for an NP.[44] These differences matter, and the high-quality scientific data confirms as much.[45]

---

34  Pines JM, Zocchi MS, Ritsema T, et al. The impact of advanced practice provider staffing on emergency department care: productivity, flow, safety, and experience. Available at: https://onlinelibrary.wiley.com/doi/full/10.1111/acem.14077. Accessed July 8, 2022.

35  Lohr RH, West Colin P, Beliveau M, et al. Comparison of the quality of patient referrals from physicians, physician assistants, and nurse practitioners. Mayo Clin Proc 2013;88(11):1266-71. Available at: https://pubmed.ncbi.nlm.nih.gov/24119364/. Accessed July 8, 2022.

36  Loeb DF, Bayliss EA, Candrian C, deGruy FV, Binswanger IA. Primary care providers' experiences caring for complex patients in primary care: a qualitative study. BMC Family Practice 2016. Available at: https://bmcfampract.biomedcentral.com/articles/10.1186/s12875-016-0433-z. Accessed July 8, 2022.

37  Rising Obesity in the United States Is a Public Health Crisis. Available at: https://www.commonwealthfund.org/blog/2018/rising-obesity-united-states-public-health-crisis. Accessed July 8, 2022.

38  National Research Council (US) Panel on Statistics for an Aging Population, Gilford DM, eds. The Aging Population in the Twenty-First Century: Statistics for Health Policy. Washington (DC): National Academies Press (US); 1988.

39  $6.1M Oklahoma Medical malpractice verdict for death of 19-year-old in ER. Available at: https://medicalmalpracticelawyers.com/6-1m-oklahoma-medical-malpractice-verdict-for-death-of-19-year-old-in-er/. Accessed July 8, 2022.

40  Use of Terms Such as Mid-level Provider and Physician Extender. Available at: https://www.aanp.org/advocacy/advocacy-resource/position-statements/use-of-terms-such-as-mid-level-provider-and-physician-extender. Accessed July 8, 2022.

41  Use of Terms Such as Mid-level Provider and Physician Extender. Available at: https://www.aanp.org/advocacy/advocacy-resource/position-statements/use-of-terms-such-as-mid-level-provider-and-physician-extender. Accessed July 8, 2022.

42  https://www.newsnationnow.com/investigation/transparencyinhealthcare/ Interview at 15:47 with Sophia L Thomas, president of the American Association of Nurse Practitioners

43  The inside joke among doctors is that the best way to find the actual doctor nowadays is finding the one person *not* wearing a white coat.

44  *Patients at Risk—The Rise of the Nurse Practitioner and Physician Assistant in Healthcare.*

45  Credit to reddit.com/r/Noctor for this *excellent* compendium of studies demonstrating worse outcomes with mid-levels: https://www.reddit.com/r/Noctor/comments/j1m7d2/research_refuting_midlevels_copypaste_format/

- **You may experience retaliation for speaking out.** One underappreciated fact about being a doctor is that you are rarely the "boss." Yes, you're the leader of the healthcare team, but this doesn't grant you any administrative authority. Nurses don't work for you. You can't fire them. Instead, your job is at the mercy of hospital administration. Therefore, you can absolutely get fired for expressing good-faith, reasonable critiques of expanding mid-level scope of practice:

"The last thing Steven Maron, MD, expected when he was called into his administrator's office was to be fired. The Arizona pediatrician said he had never faced any disciplinary actions throughout his 10 ½ years with the organization, and although he had written an opinion piece about nurse practitioners (NPs), he had expressed nothing but admiration, calling them "well-trained, dedicated, popular with patients, and intelligent."

Which is why the veteran physician of 31 years was stunned when he was abruptly terminated from a Federally Qualified Health Center (FQHC) just days after the article was published in the Green Valley News.

Maron told me he was specifically told he was being terminated because "my article stood in opposition to the principles of the organization, specifically the principle of mutual respect."[46]

Nurses will typically outnumber you in the practice setting. They often hold significant clout with administration. Take extra caution not to make any enemies at work—even if you feel that you're doing the right thing by looking out for patient safety.

- **Things will probably only get worse.** This trend is projected to worsen, with a 173% increase in the NP workforce from 2010 to 2020 compared to a 20% increase for physicians.[47] Meanwhile, at the same time as mid-levels gain easier access to practicing medicine, physicians across multiple specialties face increased pressure for additional training.
  - Pediatrics is now requiring a "pediatric hospitalist" fellowship in order to independently practice hospital pediatrics—even though most of pediatrics residency is already hospital-based.[48]
  - Many internal medicine residents are heavily pressured to do an additional "chief year"[49] to make themselves competitive for certain subspecialties (e.g., cardiology, gastroenterology).
  - Many general surgery programs essentially require two additional years of research – particularly so if you are planning on a competitive fellowship (e.g., pediatric surgery).[50]
  - Virtually all radiologists[51] and pathologists[52] are *de facto* forced to do a fellowship (or two) to make themselves competitive in the job market. Most orthopaedic surgeons[53] feel the same way, and a similar trend is developing in radiation oncology.[54]
- **The lay public will not be on your side.** Public perception of doctors has decreased over the past few decades, with 34% of Americans in 2012 citing "great confidence" in physicians compared

---

[46] Bernard R. Physicians face punishment for speaking out about non-physician care. Available at: https://www.medicaleconomics.com/view/physicians-face-punishment-speaking-out-about-non-physician-care. Accessed July 8, 2022.

[47] *Patients at Risk—The Rise of the Nurse Practitioner and Physician Assistant in Healthcare*, Loc 195.

[48] Eniasivam Archna (Introduction Weijen Chang), Monash B, Feldman LS. Why Required Pediatric Hospital Medicine Fellowships Are Unnecessary. Available at: https://www.the-hospitalist.org/hospitalist/article/121461/pediatrics/why-required-pediatric-hospital-medicine-fellowships-are. Accessed July 8, 2022.

[49] Singh D, McDonald FS, Beasley BW. Demographic and Work-Life Study of Chief Residents: A Survey of the Program Directors in Internal Medicine Residency Programs in the United States. J Grad Med Educ. 2009 Sep; 1(1): 150 -154. Available at: https://www.ncbi.nlm.nih.gov/pmc/articles/PMC2931204/. Accessed July 8, 2022.

[50] Bhattacharya Syamal D, Williams JB, de la Fuente SG, Kuo PC, Seigler HF. Does Protected Research Time During General Surgery Training Contribute to Graduates' Career Choice? Am Surg 2011;77(7):907 -910. Available at: https://www.ncbi.nlm.nih.gov/pmc/articles/PMC3720679/. Accessed July 8, 2022.

[51] 98% of radiology residents intend to pursue a fellowship. Available at: https://www.radiologybusiness.com/topics/leadership/98-radiology-residents-intend-pursue-fellowship. Accessed July 8, 2022.

[52] DO EM, Prystowsky MB, Fox AS. How to Succeed in Fellowship Acquisition: A Survey of Pathology Residents. Academic Pathology 2019;6. Available at: https://doi.org/10.1177/2374289519884711. Accessed July 8, 2022.

[53] Daniels AH, DiGiovanni CW. Is Subspecialty Fellowship Training Emerging as a Necessary Component of Contemporary Orthopaedic Surgery Education? J Grad Med Educ. 2014 Jun; 6(2): 218 -221. Available at: https://www.ncbi.nlm.nih.gov/pmc/articles/PMC4054719/. Accessed July 8, 2022.

[54] Wallner PE, Rosenzweig KE, Vapiwala N. Caveat Emptor: Fellowship Training in Radiation Oncology; What, But More Importantly, Why? Int J Radiat Oncol Biol Phys 2020;106(1):47-49 Available at: https://pubmed.ncbi.nlm.nih.gov/31647970/. Accessed July 8, 2022.

to 73% in 1966.[55] At the same time, nurses have enjoyed rising status in the public spotlight. A 2014 Gallup poll revealed that 80% of Americans believed nurses have a "very high" or "high" standard of honesty and ethics, compared to 65% of Americans for doctors.[56] During this period, the media has exploded with explorations into rising healthcare costs and errors in medical care—often placing the blame on physicians and their high salaries[57] and poor bedside manner.[58] At the same time, vocal nursing organizations such as the AANP and American College of Nurse-Midwives have launched public campaigns aimed at escalating the perception of nurses as the under-appreciated clinicians in doctors' overbearing shadows. A salient example of this is the "brain of a doctor, heart of a nurse" campaign for nurse practitioners that implies that doctors lack the heart of nurse practitioners.[59]

## 41.4 "Physicians Have a Doctoral-Level Understanding of Their Craft. I Want to Both Excel at Patient Care at the Bedside and Revolutionize Treatment as a Whole through Research. Along the Way, I'd Like to Find and Establish a Niche for Myself in an Area of Medicine that Truly Inspires Me"

This is mostly true, and "being good at what [you] do" is frequently cited as the "most rewarding" part of being a physician.[60] Many people experience a deep sense of satisfaction in honing a craft over a lifetime, and being a physician allows you to do that professionally. This is especially evident in procedural fields such as surgery or any interventional subspecialty (e.g., interventional radiology, critical care, gastroenterology), but the cognitive processes of diagnosis and treatment are also skills that one can artfully hone over a career.

In addition, medical training provides a very unique perspective for scientific research. First of all, the scientific curriculum is sufficiently rigorous for intelligently engaging with the most cutting-edge basic science done by PhD researchers. As a personal example, I had worked full-time doing bench work at the NIH for a year before starting medical school. During that year, I immersed myself in the basic literature on immunology, and I had thought myself reasonably knowledgeable by the end. After medical school immunology, it became painfully clear to me how little I had actually understood the material because *three weeks* of accelerated study in medical school taught me more than an entire year with the material as a researcher.

Beyond the scientific rigor is the clinical context you obtain by being a physician on the front lines. There is probably an infinite number of interesting hypotheses to test in biomedical science, but grant money is limited. As such, the crucial clinical context obtained by actually working in patient care allows you to identify the scientific questions that are most relevant and directly applicable to improving patient care—a tremendous advantage in determining *which* questions to study when applying for grants. This is exactly what is meant by "bench to bedside" and vice versa. The paradigmatic physician scientist has *both* the clinical experience to identify gaps in our understanding of medicine *and* the scientific expertise to generate plausible testable hypotheses.

55 Blendon RJ, Benson JM, Hero JO. Public Trust in Physicians–U.S. Medicine in International Perspective. N Engl J Med 2014;371:1570-1572. Available at: https://www.nejm.org/doi/full/10.1056/NEJMp1407373#t=article. Accessed July 8, 2022.

56 Riffkin R. Americans Rate Nurses Highest on Honesty, Ethical Standards. Available at: https://news.gallup.com/poll/180260/americans-rate-nurses-highest-honesty-ethical-standards.aspx. Accessed July 8, 2022.

57 Price G, Norbeck T. Debunking Myths: Physicians' Incomes Are Too High and They Are the Cause of Rising Health Care Costs. Available at: https://www.forbes.com/sites/physiciansfoundation/2017/11/27/debunking-myths-physicians-incomes-are-too-high-and-they-are-the-cause-of-rising-health-care-costs/?sh=20999d241400. Accessed July 8, 2022.

58 White T. Medical errors caused by doctors not examining their patients. Available at: https://scopeblog.stanford.edu/2015/12/21/medical-errors-caused-by-doctors-not-examining-their-patients/. Accessed July 8, 2022.

59 Harris PA. Open Letter to the AMA: Where is the Public Campaign Advocating for Physicians? Available at: https://www.aaemrsa.org/current-news/open-letter-to-the-ama-where-is-the-public-campaign-advocating-for-physicians. Accessed July 8, 2022.

60 https://www.medscape.com/slideshow/2020-compensation-overview-6012684

Medicine also shines in that academic physicians are actively encouraged to identify a niche in this manner: to focus on a particular subset of patients and to actively work toward science-based solutions to improving their care.[61] This also has the advantage of giving you something intellectually engaging in your day-to-day work once the bread-and-butter of your specialty becomes routine. As difficult as it is to conceptualize now, even saving the lives of patients with heart attacks and brain bleeds becomes routine over time. Actively working toward improving clinical outcomes, i.e., patients' lives and well-being, adds an additional level of meaning to work that keeps physicians engaged throughout their careers.

That said, it has been suggested that budding physician scientists will likely face tremendous pressure to publish large quantities of low-quality research using questionable research methods that are unlikely to ever be cited.[62] A major reason for this is that "number of abstracts, presentations, and publications" is used by many residency programs as a metric for the applicant's research productivity—especially for the most competitive specialties. Indeed, in 2020, the average number of abstracts, presentations, and publications for matched applicants in dermatology, neurosurgery, plastic surgery, otolaryngology, and radiation oncology was 19, 23.4, 19.1, 13.7, and 18.3.[63] You read that correctly—*the average successful neurosurgery applicant churned out 23.4 abstracts, presentations, and publications.* While it's true that higher *quality* publications benefit the applicant, it's harder for programs to objectively measure publication quality between applicants. It's much easier for residency programs to simply stratify applicants by a numerical metric like "number of publications." In addition, it's generally easier for a medical student to simultaneously work on multiple "chart review" projects and perform questionable research methods like "p hacking"[64] until *any* significant findings are found—even if by random chance—than to work hard at a single clinical question that may yield a higher-quality paper. Then, the student simply writes a paper about the significant findings while generating seemingly plausible *post hoc* explanations for the results while inviting other researchers to perform "additional analyses to validate/explore the findings." Of course, this emphasis on the *number* of publications is not unique to medicine,[65] but it's an unfortunate reality of the residency application process that applicants to competitive residency programs are *strongly* incentivized to churn out massive quantities of poor-quality research.[66]

## 41.5 "Becoming a Physician Is a Fairly Straightforward and Reliable Way to a Comfortable Income that's Recession-Proof"

This is completely accurate, and it is a *major* selling point of becoming a physician. In fact, the psychological safety in knowing that you're essentially guaranteed an upper-middle to upper-class lifestyle that's recession/pandemic-proof and secures employment worldwide is virtually unbeatable. A medical degree from the United States also offers significant career capital through signaling effects: employers can be reasonably confident that you're an intelligent professional who can work hard over many years. As a result, if you desire a career outside of traditional clinical medicine, you can use your medical degree to leverage high-level positions in other industries, e.g., finance, biotech, public health, etc.

In addition, the path to doing so—while demanding—is fairly straightforward: simply ace the pre-reqs in college, do well on the MCAT, check off the "required" extracurriculars, say the right things on the interview, and work hard throughout training for many years until you're an attending. In contrast, other careers that allow similar financial rewards, e.g., finance, tech, and law, have much more subjective

---

[61] Gupta A. Finding Your Niche in Medicine: Not a Straight Path. Available at: https://www.tctmd.com/news/finding-your-niche-medicine-not-straight-path. Accessed July 8, 2022.

[62] Wickramasinghe DP, Perera CS, Senarathna S, Samarasekera DN. Patterns and trends of medical student research. BMC Medical Education. Available at: https://bmcmededuc.biomedcentral.com/articles/10.1186/1472-6920-13-175. Accessed July 8, 2022. Sharp E. Research waste is still a scandal –especially in medical students. BMJ 2019;364:l700. Available at: https://www.bmj.com/content/364/bmj.l700.full. Accessed July 8, 2022.

[63] The Match®. Available at: https://www.nrmp.org/wp-content/uploads/2020/07/Charting-Outcomes-in-the-Match-2020_MD-Senior_final.pdf. Accessed July 8, 2022.

[64] Adda J, Decker C, Ottaviani M. P-hacking in clinical trials and how incentives shape the distribution of results across phases. Available at: https://www.pnas.org/content/117/24/13386. Accessed July 8, 2022.

[65] Ritchie S. How Fraud, Bias, Negligence, and Hype Undermine the Search for Truth. Available at: https://us.macmillan.com/books/9781250222695. Accessed July 8, 2022.

[66] Ioannidis JPA. Why Most Clinical Research Is Not Useful. Available at: https://journals.plos.org/plosmedicine/article?id=10.1371/journal.pmed.1002049. Accessed July 8, 2022.

(i.e., reliant on networking), variable, and "luck-based" trajectories. Indeed, medicine is closer to a "meritocracy" on that spectrum (although obviously not close to perfect) in the traditional sense as long as you have an aptitude for standardized tests and hard work over many years.

Yes, it's true that the "golden age" of physician wealth is behind us. Physician salaries have generally held constant or declined, and the expectation is that they will continue to do so in light of reimbursement reform by the government.[67] In addition, the expanding mid-level scope of practice will likely threaten physician incomes as healthcare systems continue to justify paying mid-levels to do the same jobs as physicians at lower salaries (thereby lowering demand for physician labor).[68] The cost of attendance for medical training also continues to rise well beyond the rate of inflation without any signs of slowing down.

In addition, the increasing corporatization of medicine will likely continue to lower physician salaries in the future.[69] In the past, it was easier for physicians to work as their own bosses, e.g., as solo owners or partners in physician-managed groups. Increasing medicolegal requirements, however, make it increasingly harder to practice medicine without the resources available to large healthcare organizations. As a result, physicians increasingly find themselves as salaried employees beholden to administrators who sometimes lack medical training. In these practice settings, it becomes much harder for physicians to negotiate reimbursement, for example. In addition, physicians are *not* "the boss" in these settings. Nurses, mid-levels, and ancillary staff answer to administrators.

Despite all these changes, it remains the case that even the lowest paying medical specialty—pediatric infectious disease—yielded a median salary of $185,892 in 2018, placing you at the 95th percentile for income in the United States. Anesthesiology is similarly competitive and yields a similar median salary of $405,000, placing you deep in the 99th percentile for income.[70]

That said, it's important to remember that income isn't the whole story; your overall *net worth* includes income, debts, and assets. First, consider the time it takes to pay back loans. To illustrate the burden of medical school debt, let's walk through the hypothetical of an average medical school graduate going into internal medicine—one of the most common specialties that has a 98% match rate for US MD applicants.[71] The median salary is $264,000,[72] and the average debt burden is $241,600 (assuming interest rate of ~7%, as it was at the time of this chapter).[73] Let's assume they live in Virginia, a state with a middle-of-the-pack tax burden.[74] *Take-home pay* will be $157,771 per year.[75] By the end of internal medicine residency, their debt burden will have increased to $295,235 due to compound interest. It will take them 4 to 26 years to pay off their loans depending on how frugally they want to live. Paying back $25,000 yearly (and living off of $132,771 yearly) would take about *26 years* to pay off loans against compound interest, whereas paying back $100,000 yearly (and living off of $57,771 yearly) would only take 4 years. This—of

[67] Levins H. Physician Income in The New Age of Health Reform Frugality. Available at: http://ldihealtheconomist.com/he000024.shtml. Accessed July 8, 2022, Morris SS, Lusby H. The Physician Compensation Bubble Is Looming. Available at: https://www.physicianleaders.org/news/physician-compensation-bubble-looming. Accessed July 8, 2022.

[68] https://www.medpagetoday.com/special-reports/exclusives/83576 At least 15 physicians have been fired from Edward-Elmhurst Health as the suburban Chicago-based health system moves to cut costs, sources told MedPage Today. The doctors, who worked across its seven "Immediate Care" or urgent care sites, will be replaced by advanced practice nurses, according to an email sent by hospital leadership that was shared with MedPage Today.

[69] Private equity, burnout, decreasing revenue affect private practice. Available at: https://www.healio.com/news/dermatology/20200128/private-equity-burnout-decreasing-revenue-affect-private-practice. Accessed July 8, 2022, Howard B. Fleishon, Arvind Vijayasarathi, Robert Pyatt, Kurt Schoppe, Seth A. Rosenthal, Ezequiel Silva III. White Paper: Corporatization in Radiology. JACR 2019;16(10):1364-1374. Available at: https://www.jacr.org/article/S1546-1440(19)30823-3/fulltext. Accessed July 8, 2022.

[70] 2019 Doximity Physician Compensation Report; U.S. Census Bureau 2019.

[71] Match Data & Report Archives. Available at: https://www.nrmp.org/wp-content/uploads/2018/06/Charting-Outcomes-in-the-Match-2018-Seniors.pdf. Accessed July 8, 2022.

[72] 2019 Physician Compensation Report. Available at: https://s3.amazonaws.com/s3.doximity.com/press/doximity_third_annual_physician_compensation_report_round4.pdf. Accessed July 8, 2022.

[73] Hanson M. Average Medical School Debt. Available at: https://educationdata.org/average-medical-school-debt. Accessed July 8, 2022.

[74] States with the Highest & Lowest Tax Rates. Available at: https://wallethub.com/edu/best-worst-states-to-be-a-taxpayer/2416. Accessed July 8, 2022.

[75] Salary paycheck calculator. Available at: https://www.adp.com/resources/tools/calculators/salary-paycheck-calculator.aspx. Accessed July 8, 2022.

course—assumes that they have no other outstanding debts or expenses, credit card debt or the extremely high costs of raising a family or living in a high cost-of-living area.

We also need to consider the significant opportunity cost in saving for retirement. A "traditional applicant" physician won't start earning any income until around age 28, versus most college graduates who enter the workforce at age 22 to 23. One of the most important principles in saving for retirement is starting early and taking advantage of compound interest. At the same time, while physicians won't be able to contribute to retirement until later in life, they will have much more available income to invest into retirement savings. The mathematical models of early vs. late retirement savings across varying levels of income are complicated and beyond the scope of this chapter, but we bring them up to highlight that the opportunity cost and debt burden of becoming a physician significantly complicate the income advantages of a medical career. For additional analysis on this topic, we defer to *The White Coat Investor*,[76] an excellent book and website with high-level financial discussion for physicians.

That said, the consequences of delayed retirement saving are so severe that some even argue delaying matriculation to medical school just to get the ball rolling for retirement (although this is probably too extreme).[77] We also need to consider that the physician who starts to pay back loans as an attending may feel inclined to place a large portion of his income into retirement accounts, further delaying the time to paying back loans (i.e., the internal medicine physician in our example may take even longer than 4–26 years as we described)

On the topic of loans, the **Public Service Loan Forgiveness (PSLF)** program deserves its own mention, as it essentially works as a "get out of jail" card for medical trainees with high amounts of debt. PSLF allows federal loans to be completely forgiven after working for a nonprofit for 120 nonconsecutive months. *Residency and fellowship training count as employment, and most residency and fellowship programs are at nonprofits.* Therefore, a neurosurgeon would have 7 years qualified simply by virtue of training. There is also no limit to how much debt can be forgiven; as of now, a physician with $600,000 in loans could legally expect all of his debt to be forgiven under this program. This also has the unintended effect of encouraging profligate spending among loan borrowers; $200,000 vs. $250,000 will be forgiven all the same after 120 months of nonprofit work, so there's really no pressure to live frugally throughout training.

That said, it's said that "if it's too good to be true, it probably is." There are two serious concerns about PSLF.

First, various politicians have discussed capping the maximum amount that can be forgiven.[78] The motivations for this are multifactorial. First, capping forgiveness would likely discourage the reckless borrowing and spending that is incentivized under the current system of unlimited forgiveness.[79] Another reason is that the program was intended to relieve the "typical" low-income nonprofit employee (e.g., public school teacher).[80] High-earning physicians were never the intended beneficiary. That said, we—including the author of this chapter—are certain that any federal loan borrower who was eligible for PSLF at the time of loan disbursement will continue to have the full-forgiveness option available. This is because you sign a legally binding document called a Master Promissory Note (MPN) when you take out a federal loan that is tightly enforced by contract law.[81] This is evidenced by the fact that all proposed legislation modifying PSLF explicitly excluded current borrowers. In addition, there is an example of US case law establishing the precedent that the conditions of PSLF cannot be reversed.[82] In any case, serious adjustments to PSLF down the line would have life-altering effects on borrowers, e.g., potentially forcing them to reconsider working at a for-profit institution that they otherwise passed up to qualify for PSLF.

---

[76] Retirement. Available at: https://www.whitecoatinvestor.com/category/retirement/. Accessed July 8, 2022.

[77] De M. Why medical school should start at age 28. Available at: https://www.statnews.com/2020/02/17/why-medical-school-should-start-at-age-28/. Accessed July 8, 2022.

[78] Farrington R. What Does The PAYE Expansion Proposal Really Mean? Available at: https://www.forbes.com/sites/robert-farrington/2015/07/17/what-does-the-paye-expansion-proposal-really-mean/. Accessed July 8, 2022.

[79] Delisle J. The coming Public Service Loan Forgiveness bonanza. Available at: https://www.brookings.edu/research/the-coming-public-service-loan-forgiveness-bonanza/. Accessed July 8, 2022.

[80] Taylor C. This Loan Forgiveness Program Promised To Help Teachers and Police Officers. Then It Denied 99% of Their Applications. Available at: https://fortune.com/2019/12/02/this-loan-forgiveness-program-promised-to-help-teachers-and-police-officers-then-it-denied-99-of-their-applications/. Accessed July 8, 2022.

[81] Will I qualify for PSLF? Available at: https://www.benwhite.com/finance/will-i-qualify-for-pslf/. Accessed July 8, 2022.

[82] 3 Borrowers Win Case on Eligibility for Public Service Loan Forgiveness. Available at: https://www.nytimes.com/2019/02/23/your-money/public-service-loan-forgiveness-lawsuit.html?ref=oembed. Accessed July 8, 2022.

Contract law attorneys would have a field day pursuing lawsuits against the federal government if the rug were pulled out on borrowers.

Second, as of 2020, only 1.8% of the 174,495 PSLF applications had been approved. While this may appear discouraging, we are still optimistic for several reasons. First, ~80% of the rejected applications in 2019 simply did not meet the requirements (120 months at a nonprofit) or had incomplete paperwork.[83] Next, there are multiple physician success stories of loan forgiveness through PSLF that validate the program's promises.[84] Therefore, our takeaway is that PSLF absolutely works, but you need to keep *meticulous records* of employment and qualifying payment over the 120 months—ideally multiple secured physical copies.

So there you have it. Becoming a physician is still essentially a guaranteed financial win (see Chapter 37, Financial Aid for further information). All of this, however, comes with significant sacrifice and opportunity cost that may simply be *unbearable* if you're not otherwise highly passionate about medicine. Yes, you've probably heard ad nauseum that medical school and residency are grueling, but we emphasize that it's really difficult to understand *exactly* how defeated you will feel day-in and day-out if you're not reasonably interested in and passionate about the profession.

## 41.6 Ok, I Get It. Residency Is Hard. But How Bad Can It Really Be?

Let's start with the obvious offender: residents work insane hours. In most residency programs (notable exceptions being dermatology, psychiatry, diagnostic radiology, physical medicine and rehabilitation, radiation oncology), you are expected to work 6 days a week from 6 AM to 6 PM most months, and you will frequently have to stay beyond 6 PM to finish up work piled on at the end of the day (e.g., new admission shortly before shift change, add-on surgery). Every once in a while, you will treat yourself to a *golden weekend*: 2 whole days off in a row (aka a normal weekend, as is seen in virtually every other profession). Many programs still have 30-hour shifts. Before work-hour caps, residents had logged working 136 out of the 168 **total** possible hours in a week.[85] After a tragic patient death,[86] work hour cap restrictions were set in place, which generally reduced the hour burden, although it occasionally incentivized residents to lie about their hours to maintain compliance.[87] These hours are directly linked to chronic sleep deprivation among residents, with 20% reporting sleeping an average of < 5 hours per night and 66% reporting an average of < 6 hours per night.[88] This sleep deprivation is linked with a significantly higher risk of car accidents when driving home after shifts.[89] Being awake and alert for > 24 hours has a similar effect on hand-eye coordination as a blood alcohol content of 0.10%[90]; the legal cutoff for a DUI is 0.08% (guess which of the two would get you suspended from your residency program!)

This begs the question: *why* do residents work so many hours and deal with sleep deprivation? Some data suggests that reducing resident hours may actually compromise patient safety by forcing more patient "handoffs,"[91] or transfer of care of a patient from one physician leaving a shift to another physician

83 Hornsby T. Why the PSLF Success Rate Will Hit Over 50% by 2024. Available at: https://www.studentloanplanner.com/pslf-snowball-effect/. Accessed July 8, 2022.

84 A Public Service Loan Forgiveness Success Story-Podcast #176. Available at: https://www.whitecoatinvestor.com/pslf-success-story-podcast-176/. Accessed July 8, 2022.

85 Medical Residents' Work Hours. Available at: https://web.archive.org/web/20070310201116/http://www.internetfreespeech.org/print_article.cfm?ID=6666. Accessed July 8, 2022.

86 Asch DA, Parker RM. The Libby Zion Case. N Engl J Med 1988; 318:771–775.

87 Fargen KM, Rosen CL. Are duty hour regulations promoting a culture of dishonesty among resident physicians? J Grad Med Educ 2013;5(4):553–5. Available at: https://pubmed.ncbi.nlm.nih.gov/24454999/. Accessed July 8, 2022.

88 Baldwin Jr. DeWitt C, Daugherty SR. Sleep deprivation and fatigue in residency training: results of a national survey of first- and second-year residents. Sleep 2004;27(2):217–23. Available at: https://pubmed.ncbi.nlm.nih.gov/15124713/. Accessed July 8, 2022.

89 Mak NT, Li J, Wiseman SM. Resident Physicians are at Increased Risk for Dangerous Driving after Extended-duration Work Shifts: A Systematic Review. Cureus 2019;11(6):e4843. Available at: https://www.ncbi.nlm.nih.gov/pmc/articles/PMC6684113/. Accessed July 8, 2022.

90 Dawson D, Reid K. Fatigue, alcohol and performance impairment. Nature 1997;388(6639):235. Available at: https://pubmed.ncbi.nlm.nih.gov/9230429/. Accessed July 8, 2022.

91 Reducing Work Hours for Medical Interns Increases Patient 'Handoff' Risks. Available at: https://www.hopkinsmedicine.org/news/media/releases/reducing_work_hours_for_medical_interns_increases_patient_handoff_risks. Accessed July 8, 2022.

starting a shift. After all, if physicians work fewer hours in a row, then there will need to be more, shorter shifts worked by the collective resident pool to cover all hours.

Interestingly enough, the conversation has broadened with the publication of a landmark study that found no difference in patient safety with shorter shifts compared to longer shifts.[92] Sadly, the takeaway from this was, "We can continue to make residents work long shifts, and it won't compromise patient safety!" instead of "We can allow residents to work more humane hours without compromising patient safety." After all, there is no compelling evidence that working superhuman hours leads to better training. Instead, much of the justification for the status quo appears to be related to modifiable safety concerns.

Also consider that you will be doing all of this for about $60,000 per year.[93] Other professional careers with comparable hours for new graduates tend to pay *much more*, e.g., big law ($190,000 yearly starting out)[94] and investment banking ($150,000–$200,000 in the first year).[95] Also consider that you will be working these hours for minimal pay in the "prime years" of your life, and you will likely experience a significant sense of envy toward others in your peer group working 40 to 50 hours a week making reasonable salaries and enjoying regular vacations. You will also be expected to find time to study and potentially work on research projects in your off-time. Depending on your specialty, you may also experience the low-key constant stress of making yourself marketable to a competitive fellowship specialty (e.g., cardiology, gastroenterology, plastic or pediatric surgery).

Because of these demands on your time, you will have to significantly budget your time and cut out a lot of personal hobbies and exploration of nonmedical things. In our experience, most people who thrive in medicine prioritize studying and actively maintaining their physical and mental health. With their remaining time, they *may* be able to continue sustained commitment to one to two other nonmedical hobbies.

Much of your day will also be unpredictable and at the complete whim of your supervisors. With rare exceptions (e.g., shift work specialties such as emergency medicine and radiology), your day officially ends when all the i's are dotted and t's crossed. If a new patient is admitted or a new operation is added shortly before closing time, you better expect to stay at work for several more hours. You are also a perpetual trainee who very slowly gains confidence in your abilities. Imposter syndrome is very real in residency because you will feel clueless throughout much of the process—even though you are frequently dealing with high-stakes scenarios.

You will also have very limited bargaining power to improve your working conditions. Residents cannot easily leave their positions for a program with better working conditions, as is seen in other industries.[96] This lowers competitive pressure for residency programs to improve working conditions. While there is great incentive for programs to *advertise* a commitment to resident well-being at recruitment events during the interview trail, there is much less incentive to follow through on these commitments because residents who are matched rarely leave.

Residents also have a significant loan burden, and their best chance at overcoming that burden is advancing through residency to make an attending salary. As a result, they face the *collective action problem*[97]: while working conditions for residents would likely improve if *everyone* banded together (e.g., through unionization—as has been done successful at programs like the University of Michigan[98]),

[92] Silber JH, Bellini LM, Shea JA, et al. Patient Safety Outcomes under Flexible and Standard Resident Duty-Hour Rules. N Engl J Med 2019;380:905-914. Available at: https://www.nejm.org/doi/full/10.1056/NEJMoa1810642. Accessed July 8, 2022.

[93] Gooch K. Average resident salary by specialty. Available at: https://www.beckershospitalreview.com/compensation-issues/average-resident-salary-by-specialty.html. Accessed July 8, 2022.

[94] Lane R. Big Law: What It Is and What Salary You Should Expect. Available at: https://www.nerdwallet.com/article/loans/student-loans/big-law-salary. Accessed July 8, 2022.

[95] DeChesare B. The Investment Banking Analyst: Job Description, Hours, Salaries and More. Available at: https://www.mergersandinquisitions.com/investment-banking-analyst-job/. Accessed July 8, 2022.

[96] Park R. Why So Many Young Doctors Work Such Awful Hours. Available at: https://www.theatlantic.com/business/archive/2017/02/doctors-long-hours-schedules/516639/. Accessed July 8, 2022.

[97] THE COLLECTIVE ACTION PROBLEM. Available at: https://spot.colorado.edu/~mcguire/collact.html. Accessed July 8, 2022.

[98] Greene J. University of Michigan health system residents approve new union contract. Available at: https://www.modernhealthcare.com/labor/university-michigan-health-system-residents-approve-new-union-contract. Accessed July 8, 2022.

*individual* residents have too much to risk by being the gadfly who stirs the pot. Medical specialties are small communities, and the risk of tarnishing your reputation by annoying higher-ups is too great for most individual residents to fight back against intolerable working conditions. Since (1) residency is temporary, (2) attending-hood is the rest of your life, and (3) graduating residency with a stellar reputation is optimal for attending-hood, many residents would prefer to grit their teeth and take the pain. In addition, as we've emphasized many times over, there are real and perceived risks to seeking mental healthcare, even though residency training introduces many severe stressors that may introduce or exacerbate mental health issues in its trainees[99] (see Chapter 18, Self-Care and Wellness).

Fortunately, the lifestyle is essentially guaranteed to improve once you're an attending. Even in the work-heavy specialties (i.e., surgery), you can still tailor your individual practice to be more lifestyle-friendly, albeit at a cost (typically income). Many attendings also speak of a significant sense of pride in their work, as they finally make use of their years of training to make the conclusive expert decisions for difficult clinical encounters. Attendings also experience a dramatic improvement in their quality of life due to suddenly making hundreds of thousands of dollars, as well as the newfound earned respect of being on top of the medical hierarchy.

We don't highlight these points to scare you out of becoming a doctor. Yes, residency can be ruthlessly soul-crushing at times. Depending on where you train, it may consistently be an unpleasant experience for 3 to 7 years. Fortunately, the culture of medicine does actively seem to be improving to embrace more humanity and evidence-based working conditions. If you genuinely believe that medicine is your best career path, then you will have the best odds of weathering training. Just be mindful that it can and *will* be a lot worse than anything you have ever imagined. Take care of yourself physically and mentally, and keep a close circle of confidants for emotional support.

Along the way, we encourage you to go the extra mile to make the journey more tolerable for the next generation. Go out of your way to make the medical students feel valued on the team. Grab them chairs to make sure they're not awkwardly standing during team meetings or in the clinic. Help them out by reviewing high-yield learning material for their shelf exams. Let them go home early if they're stuck at the hospital not doing anything of educational value. Roll up your sleeves and help your new interns with difficult logistical material (e.g., navigating the EMR) when you're the senior on the team. It sounds clichéd, but medicine is a small enough community that *you can genuinely be the change that you want to see*. Please be a kind human—not only for your colleagues' sake, but also for your own well-being.[100]

---

[99] https://pubmed.ncbi.nlm.nih.gov/31299659/... "It is the very nature of medical education and training that contributes to these high rates of emotional distress, since students entering medical school score better on indicators of mental health than similarly aged college graduates."

[100] Why Being Kind Helps You, Too–Especially Now. Available at: https://www.wsj.com/articles/why-being-kind-helps-you-tooespecially-now-11597194000. Accessed July 8, 2022.

# 42 Real Talk on the Medical School Experience

*Ray Funahashi and Joel Thomas*

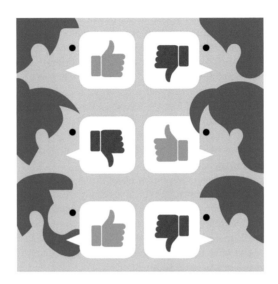

Many pre-meds are completely preoccupied by the mission to get into medical school and aren't overly concerned with what medical school is *actually like*. This isn't unreasonable; if you can't get into medical school, then there is no point in worrying about what the process is like to get through it. In addition, you can't skip medical school, so it's easy to conclude, "I just know I want to be a physician—I'll do whatever it takes." Having gone through the medical school experience, we can confidently say this is a huge mistake for two reasons. First, knowing what the medical school experience is like should absolutely play a role in deciding on pursuing a career in medicine. Second, knowing what is coming ahead will help you start habits as a pre-med that will be both immediately useful and help you become a more competitive and competent medical student.

In this chapter, we will give you the inside scoop on what medical school is *actually* like because it's easy to be influenced by the romanticized perspectives offered by the ADCOM and inspirational media (i.e., YouTube and Instagram personalities). In doing so, we will pay particular attention to the mundane, boring aspects of medical school that will occupy most of your time.

Keep in mind that the medical school experience can vary tremendously depending on where you are (e.g., due to cultural differences by location, curriculum) and who you are (e.g., your ability to deal with b*llshit, your baseline tendency toward depressive outlooks). In addition, this chapter only reflects the experiences of the authors and their personal circle of colleagues at select other institutions. That said, our experience seems consistent with that of our colleagues at other institutions. Therefore, we're confident that this chapter will give an accurate taste of things to come.

## 42.1 Medical School in a Nutshell

Medical school is hard, and you will underestimate how difficult it is. The pace and volume of information will come at you hard, so you will have to study a lot. You will also need to retain almost all of this material *cold* for years at a time; you can't simply cram and regurgitate as you may have done in undergrad. This is because the curriculum is (ideally) distilled to only cover material that has direct clinical utility. To promote retention and application of the material in a clinical context, you will likely be "pimped"[1] on your knowledge throughout your training. This is when a more senior member of the healthcare team

---

[1] Detsky AS. The Art of Pimping. JAMA 2009;301(13):1379–1381. Available at: https://jamanetwork.com/journals/jama/article-abstract/183639. Accessed July 8, 2022.

(e.g., intern, resident, fellow, or attending physician) sequentially asks you questions about a topic in a Socratic fashion until you get something wrong. This is done to expose the limits of your understanding so that you can focus your studying toward your knowledge gaps. In addition, it's believed that getting the question wrong in a "safe" but fairly high-pressure environment will make sure you never forget it down the line in a more critical situation (e.g., crashing patient). For example, in your third year pediatrics clerkship, you may be asked point-blank about one of the thousands of facts you learned in biochemistry in your first year of medical school, e.g., "What is the clinical significance of glucose 6-phosphatase?" If you get it right, the attending may follow up with, "What substrate accumulates if this enzyme is deficient?" "What disease is characterized by a deficiency of this enzyme?" "What is the treatment for this disease?" "What is the mode of inheritance of this disease?" "How do patients with this disease clinically present?" "How does lack of this enzyme lead to the clinical manifestations?" etc.

There are many analogies that describe this process. Our favorite is the "stack of pancakes" analogy: medical school is like eating a stack of pancakes every day for 4 years. Most people like pancakes. Heck, I'd be thrilled to eat a warm, fluffy stack of pancakes today. Likewise, medicine is really interesting, and I'd be stoked to learn about rare diseases and physiology for a day. But what about tomorrow? And the day after that? And the day after that repeat ad nauseum? You get the idea. Eventually, you'll get sick of pancakes. And the worst part is that you still have to eat whatever pancakes you didn't finish. So if you slack off for a few days, you might be looking at eating 40 pancakes in a single day. Not nice.

And yet, you will get used to it. You wouldn't have gotten into medical school if you couldn't handle it (generally). Indeed, there's a reason why US medical schools care so much about admitting applicants with the highest GPAs and MCAT scores. Getting through medical school is an inherently difficult process, but the data and years of experience show that the students who matriculate get through it with nearly a 100% success rate.[2]

Socially, it will feel like a weird mix of college, the workplace, and the military. You will get to know new classmates all over again and experience new highs and lows with them. You will be enthralled by the amazing humans you call your classmates and their backstories and accomplishments. You will be surrounded by world-class athletes, accomplished musicians, and former high-level professionals in other careers—all of whom are also extremely intelligent and driven students.[3] Self-care will be much harder, but you will find your own way of managing. In order to be competitive for various specialties you will be involved in extracurricular activities like research and publishing papers throughout med school.

You will eventually hit the wards and help take care of patients. You will feel incompetent a lot, as you are understandably incompetent but expected to take histories and perform physical exams on actual patients in a real healthcare setting. Your imposter syndrome[4] will probably get worse as you start working in the wards and are surrounded by clinicians and residents who know *way* more than you. You'll study for shelf exams as best you can, even though you will be exhausted from being at the hospital nearly every day. In addition, you'll be frustrated to find that much of what you spend studying for shelf exams will be random minutiae that is not relevant to your day-to-day experience on the wards (e.g., obscure parasitic diseases, outdated antibiotics). Your grades will be a mix of objective shelf exams and residents' and attendings' subjective judgment. Sometimes you will feel slighted and believe you deserve a better grade. At some point, the electronic health record (EHR) will overwhelm and anger you. You will find flaws in medicine and how we practice it. You will have horrible moments like your patient dying, making a mistake, or being berated by someone for no apparent reason. You will feel exhausted after night shifts or extended hour shifts—especially when you feel like you're only there to take up space. You will miss holidays, weddings, and friends' outings, and they will not understand why you can't take the day off. Planning for the future will be harder than ever, as your schedule is rarely available to you ahead of time, and is subject to high variability even on a day to day basis.

---

[2] Moon K. Will Attending Medical School In The Caribbean Hurt My Chances Of Becoming A U.S. Doctor? Available at: https://www.forbes.com/sites/kristenmoon/2020/05/11/will-attending-medical-school-in-the-caribbean-hurt-my-chances-of-becoming-a-us-doctor/?sh=61e36f66676a. Accessed July 8, 2022.

[3] One of my most memorable interactions with a classmate was when she randomly mentioned an experience from her PhD program. None of us knew she had a PhD; she just nonchalantly brought it up.

[4] Imposter Syndrome. Available at: https://students-residents.aamc.org/attending-medical-school/article/imposter-syndrome/. Accessed July 8, 2022.

But you will also have privileged moments and milestones like having a patient praise you specifically during team rounds, diagnosing something your superiors missed, and flawlessly performing a procedure. If patient care is sufficiently rewarding to you, these things will sustain you. If it isn't, then you may end up depressed.

In fourth year you will decide what specialty to apply to for residency (more in Chapter 44, A Peek at the Residency Application Process), i.e., decide what kind of doctor you want to be. This will either be an easy or agonizing process. If you're aiming for a very competitive speciality (e.g., orthopaedic surgery, otolaryngology, neurosurgery, integrated interventional radiology, dermatology, urology), then you will go to other medical schools to do away rotations to impress them. Along the way, you will take USMLE Step 2; in the past, this was simply a formality, albeit a stressful one. In the wake of Step 1 being made pass/fail, we predict that studying for Step 2 may become the hyper-stressful gauntlet that determines your career—moments before you even apply to your specialty of choice.

And with that, the most stressful parts are mostly done. You collect recommendation letters and before you know it, it's deja vu—applying to residency feels a little like applying to medical school again. Interview invites and interviews. Traveling. Ranking which programs you like and submitting them. You anxiously await where you will match while you complete elective rotations. Finally in March you find out where you are going for residency! Or if you're unlucky, not going. It's party time until graduation in May. Say goodbye to your friends. You will keep in touch with some of them. Catch a well-deserved breath because residency starts a few months later.

## 42.2 Medical School Hot Takes

Before we delve into the details above, here are some key insights that will help you understand what med school is like.

### 42.2.1 Memorization Is King but not Enough

- **Expectations:** "Memorization" just comes down to *understanding* medical concepts. If you can conceptually understand the first principles, then you can solve any problem. If you don't know something, you can always look it up. After all, we live in the modern world of smartphones and databases.
- **Reality:** Doing well on the Step exams and the wards requires you to memorize a ton of stuff. There is a surprising amount of the information you study that you will need to know cold. Yes, it's all stuff that you could theoretically look up at any given time, but a competent physician practicing at the top of their game will *already* be looking up a ton of stuff at work, even after having memorized all this baseline knowledge.
  - At the same time, memorization isn't enough. If you try to memorize things that you don't understand at baseline, you will not break into the upper echelon of test performance because the hardest questions apply second- and third-order thinking to obscure minutiae that you have to know cold.
- **What it feels like:** Utterly overwhelming. You will always feel like you don't know enough because it's probably impossible to know everything you need to know. You will feel guilty for procrastinating or skipping studying for something else because there is always an opportunity to study even more. In fact, because the material is not particularly conceptually challenging, outperforming your classmates (and scoring the highest percentiles on the standardized board exams) simply requires putting more hours into studying. Indeed, one of the best predictors of high scores on USMLE Step 1 appears to be the sheer number of flash cards and practice problems completed.[5] Over time you will figure out what information is extraneous and not necessary to commit to memory. Highly rated third-party materials generally do a great job of highlighting which information you will need to retain, but you may become overwhelmed by the number of different options available (e.g., UWorld, NBME exams, AMBOSS, Online MedEd, Pathoma, First Aid, SketchyMedical, Boards and Beyond, Anki, Memm, etc.). Everyone has

---

5 Deng F, Gluckstein JA, Larsen DP. Student-directed retrieval practice is a predictor of medical licensing examination performance [published correction appears in Perspect Med Educ. 2016 Nov 18]. Perspect Med Educ. 2015;4(6):308–313. Available at: https://www.ncbi.nlm.nih.gov/pmc/articles/PMC4673073/. Accessed July 8, 2022.

different methods and systems that they develop, but this process requires self-experimentation. The knowledge anxiety drops off briefly after Step 1, only to shoot back up after you hit the wards. It will also build up to Step 2 and the drop off again until residency approaches!

- **Our recommendation:** *Use the exact same high-quality methods we recommend for undergrad.* Spaced repetition and active learning are key here. Obtain a deep conceptual understanding of the material first, and then use spaced repetition to retain the understanding for years at a time. Do practice problems to integrate your knowledge across disciplines and to approach it from different angles. We will discuss more in Chapter 43, Real Talk on Succeeding in Medical School, but the nuts and bolts are to do several hours of studying most days for several years. *Consistency is key.*
  - Treat studying like a full-time job, not as something you simply have to get out of the way. Learn to embrace it and find joy in the process of expanding your ever-growing web of medical knowledge. That said, you will probably still do much studying on weekends, especially if you're aiming for a competitive specialty.
  - **Realistically, expect to spend 5 to 10 hours** *each day,* **5 to 7 days a week studying in the first 2 years.**[6]

## 42.2.2 School Material Alone Is often Inadequate to Succeed

- **Expectations:** The lectures the school provides and the associated material will give you everything you need to know to do well on the Step exams and shelf exams.
- **Reality:**
  - Your school may provide you with a "syllabus" for each course (or just sections from a textbook to read). In undergrad, the syllabus was simply a reference document that summarized grading and course expectations. In medical school, the syllabus is a several hundred-page "textbook" that contains all of the information you will need to know for the course. It is a faculty created document meant to be paired with lectures. These syllabi consolidate decades of medical research into an organized web of knowledge. A given course may be taught by 30 to 50 different faculty members (e.g., the GI block may have lectures from experts in pancreas disease, liver disease, stomach disease, etc.).
  - Ideally, it contains only the minimum amount of information required to give you a comprehensive understanding of the basic science. In reality, it will probably still contain low-yield extraneous minutiae.
  - In addition, many instructors are not that great at teaching (some PhD lecturers are notorious for this), and frequently give you a disproportionate focus on information on which they are specialists. You will quickly realize that you will have to budget your attention between knowing material to pass your school's exams, the "high-yield" material that's emphasized on boards, and actually clinically useful material. In an ideal world, these three things would overlap completely, but the reality is that they don't. A lot of schools now stream their lectures so many students choose not to attend them. This is especially true with lecturers who don't have a great teaching reputation. As a result, many students at true pass-fail schools completely ignore their school's lectures and study entirely for boards with third-party material.[7] These materials tend to be good enough that the students can pass—but maybe not excel at—their school exams.
  - Exams tend to be mix of both high-yield, big-picture material (that everyone needs to know to be a competent physician), as well as super-specific nitty-gritty info (that may not even be that relevant to clinical practice, e.g., PhD researcher minutiae) to separate the cream from the wheat.
  - You're now an adult learner. There is greater freedom to "choose your adventure" in terms of how you budget your time (e.g., research, shadowing, appropriate time off).
  - You will spend a lot of time in a mental fog only to experience paradigm shifts of clarity down the line. This is because **medical education places a lot of emphasis on granular detail, and it's easy to miss the forest for the trees.** Over time, the material across multiple subjects will interlock, and you will gradually develop a fundamental shift in your sense of identity as you adopt a new role as a physician.

---

[6] https://revisingrubies.com/how-many-hours-a-day-do-medical-students-study/, https://www.mededpublish.org/manuscripts/1506

[7] Murphy B. Why some medical students are cutting class to get ahead. Available at: https://www.ama-assn.org/residents-students/medical-school-life/why-some-medical-students-are-cutting-class-get-ahead. Accessed July 8, 2022, Farber ON. Medical students are skipping class in droves, and making lectures increasingly obsolete. 2018. Available at: https://www.statnews.com/2018/08/14/medical-students-skipping-class/. Accessed July 8, 2022.

- **What it feels like:** Frustrating. You may be spending tens of thousands of dollars toward a formal medical education, only to do most of your learning from third-party material that you have to spend an additional several hundred dollars on.
- **Our recommendation:** You will get mixed opinions. Here are our recommendations:
  - **Ray Funahashi:** Stick with the third-party materials. It sucks to spend the extra money so be judicious on choosing only a few. Most schools have moved to a pass-fail system. Focus on learning and doing well with question banks. Especially NBME exams to test your knowledge.
  - **Joel Thomas:** I made heavy use of third-party materials and prioritized doing well on the Step exams. At the same time, I felt that my school's materials were very good at tying the disparate facts from third-party materials into a cohesive web of knowledge that integrated multiple disciplines. I also valued a deep scientific level of understanding for its own sake. I don't know what the counterfactual scenario would have been like (i.e., if I had only used board prep material), but I felt that the intellectual framework I got from my school's syllabi gave me a stronger level of understanding compared to that of my peers who only used third-party material. Therefore, I recommend using both your school's and third-party materials *if you have the time and care about this level of understanding.* If you simply want the most time-efficient way to learn the highest yield material, third-party materials alone is probably the best approach.
  - **Phillip Wagner:** I mostly avoided third-party materials during the preclinical years, although I didn't begrudge people that focused on them. The material provided by the school was more comprehensive, and I generally thought it was more helpful in building an initial conceptual framework for the content. When classes were taught particularly poorly (or more often just not done in a way that was easy for me to retain), it was pretty helpful to transition to better organized third-party material. By the time I got ready to study for step 1, however, the school material was just too unwieldy for efficient review, and I focused exclusively on third-party review materials. By the time I was in my clinical years, it was my experience that content was most delivered on a patient-centered basis while on the job (you relearn applied physiology and pathology when you read about your specific patients and their problems), or via third-party question banks that are marketed specifically for medical students. As my clinical career progressed, third-party materials are gradually getting replaced by primary research articles, meta-analyses, society guidelines, reference material meant for medical professionals, and podcasts and opinion pieces by experts. Learning on the job to cater to your patients' specific needs is the primary driving force for this continued learning.

## 42.2.3 Extracurriculars—Aside from Research—Don't Really Matter as much in Medical School

- **Expectations:** I will have to balance extracurriculars and academics all over again like in undergrad.
- **Reality:** Extracurricular activities can matter a little less for residency programs than they did when applying to medical school. Across all medical specialties, residency program directors rank extracurricular experiences in the bottom half of variables considered when evaluating applicants.[8] That said, they can be used to continue to build your narrative, or—*GASP!*—just for sheer enjoyment (you know—like normal people do?). Research is extremely important for competitive specialties, as described in Chapter 41, Real Talk on a Medical Career.
- **What it feels like:** Freeing. You no longer have to split your attention across so many things. Instead, you can focus deeply on studying and pursue extracurriculars as you see fit. The exception being research, of course. If you're going for a competitive specialty, then it is in your best interest to spend as much time as you can on research projects aimed at producing abstracts, presentations, and publications to pump up your numbers.
- **Our recommendation:**
  - **If your school isn't pushing research or you're not interested in a competitive specialty:** Do whatever extracurriculars genuinely interest you. As a medical student, you tend to have much more influence in extracurricular organizations—especially if there are other schools at your university. You

---

[8] Results of the 2018 NRMP Program Director Survey. Available at: https://www.nrmp.org/wp-content/uploads/2018/07/NRMP-2018-Program-Director-Survey-for-WWW.pdf. Accessed July 8, 2022.

can meaningfully participate in clinical volunteering because you have actual clinical skills. You can participate in political activism with more clout behind your actions because of your perceived expertise as a future physician. Follow your passion.

- **If you're even remotely interested in a competitive specialty:** If you're starting medical school interested in dermatology, find a research mentor in dermatology ASAP (ideally one who has yielded many publications with medical students in the past). Get involved with research and spend whatever time you can with that mentor churning out abstracts, presentations, and publications. If you change your mind about dermatology and pick a less competitive specialty down the line, your research experience will still go a long way. On the other hand, if you did research in the less competitive specialty but ultimately chose dermatology, you would be at a disadvantage because dermatology (and other competitive specialties) value research in their field.
- **If you decide late on a competitive specialty:** Speak with a faculty advisor in that field and determine whether you need to take time off to pursue a research year in that field. This is an increasingly common strategy in competitive fields.[9]
- **Do extensive shadowing across basically every field in your preclinical years:** It's extremely easy to shadow as a medical student. Oftentimes, you can just cold-email faculty, and they'll invite you to shadow in the next few days. I even got a full tour of a department from the chairman by emailing him, asking to shadow. We recommend shadowing early in medical school to get a better sense of what field you want to pursue; you might discover early on that you're energized by a more competitive field, and you may be moved to pursue research in that field.

## 42.2.4 You Might Run into Some Hypercompetitive "Gunners," but Overall the Environment Tends to be Collaborative

- **Expectations:** Getting into medical school felt like The Hunger Games. It's only going to get worse in medical school because I will be surrounded by the best and brightest of those people.
- **Reality:** Medical school generally has a less malignant culture than pre-med culture. Pass-fail curriculums of med schools tend to help foster more collaboration and less gunning. It's not uncommon for classes to have a shared Google drive of study materials. Class Facebook groups often help facilitate info that is helpful about upcoming events. In addition, medical students tend to realize that the vast majority of their competition for residency is coming from *other schools*. Therefore, students at any particular school have it in their best interest to help each other out to do better than the vast majority of their competition elsewhere.
- **What it feels like:** Generally, people are willing to help each other. Going to medical school is kind of like joining the military. You go through tough training with your classmates, so there is a sort of kinship that develops that will continue through med school and beyond.
- **Our recommendation:** Lead by example and be a helpful classmate. Your medical school class is a small community, so your individual efforts to foster the group dynamic will go a long way. For example, if you share a helpful study guide that you made, it may encourage someone else to do the same for the next class.

## 42.2.5 Grading Can Be Hit-or-Miss at Times

- **Expectations:** My grades will be a reflection of how hard I work, my knowledge, and professionalism.
- **Reality:** While your grades during your first years studying basic science will be objective and based on how hard and efficiently you learn and apply concepts, your grades in rotations will have a significant subjective component. Indeed, the subjectivity of clinical evaluations has come under scrutiny for potentially perpetuating societal biases.[10] In addition, being on a good team and having a great attending physician makes a tremendous difference on your experience of clerkships. Unfortunately, a lot of this is based on luck. Your clerkship grades still do have an objective component with the shelf

---

[9] Bram JT, Pirruccio K, Aoyama JT, Ahn J, Ganley TJ, Flynn JM. Do Year-Out Programs Make Medical Students More Competitive Candidates for Orthopedic Surgery Residencies? J Surg Educ 2020;77(6):1440–1449. Available at: https://pubmed.ncbi.nlm.nih.gov/32505668/. Accessed July 8, 2022.

[10] Medicine@Browon. Available at: https://medicine.at.brown.edu/article/isnt-she-lovely/. Accessed July 8, 2022.

exams so if you do well on those it will help tremendously. The USMLE Step exams also are objective and have a huge role in your overall academic standing.

- **What it feels like:** Occasionally you will be in the right place at the right time and it will feel awesome. You catch a heart murmur or diagnosis the team missed, and you get recognized for it. You might also work and get along with attendings and residents that you "click" with. Your grades will often reflect this. The opposite can sometimes happen too. Your subjective grades will be heavily based on how you present your patient orally, come up with differential diagnoses, come up with a diagnostic and treatment plan, write patient notes, answer on-the-spot knowledge questions (aka pimp questions), and perform clinical exams and procedures.

- **Our recommendation:**
  - While clinical evaluations will always have a subjective component, you can maximize your odds of doing well with our recommendations. We recommend following the **3 A's**. Be available, affable, and able (in that order).
    - **Available:** This means that you should show up to everything a little early and stay as late as you can. This means reading between the lines for "trick scenarios". If the resident tells you, "we have a new admit coming soon, but you can go home if you want," you should absolutely stay longer to see the new admit. On the other hand, if the resident tells you point blank, "Go home," do *not* test their patience by sticking around. In general, medical students should see new patients (e.g., admissions and consults), but if the rest of the team is just sitting around working on notes, then it's probably fine for you to go home if offered. You should *not* ask, "Can I go home?" Instead, ask, "What can I help you with?" *This is socially acceptable code-speak for "Can I go home?".* If there's nothing for you to do, the resident will say "Nothing, go home." This way, you can go home, *and* you've demonstrated that you're willing to help the team.
    - **Affable:** This means that you should generally be outwardly pleasant. Don't brown-nose the team—it's incredibly cringe-worthy and generally obvious. Don't volunteer to go out of your way to get people coffee and snacks. Don't go out of your way to bake goods for the team. That said, laugh at people's jokes, even if they're not particularly funny; people are trying to lighten the mood, and showing social reciprocity goes a long way in a stressful clinical environment. Make appropriate casual conversation with the team, but don't be overly familiar. Do *not* initiate inappropriate jokes or off-color conversation. Read the room—the socially inept will struggle in clinical environments, unfortunately.
    - **Able:** Demonstrate your medical knowledge when it's appropriate to do so. Knock your presentations and notes out of the park. Stun the team with your medical knowledge when you are being pimped. Impress the team with the depth and nuance of your clinical questions; most of your seniors will enjoy intellectually stimulating conversation, and you can contribute to this by posing thoughtful questions about clinical practice (e.g., "I learned that you shouldn't drink alcohol when taking metronidazole, but it seems like there's randomized controlled trial data disproving this.[11] How should we counsel patients?"). Be careful with your questions, as they can leave impressions about your (lack of) knowledge. Never ask someone something that can be easily Googled. Instead, use your questions to demonstrate that you've done baseline research (e.g., "I was reading that some providers prefer to use the X method for this disease, instead of the Y method we're using. What are your thoughts on the X method?").
  - Study hard with third-party materials (more in Chapter 43, Real Talk on Succeeding in Medical School).
  - Before starting clerkships, have a fourth year medical student teach you (in order of priority) the basics of navigating the EMR, oral presentation, note-writing, and physical exam.
  - Know everything about your patient's cold. You only have a few of them where the rest of the team has many more. You should know them better than those senior to you.

---

[11] Paauw DS. Alcohol and Metronidazole Interaction: Real or Fake? Available at: https://www.medscape.com/viewarticle/917065_2. Accessed July 8, 2022, Visapää JP, Tillonen JS, Kaihovaara PS, Salaspuro MP. Lack of disulfiram-like reaction with metronidazole and ethanol. Ann Pharmacother 2002;36(6):971–974. Available at: https://pubmed.ncbi.nlm.nih.gov/12022894/. Accessed July 8, 2022.

- Never lie. If someone asks you about an obscure part of the patient's history that you didn't ask about, go back and ask them. Don't make something up.
- Be eager to do whatever your senior asks you to do[12] and appear enthusiastic about doing it.
- Recognize that **at** the end of the day—you can "do everything right" but still not get "honors" due to bad luck (i.e., not clicking with your resident or attending because of fundamentally different personalities, your supervisors having difficult circumstances in their life when they evaluated you, etc.).

## 42.2.6 Altruism, Passion, and Empathy Aren't Enough to Ward against Burnout

- **Expectations:** Altruism, passion, and empathy are all you need to get through medical school other than studying hard.
- **Reality:** The practice of medicine has many components you can't appreciate from shadowing doctors as a student. While altruism, passion, and empathy are essential for being a great clinician, the grinding work schedule, the emotional investment in patient care, bureaucracy, the inefficiencies of hospital operation and electronic medical record, occasional malignant personalities, and social sacrifice can play a role in burnout for anyone. Indeed, many students will slowly develop a sense of cynicism toward clinical medicine—compounded by the fact that much of what kept you going through the hard work of getting into and surviving medical school was based on noble ideals. Samuel Shem's *House of God* poignantly and profanely depicts this point of view shift experienced by many medical trainees.[13]
  - Strictly speaking, you learn how to be a *doctor* in residency. Medical school prepares you to be a functional resident (i.e., having a basic, broad scientific knowledge of medicine, seeing the division of labor in a hospital, interacting with an EMR, understanding and coming to terms with the process of identity formation, etc.).
- **What it feels like:** How people deal with the stress of medical school and medical practice will vary. Luck also sometimes plays a role in good vs bad experiences. Also, despite what people may say, it is possible to be altruistic, passionate, and empathetic, and still end up not liking the practice of direct patient care.
- **Our recommendation:** Deeply consider all the information out there on the practice of medicine and understand the actual sacrifices involved with a career in medicine before committing to applying to medical school. During medical school, make it a priority to invest in self-care and mental health care. Maintain a professional and positive attitude as much as possible.
  - Seek mentors early. Mentors should be both upper class medical students (preferably third and fourth year students) as well as faculty. Get frequent advice and invest in those mentor-mentee relationships throughout medical school.
  - If you conclude at the end of clerkships that you would not be happy spending the rest of your life in direct patient care, *speak to your academic advisors*. Revisit the same rotations as a fourth year—your perspective may shift dramatically after a year of clerkships, and the expectations and pressures of a fourth year rotation are much more like residency (e.g., no shelf exams, greater integration into the team). Explore as many specialties as you can, including ones with less direct patient care (radiology and pathology). If even these don't appeal to you, consider nonclinical opportunities after medical school (more in Chapter 46, Nonclinical Careers).

## 42.2.7 Self-Care Is Harder but Still Non-negotiable

- **Expectations:** I will be sleep deprived and incredibly stressed. I will keep in contact with people outside of medicine.

---

[12] Within reason, of course. Don't do anything that's clearly demeaning. If you're in doubt about something that happened on a clerkship, discuss with your peers and consider bringing it to a clerkship director or whatever mechanism your school has for reporting inappropriate clerkship behavior. Many schools have anonymous reporting mechanisms.

[13] ACP Hospitalist is available exclusively to ACP Members. Available at: https://acphospitalist.org/archives/2008/10/book.htm. Accessed July 8, 2022.

- **Reality:** *You need to continue the self-care strategies you developed in undergrad* (see Chapter 18, Self-Care and Wellness) *throughout medical school.* This will be **much** harder because your time will be greatly limited and much more regimented. The medical school schedule can also often place a lot of strain on relationships.
- **What it feels like:** It heavily depends on your self-care, disposition, support systems, and mental health at baseline. It also depends on whether you want to pursue a highly competitive residency program; students interested in very competitive specialities will face much more pressure to work longer hours to receive the highest grades.
  - You will probably experience some resentment and disappointment in having to give up so much of your freedom and being forced to regiment your time so carefully. Realistically, you won't have as much spontaneity in your life as you did in college (e.g., randomly going out with your friends on weekdays, spontaneous weekend trips out of town).
  - Your friends and family outside of medicine may do their best to understand your world, but at the end of the day, they won't really understand your struggles. You will gravitate to your classmates who understand your concerns on a deeper level.
  - You probably will not be very sleep-deprived. Night shifts are relatively rare in medical school, and it's not uncommon to get 6 to 8 hours of sleep almost every night in medical school, although that may not be true for certain rotations.
  - Self-care is generally easier in the preclinical years, especially if you don't go to lectures. Yes, you have to spend a lot of time studying, but you can do this at your own schedule. This can be a great time to implement a system of self-care (e.g., meditation in the AM, gym at noon, calling friends and family at night) that you will learn to modify during clerkships.
    - Self-care becomes dramatically harder during clerkships because your time is no longer your own. You have to report to your clinical site at a specific time (often very early), and you cannot go home until you are excused. On some clerkships, you may be at the hospital from ~6 AM to 6 PM *6 days a week*. On top of that, you are expected to spend time studying for your shelf exam. It's more common to have absolutely no life other than medical school and self-care (i.e., working out every few days, sleeping 6–8 hours a night) on a surgery or medicine rotation.
  - Believe it or not, people do manage to become pregnant and raise children in medical school. You will definitely have to be *even stricter* about discipline, but it can be done. You don't have to put your life on hold for your career.
    - At the same time, some institutions are much more accommodating about family life than others (e.g., offering paternity leave, lactating rooms during medical school and residency). It's unfortunate that not all programs do this, but it's in your best interest to seek out institutions that facilitate optimal family planning.
  - Some schools will be more flexible and allow you to change things around in your educational timeline (e.g., delay Step, delay clerkships, take educational leave of absence to pursue other interests/degrees/research fellowships, etc.). These things are rarely advertised up-front. You should discuss with trusted advisors and upperclassmen about whether these are possibilities that your school offers if you feel that you would benefit.
- **Our recommendation:** Make a conscious effort to practice the self-care habits we recommend in Chapter 18, Self-Care and Wellness. Check in with yourself every month or so to systematically assess your well-being across each dimension in that chapter. Try to Zoom or call friends and family outside of medicine at least once every month (schedule it in your personal calendar).
  - We encourage you to regularly engage with at least one hobby that's genuinely enjoyable for you. If you were an artist or a musician before medical school, keep this up if you can. You might experience disappointment in not being able to perform at the same level, but you should continue to unwind with whatever made you happy before medical school—even if it's just a few minutes a day.
  - Really tune into your mental health and overall well-being at various points throughout the process. *Be honest with yourself.* Understanding what genuinely bothers you and what genuinely makes you happy is **crucial** for determining which specialty you want to work in day-in and day-out for the rest of your life. Most medical students will entertain *many* different specialties at various points throughout medical school, and many students will change their mind after career plans even late in

medical school.[14] Many people don't fully decide on their specialty until their fourth year of medical school, and are often considering widely disparate specialties before that.

- Take the time to figure out what's truly important to you. Many people in medicine are so used to the hypercompetitive rat race because it's what was encouraged as a pre-med. You don't *have* to continue down this track by matching at the most prestigious specialty/program you can get. Instead, you can now take the time to reassess what will genuinely make you happy. If you genuinely feel that becoming a psychiatrist would be more fulfilling to you than going into surgery—even though your parents would brag more about having a brain surgeon as a child—then *become a psychiatrist.* If you genuinely feel that going to a less prestigious residency program in a location that makes you happier would be the right move, then it's ultimately on you to make that decision. **Don't blindly chase prestige and work yourself to death because it's been expected of you for so long.**

## 42.2.8 The Social Scene Is Very Unique

- **Expectations:** The social scene in medical school will be like college all over again!
- **Reality:** Socially, while the vibe is more professional than undergraduate, there are definitely some high school vibes since the first years everyone attends the same classes with cliques inevitably forming. Likewise, classmates at many schools tend to have parties in the preclinical years after exams, as everyone's generally on the same schedule. It becomes much harder to socialize during clerkships because students are working at different schedules (e.g., you might be working 6 AM–6 PM 6 days a week on internal medicine, while your best friend is working 8–5 M-F on family medicine).
  - Many of your classmates will also be in serious relationships or will have families to take care of. They simply will not prioritize making or maintaining new friendships when the schedule becomes dramatically more demanding (e.g., clerkships).
- **What it feels like:** Topics that dominate conversations with your friends will be about medical school, gossip, upcoming tests, and pros and cons of various specialties. You might also feel isolated during clerkships—especially during the winter when fewer people are socializing outside.
- **Our recommendation:** Making an extra effort to be social in the first 2 years of medical school is your chance to create solid friendships that will help support you because everyone is more or less on the same schedule. Make an effort to continue your friendships outside of medical school because it will be easy to lose them. Sometimes when medical school gets tough and all of your medical friends are too busy to hang out or chat, your friendships outside of medicine will help support you.

## 42.2.9 You May Experience (Covert) Harassment, and It Is *not* Ok or "Just Part of the Process"

- **Expectations:** Medicine is a stressful environment, and you simply have to toughen up and deal with harsh criticism.
- **Reality:** That expectation may be true, but it should not apply to emotional abuse, sexual harassment, and other forms of discrimination and mistreatment are unfortunate realities in medical training.[15] They are absolutely unacceptable, and everyone has an active role to play in making sure it doesn't continue. In addition, much of learner mistreatment may not be overt macroaggressions but instead microaggressions that grant plausible deniability to the offender.[16]

---

[14] Jones Jr. MD, Yamashita T, Ross RG, Gong J. Positive predictive value of medical student specialty choices. BMC Med Educ 2018;18:33. Available at: https://www.ncbi.nlm.nih.gov/pmc/articles/PMC5845137/. Accessed July 8, 2022.

[15] Binder, Renee MD; Garcia, Paul MD; Johnson, Bonnie MSW; Fuentes-Afflick, Elena MD, MPH Sexual Harassment in Medical Schools: The Challenge of Covert Retaliation as a Barrier to Reporting, Academic Medicine: December 2018 - Volume 93 - Issue 12 - p 1770–1773 doi: 10.1097/ACM.0000000000002302, https://www.npr.org/sections/health-shots/2020/06/16/876279025/racism-hazing-and-other-abuse-taints-medical-training-students-say

[16] Commit to Confronting the Microaggressions That Are Affecting Your Learners. Available at: https://accelerate.uofuhealth.utah.edu/explore/commit-to-confronting-the-microaggressions-that-are-affecting-your-learners. Accessed July 8, 2022, Sandoval RS, Afolabi T, Said J, Dunleavy S, Chatterjee A, Ölveczky D. Building a Tool Kit for Medical and Dental Students: Addressing Microaggressions and Discrimination on the Wards. MedEdPORTAL 2020;16:10893. Available at: https://www.ncbi.nlm.nih.gov/pmc/articles/PMC7187912/. Accessed July 8, 2022, Lacy T. Microaggressions and Medical Education. Available at: https://medicine.uic.edu/microaggressions-and-medical-education/. Accessed July 8, 2022.

- **What it feels like:** Harrowing and isolating. Many times, abuse in medical training is not clear cut. You may simply think that you're not thick-skinned enough and that your supervisor was just giving you "tough love." On the other hand, you may experience or witness harassment but decide that the costs of reporting it are simply too high. For example, if you were the only medical student working with your surgery attending in June, you might worry that an "anonymous" complaint by the medical student in June would not be anonymous at all and that you might experience retaliation by that attending (e.g., he might tarnish your reputation with his colleagues down the line come residency application season). Indeed, many medical students fear reporting harassment out of concerns that their supervisors would ruin their careers—even in supposedly anonymous reporting environments.[17]
- **Our recommendation:** In general, we'll state the obvious that emotional abuse and harassment have no place in medical training. At the same time, we recognize that there are real concerns about reporting mistreatment. We encourage you to speak with upperclassmen and trusted advisors about the mechanisms in place at your medical school to anonymously report mistreatment and to make sure that bad actors are appropriately disciplined. If there are not appropriate avenues for reporting mistreatment, be active about getting these established at your school (and **communicate this clearly to applicants to your school,** e.g., "What would you change about your school/what do you dislike about your school?"; it is an **enormous** red flag if a medical school does not have working opportunities to rectify learner mistreatment).

## 42.3 Medical School: A Class-by-Class Breakdown

Let's now go through the medical school experience in chronological order. This is rapidly changing from school to school, so it's best to think of it as "basic sciences" in the first 2 years versus "clinical" in the second 2 years. At most schools, the workload is lightest in the first year (but still orders of magnitude greater compared to college). Get it into your head that much of your career will be shaped by your scores on various exams that test in-depth memorization and understanding of years' worth of material. It's ultimately a marathon, not a sprint. You should learn to appreciate the journey and not just the destination.

### 42.3.1 Year 1: Basic Sciences

As described earlier, many schools are experimenting with different curricula. The most basic model is the traditional "2 + 2 model" of 2 years of basic science, with year 1 being "normal" basic science, (i.e. normal anatomy, physiology, immunology, etc.) and year 2 being "abnormal" pathology in each organ system, (i.e., cardiology, renal, pulmonology, etc.) Another model is the integrated curriculum, in which you may go through each organ system sequentially but do normal and abnormal by each system (e.g., starting with normal cardiac anatomy and physiology, followed by various diseases). Some schools are also experimenting with truncated, accelerated curricula that reportedly remove the redundancies/overlapping material covered in 2 years of education. In addition, as with virtually all of medical school, **you will forget (and relearn) most of the material in every course. It's critical to deeply learn the material the first time so that you can easily relearn it down the line.** All this considered, these are the courses you will probably take at every medical school:

### Gross Anatomy

This is the quintessential medical school class. It's the first class at many schools—the rite of passage into the medical profession. There is a strong performative aspect to it, as you will don the protective equipment and wield the scalpel to gracefully explore the depths of the human form. You will pay deep respects to the donors who made the ultimate sacrifice for science. You will be overwhelmed by the sheer amount of material there is to know about the body. You will be shocked to discover that there can be as much variation *inside* bodies as there is on the outside (e.g., aberrant blood vessels, abnormal placement

---

[17] Chung MP, Thang CK, Vermillion M, Fried JM, Uijtdehaage S. Exploring medical students' barriers to reporting mistreatment during clerkships: a qualitative study. Med Educ Online. 2018; 23(1): 1478170. Available at: https://www.ncbi.nlm.nih.gov/pmc/articles/PMC5990956/. Accessed July 8, 2022.

of organs). You may actually form deep friendships with your classmates in your dissection group. Unfortunately, you may also discover that much of the *time* you spend in anatomy lab is low-yield dissection of fascia and fat. This may be more appealing if you're surgically inclined. Many students, however, may ultimately find themselves avoiding anatomy lab whenever possible to study out of textbooks (e.g., Netter's and Rohen's) and online cadavers that have been previously dissected. Indeed, many schools are attempting to revitalize the first-year anatomy curriculum because of conflicting perspectives on the utility of traditional dissection.[18] In addition, in our experience, much of gross anatomy was fairly low-yield for board examination purposes.

## Biochemistry + Genetics

These are considered one of the hardest subjects in medical school, especially if you did not learn biochemistry well the first time in undergrad. Board exams love to test you on it because it's an easy way to stratify the best test-takers. The pace is grueling, as well. Covering a *year's* worth of undergraduate biochemistry in 3 weeks is not uncommon. The emphasis is also different. While you will no longer cover the highly theoretical, basic elements (e.g., Gibbs free-energy equations, protein-folding mechanisms), you will need to understand the diseases associated with defects in various biochemical pathways, as well as drugs that interact with biochemical pathways. This is particularly relevant for medical genetics and developmental pediatrics.

## Medical Microbiology

This is one of the most content-heavy courses in medical school, as you will need to learn over 100 different bacteria, viruses, fungi, and parasites, as well as basically every imaginable fact about them. Many students use "SketchyMicro" to make this easier. It's *extremely* high-yield for board examinations, and if you don't learn antibiotics well the first-time, you will likely struggle eternally in clinical practice (and probably actively contribute to antibiotic resistance among superbugs).

## Immunology

This is one of the more conceptually difficult courses. It's now also very memorization-heavy because many diseases are now being treated with monoclonal antibodies that have extremely long and difficult-to-pronounce names. There are also many molecules called interleukins that you have to know cold that are just numbers, as well as immunology-related genes associated with various diseases that are also clusters of letters and numbers.

## Pharmacology

Also very memorization heavy but also conceptually heavy because of equations related to pharmacokinetics and pharmacodynamics (i.e., determining loading and maintenance doses, understanding the clearance of drugs). Enzyme kinetics makes a return here with the infamous Michaelis-Menten equation.

You will also need to memorize a ton of drugs and their side effects, although this is much easier if you deeply understand the mechanism of action of the drug because the side effects can often be conceptually linked to the mechanism. For example, a drug that blocks pancreatic lipase in the small intestine will lead to gross, fatty stool because the fat simply leaves the gastrointestinal (GI) tract instead of being absorbed by the body at the intestine.

## Pathology and Histology

Pathology is extremely important because it's the scientific basis of disease at the microscopic level (e.g., cell death, inflammation). Students almost universally use *Pathoma* as a supplement. Histology relates to pathology, as it's microscopic anatomy (i.e., looking at slides of various tissues in health and disease). Histology can

---

[18] Memon I. Cadaver Dissection Is Obsolete in Medical Training! A Misinterpreted Notion. Med Princ Pract. 2018;27(3): 201–210. Available at: https://www.ncbi.nlm.nih.gov/pmc/articles/PMC6062726/. Accessed July 8, 2022.

be interesting, but very few specialites will have to look at slides in day-to-day clinical practice (except pathology and dermatology—some surgeons may choose to look at the slides with pathologists, and some radiologists may participate in radiology-pathology concordance sessions.). Instead, most specialties that interface with pathologists simply read and interpret the pathology reports. Our experience has been that histology is very low-yield beyond Step 1—there's virtually no histology on Steps 2 and 3.

## Patient Care Courses

You will take dedicated courses that teach medical interviewing and physical exam skills in great depth. There is probably a good amount of heterogeneity in how they are taught across schools, but they are ultimately designed to allow students to pass standardized clinical encounters called **OSCE's**—objective structured clinical examinations—as well as USMLE Step 2 CS (Clinical Skills—currently on hold during COVID indefinitely). These are overall helpful on a theoretical level, but they can hold you to an artificial professional standard that's rarely seen in actual clinical practice (e.g., you're expected to ask every patient about their sexual history, but this is rarely done—for better or for worse—in routine clinical practice). They were excellent practice for having a standardized system for history-taking and physical examination for clinical practice with room for further refinement. They also promoted a framework of active listening and being openly empathetic with patients, which may not have been so heavily emphasized in medical training in the past.[19]

## 42.3.2 Year 2: Organ Blocks

In the traditional 2 + 2 model, you will spend second year going through the various organ systems, learning normal anatomy and physiology (in the language of your basic sciences, i.e., anatomy, biochemistry, genetics, histology, pathology, immunology) followed by disease. Typically, this includes the cardiovascular system, respiratory system, renal system, gastrointestinal system, reproductive system, musculoskeletal system, integumentary system, neuroscience, hematology and oncology, endocrine system, and psychiatry.

These tend to be more interesting and rewarding to study (i.e., you start to feel like a real doctor and can intelligently discuss medicine with friends, family, and other healthcare professionals), but they tend to have much more information. They will also be much harder if you don't have a strong conceptual understanding of the first-year material.

That said, you will get surprisingly little education in "diet and exercise." This is largely because there isn't any compelling, easy evidence for "what is the best diet?" and "what is the best exercise" compared to more specific clinical questions like "Which medications improve mortality in heart failure with reduced ejection fraction?"

## 42.3.3 Year 3: Core Clerkships

At most schools, you will rotate in—at minimum—adult inpatient medicine, surgery, inpatient pediatrics, psychiatry, obstetrics and gynecology, family medicine, and potentially outpatient internal medicine and pediatrics.

You will face a tension between learning and being actually useful; in general, your role on the team is to learn and to become the best future physician you can be. While you should aim to help the team whenever you can, don't stress too much if you don't feel like you can do much. Your superiors will generally appreciate that you're willing to help, even if there isn't much you can actually do.

You will also face the challenge of translating what you learned in preclinical years in an abstract sense into real-world clinical practice. You will see that there's sometimes discordance between the two and that much of the day-to-day decisions in clinical medicine don't appear to have any apparent logic behind them. This is because seasoned professionals often make intuitive, "snap" judgments[20] based on years of experience and conscious, deliberate thinking. Frustratingly, they may not verbalize their reasoning to you.

---

[19] How Medical and Nursing Schools are Teaching Bedside Manner Today. Available at: https://dailynurse.com/medical-nursing-schools-teaching-bedside-manner-today/. Accessed July 8, 2022.

[20] Kahneman D. Thinking Fast and Slow. Available at: https://www.punkt.ch/en/inspiration/library/thinking-fast-and-slow. Accessed July 8, 2022.

In addition, much of your learning will be on the first-order principles (mastering history taking and physical exam, formulating a differential, choosing the appropriate treatment, determining the diagnosis) whereas your superiors may have immediately figured out all of those things and are more focused on higher-principle issues (*why* does the patient have this particular diagnosis of a heart failure exacerbation, how do we coordinate care to minimize risk of rehospitalization, what community resources are available, how do we integrate multiple disciplines like physical therapy, occupational therapy, social work, case management). That is, your superiors' learning objectives will be very different from yours, and you may feel that your educational objectives may be irrelevant.

You will want to be competent on day 1, but this is simply impossible. Much of doing well in medicine relies on experiential knowledge and the associations that come with seeing many different patients and exposure to different clinical encounters (e.g., how to cordially interact with other professions such as nurses, physical therapists, case management, social workers). Be open to new experiences and hone your sense of pattern recognition. Medical practice is ultimately a fine balance between fast, intuitive "system 1" thinking that you appropriately modulate with slow, methodical "system 2" thinking when you feel that there's externalities or anomalies that modulate the situation. For example, as an attending physician, you will operate on autopilot to some degree by coming up with fast, intuitive differential diagnoses for chief complaints (e.g., "What are six common causes that could explain this patient's crushing chest pain?"), but you will also need to tap into your extensive knowledge and experience repository to *modulate* your automatic thinking with specifics of the particular patient encounter. ("This patient has also recently traveled abroad - how should I adjust my differential appropriately?")

There is also a hierarchy on the medical team,[21] and the degree to which this is enforced depends on the culture of the field, as well as the superiors you work with. In our experience, surgical subspecialties tended to have the more clear-cut sense of hierarchy (e.g., attending physicians only hearing about new consults from the senior resident and minimally interacting with medical students), whereas psychiatry and family medicine tended to have the most approachable attending physicians. Of course, this is completely anecdotal and varies tremendously across different settings. The point we want to communicate is to not be surprised if you find a strict sense of hierarchy. Just roll with it as long as it's not pathologic.

The biggest transitions from the preclinical years are that (1) your time is no longer your own, (2) your highs will be higher and your lows lower, and (3) your grades suddenly matter (if you went to a pass/fail school).

- **Your time is no longer your own:** You show up when you need to show up, and you leave when your resident or attending tells you to leave.
- **The highs will be high** (delivering a baby, scrubbing into a high-risk surgery and watching the surgeon tell the family everything went ok) **but the lows will be much lower** (sleep deprivation on overnight shifts, having patients receive devastating news).
- **Grades suddenly matter:** Remember that super collaborative environment in the first 2 years of medical school? That may suddenly go out the window if you work directly with another medical student. Many of us were shocked to discover that some of the most laid-back classmates from the first 2 years were the most vicious, hypercompetitive classmates imaginable on the wards. You will be judged—consciously or subconsciously—against your peers, and there is strong incentive to perform your absolute best, especially if you're trying to get into a competitive specialty. In addition, with Step 1 becoming pass/fail, clerkship grades may become even more important down the line.
  - **Shelf exams:** At the end of each clerkship, you take a standardized test called a "shelf exam" that is part of your grade for the clerkship. The percentage of your clerkship grade determined by your shelf exam score varies from school to school. These greatly add to the stress of clerkships because not only are you adjusting to the workplace demands of clinical medicine as a greenhorn, but you are also expected to intensely study for a difficult exam when you get home. In addition, much of the material covered on shelf exams is not relevant to day-to-day clinical practice and vice versa. We discuss strategies for acing shelf exams in Chapter 43, Real Talk on Succeeding in Medical School.

The following were our experiences with core clerkships at our medical school.

---

[21] Vanstone M, Grierson L. Medical student strategies for actively negotiating hierarchy in the clinical environment. Med Edu 2019;53(10):1013–1024. Available at: https://onlinelibrary.wiley.com/doi/abs/10.1111/medu.13945. Accessed July 8, 2022.

## Adult Inpatient Medicine

Rounding often starts at 9 AM. This is when the attending physician, senior resident, interns, and medical student(s) walk together to see all the patients to discuss the plans for the day. During this time, the intern or medical student "presents" the patient (i.e., what happened the day before and what our plan is for the day) to the senior resident or attending. The senior resident or attending may also do teaching during this time (e.g., demonstrating a physical exam finding, going over the pathophysiology of a disease, discussing new literature in patient management). Rounding is frequently when "pimping" occurs. There is a strict hierarchy to pimping: the resident/attending asks the most junior member of the hierarchy the question first (i.e., the medical student) and then goes *up* to the resident. *Never* answer a pimp question directed at the resident if the resident does not know the answer—this makes the resident look bad in front of the attending (obviously read the room—if the attending directly asks you, just answer, but this doesn't usually happen).

- The medical student shows up between 7ish AM to "pre-round," (i.e., check the chart for vitals, labs, events, imaging, etc.), from the previous day to incorporate into the presentation and plan for today. The medical student will also physically visit each patient to do a focused history and physical exam. The medical student may have one to four patients. The medical student is encouraged to discuss his/her plan with the intern for feedback before presenting to the resident or attending.
- Rounding typically takes 1 to 3 hours. There may be a new patient admitted during rounds, and the medical student may end up seeing this new patient after rounds.
- Rounding may be extremely boring because you're simply walking around and listening to other people present once you've presented on your patients. Of course, you may be pimped at any time, so you should not doze off. Ideally, you should be listening to and learning from others' presentations.
- After rounds, the interns will work on notes, place orders, and call consults to execute the plans decided on during rounds. You can help the interns by calling consults or obtaining additional information if suggested during rounds (e.g., calling patients' family members for collateral information).
- At lunch, you will likely attend some educational conference. **Yes, you don't even have free time to enjoy your lunch in silence**. These are really hit-or miss in terms of quality and relevance to your education.
- After lunch, you will write your notes, get more formal teaching in the form of chalk talks, interview and examine new patients, and accomplish tasks for the patients you are already taking care of (and maybe surreptitiously study for your shelf exam). If you have understanding residents, they will let you go home early if there's nothing to do. Otherwise, ask if there's "anything you can help with" (unless the attending will be coming back in the afternoon to do formal teaching—you should definitely stay for this).
  - Likewise, stay if there's an admit in the afternoon.
- Depending on how nice your seniors are, you may leave anytime from immediately after rounds (~12 PM) to sign-out in the evening (6 PM). You will be in the hospital 6 days a week.
- The shelf exam for inpatient medicine is considered the hardest one in medical school because it covers the broadest range of topics. Study hard for this. It's very similar to Step 2 CK.
- Overall, most students feel like they learn the most in this rotation.
- Pre-COVID, you would wear dress clothes with your white coat. Post-COVID, scrubs are sometimes allowed.

## Surgery

This typically has the worst hours of any clerkship, and it has a reputation for being a brutal clerkship with difficult personalities.

- Rounding can start as early as 5 AM in some places, and it's typical to have to wake up at 4 AM to get to your clinical site. Depending on your service, you would get home at 4 to 7 PM. Repeat this 6 days a week. This means that at the absolute worst, **you would be at the hospital from 5 AM to 6–7 PM for 6 days a week (if not more if you were really trying to impress your attendings and seniors)**. On top of that, you're studying for a shelf exam that covers an enormous amount of material.
- Rounding was much faster in surgery, but you typically don't do as much. You will pre-round on your patients extremely quickly by asking them if they had any bowel movements or were passing flatus and asking them how their pain was. Rounding happens at a lightning-pace (literally speedwalking most of

the time). Afterward, you will scrub into various surgeries, which would range from 2 to 10 hours of the day. You will randomly get "pimped" throughout the surgery on concepts both general to the field of surgery and specific to the surgery taking place. Depending on your team and the complexity of the surgery taking place, as well as how many other trainees are there, you may get to "assist" in the most minimal of ways.

- Throughout the day, there would be random moments of downtime, as well as seeing new consults. You may feel that many of the floor management decisions are not completely evidence-based as compared to medical services (e.g., giving docusate as a stool softener to prevent constipation[22]), but try not to focus on it.
- You generally will wear scrubs unless it's a clinic day for your surgery team.

• A lot of students have trouble standing for extended periods of time and being minimally involved, and don't necessarily feel actively engaged just shadowing in the OR all day. Not being able to use the bathroom or eat on your own schedule, and virtually having no life outside of the hospital, can also be aggravating.

- As an intern, however, it's more common to be more involved with various surgeries. This is generally more rewarding. The issue is that there's very little that a medical student can safely do on a surgical rotation, and it's not uncommon to spent much of your time day-dreaming and wishing that you had more time to study for the actual shelf exam. For people that are intensely interested in surgery, it's not uncommon for this same experience to be interesting and formative, even if they aren't doing a lot in the OR.

## Psychiatry

This often has the best hours of any core clerkship. You may be shocked and unaccustomed to the pleasantness of psychiatry. Attendings were extremely approachable. Patients were very fascinating, and there seemed to be a much heavier role for interdisciplinary care (e.g., psychologists, social work, pharmacists) than you may see in other clerkships.

• Hours tend to be business hours or slightly less (leaving mid-afternoon).

• You will complete patient histories (with supervision from the resident) and do follow-up histories on patients admitted in the hospital. You will present new patients to the attending, give your assessment, and offer a plan for further work-up and/or treatment.

• Psychiatry placed a great emphasis on a careful, broad psychiatric history - with collateral information because patients often did not give the most "accurate" histories (e.g., acutely psychotic patient having active hallucinations). This rotation gives many opportunities to obtain careful, nuanced patient history and to integrate conflicting accounts from multiple sources.

• The shelf exam is extremely easy and probably covers the least amount of material of any shelf. That said, it has historically had a very harsh grading curve, requiring students to get a near-perfect score to achieve an honors-level grade.

• Dress code is generally professional attire.

## Pediatrics

This was similar to medicine in that you show up early to round, and the structure of the rest of the day was very similar. Rounding tended to be a bit earlier than medicine (8 AM rounding vs. 9 AM in adult medicine), and there was a strong emphasis on **family-centered rounding.** This meant explaining the patient's clinical course, differential diagnosis, and plan for the day in *lay person* speech (vs. medical jargon, as was done in medicine) directed at the patient's family. The shelf exam felt slightly easier than medicine but had more emphasis on weird developmental disorders and syndromes. The residents and attendings were generally very outwardly nice and bubbly. Lots of people also wore bow-ties (toddlers grab at things), and we didn't have to wear our white coats.

---

[22] Fakheri RJ, Volpicelli FM. Things We Do for No Reason: Prescribing Docusate for Constipation in Hospitalized Adults. Journal of Hospital Medicine 2019;14(2):110-113. Available at: https://www.journalofhospitalmedicine.com/jhospmed/article/193136/hospital-medicine/things-we-do-no-reason-prescribing-docusate-constipation. Accessed July 8, 2022.

## Family Medicine (and Outpatient Medicine, Pediatrics)

These were typically 8 to 5, Monday to Friday outpatient clinic rotations in which you see patients by yourself, perform a history and physical, and then present to the attending physician what you think is wrong with the patient and what the appropriate next steps would be (e.g., transferring them to the ED, referring to a specialist, ordering more tests and imaging, prescribing a medication, or simply providing reassurance). Overall, these were relaxed rotations, but they highlighted how primary care physicians can experience burnout due to being pressured for time and having to see so many patients (often with multiple complex issues and complaints) in short 15-minute segments. The shelf exams were broad and covered similar topics as the medicine shelf.

- Dress clothes and white coat are standard.

## Obstetrics and Gynecology

This rotation van be divided into labor and delivery, gynecologic surgery, and obstetrics and gynecology clinic. This rotation has a reputation for being extremely malignant at many medical schools.[23]

- **Gynecologic surgery**—This can feel like surgery all over again: long hours, unpredictable schedule, and spending long periods of time not doing anything that feels useful. Hours will generally be surgical—6 days per week with extended days.
- **Obstetrics and gynecology clinic**—Like other outpatient rotations, this was 8 to 5 PM, 5 days a week. The workflow is the same as other outpatient clinics, and the content is often routine prenatal care of pregnant women at various points during their pregnancy. Wear dress clothes and a white coat.
- **Labor and delivery**—You will see patients in the labor and delivery triage area (basically an emergency room for pregnant women concerned that their water may have broken or about vaginal bleeding during pregnancy) or assist with emergency C-sections. Wearing scrubs is common.
- The shelf exam is fairly straightforward, but has a large scope of outpatient clinic questions as well as emergent conditions. Not to mention, you will forget a ton of this material if you're not going into OB/Gyn.

### 42.3.4 Year 4

Most of fourth year of medical school is spent on the residency application process, which is covered in Chapter 44, A Peek at the Residency Application Process.

- If you're pursuing a hypercompetitive specialty, you will do multiple **acting internships**. This is like a clerkship on steroids: you're trying to assume the role of a first-year resident in that specialty to be evaluated by faculty in that specialty. This is extremely stressful. You will typically do three acting internships: one at your medical school, as well as two at different institutions (i.e., **away rotations**) to get letters of recommendation from esteemed faculty in that field at other institutions. Most likely, you will match in one of these three institutions when you apply for residency in that field. These are extremely stressful because they're essentially like month-long interviews; if you screw up badly enough at *any point* in that month, you will tank your entire shot at matching at that institution. If you are trying to match into a less competitive specialty, just one acting internship is fine.
- Every medical student will do an acting internship in a "core" speciality (pediatrics, family medicine, surgery, or internal medicine). This is like the 3rd year clerkship but harder. You will have greater responsibility and be held to a greater standard in terms of history and physical, assessment, plan, etc. You will carry more patients, and you may even take call. Many medical students choose to do this at the end of 4th year, but we recommend doing it early (before residency applications are sent) if you're applying to a specialty that requires a separate intern year. This is because you can apply to **transitional years**, which are "cush," low-stress intern years with lots of elective rotations. These programs, however, tend to be extremely competitive, and having an "honors" in your acting internship before you apply will help you match to a transitional year.
- If you haven't already, you will need to take Step 2.

---

[23] Why does OBGYN have a malignant reputation? Available at: https://www.reddit.com/r/medicalschool/comments/80m9me/why_does_obgyn_have_a_malignant_reputation/. Accessed July 8, 2022.

- Otherwise, you will spend your 4th year taking various electives. These are *much* more relaxed compared to 3rd year rotations, as there isn't as much cut-throat competition to get honors. There is also no shelf exam. As such, you can genuinely just focus on becoming clinically competent and getting alone with the team without the pageantry that often plagues core clerkships.

### 42.3.5 Miscellaneous Years

Students at medical schools are increasingly taking additional time to graduate, e.g., paid research years, additional degrees, etc. Students that don't match in a specialty
  will also choose to delay graduating so that they can re-apply as a "medical school" senior. This is because you're at a disadvantage applying to residency programs as a medical school graduate compared to a medical school senior.

## 42.4 Summary

Medical school is difficult in ways that are hard to explain to someone that hasn't experienced it, but it's helpful to understand what you are getting yourself into. Here are some of the key takeaways:

- The pace and volume of information will come at you hard, so you will have to study a lot. You will also need to retain almost all of this material *cold* for years at a time; you can't simply cram and regurgitate as you may have done in undergrad.
- Self-care will be much harder, but you will find your own way of managing.
- Doing well requires you to memorize a ton of stuff, regardless of your ability to look things up on the job. However, if you try to memorize things that you don't understand at baseline, you will not break into the upper echelon of test performance because the hardest questions apply second- and third-order thinking.
- Spaced repetition and active learning are key here. Obtain a deep conceptual understanding of the material first, and then use spaced repetition to retain the understanding for years at a time. Do practice problems to integrate your knowledge across disciplines and to approach it from different angles.
- Realistically, expect to spend 5 to 10 hours *each day,* 5 to 7 days a week studying in the first 2 years.
- As far as what to use studying: you will have options between school material (lectures, syllabi), third-party materials (for courses as well for board review), and primary sources (research articles, expert opinion). A lot of how you study will be finding what works for you. The most common option is some degree of school material and third-party resources, depending on the quality of the school material, especially in the first 2 years. You should feel open to exploring what proportion works best for you.
- Research is essential for the most competitive specialties, but still helpful for everyone else to be competitive.
- Extracurriculars are less important in medical school (not as much need to "check a box"), so you should focus on ones that you are passionate about (when you have time).
- The environment should be collaborative. Lead by example and be a helpful classmate. Your medical school class is a small community, so your individual efforts to foster the group dynamic will go a long way.
- Grading is pretty straightforward in the preclinical years, and largely based on test performance. The situation becomes more stressful during clinical rotations as the grading becomes more subjective. While clinical evaluations will always have a subjective component, you can maximize your odds of doing well with our recommendations. We recommend following the **3 A's**. Be available, affable, and able (in that order). Incorporate feedback aggressively and rapidly.
- Many of the rotations during your clinical years have their own unique structures and expectations, which often changes how you are evaluated. While certain things will be different, you will continue to be evaluated on your test performance (keep studying), your bedside manor and ability to work within a team, and your ability to perform history and physicals, and then present those findings (and most importantly your assessment of the patient and clinical plan of management) to your superiors. If you want to differentiate yourself, focus as much as you can on the latter.
- Before rotations or new experiences, check in with an upper classman to get the details on what to expect, how to prepare, and how to excel at your specific institution.

# 43 Real Talk on Succeeding in Medical School

*Joel Thomas*

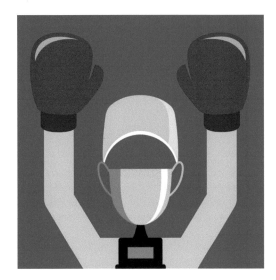

In Chapter 42, Real Talk on the Medical School Experience we explored the overall medical school experience and shared general strategies for success. In this chapter, we will discuss specific strategies for thriving in medical school.

This is rapidly changing territory, and it frankly could be a book on its own. For example, the Anki deck fervently recommended to first- and second-year medical students several years ago for acing Step 1 became outdated rapidly. Several years after that, Step 1 was made pass/fail. As such, we recommend keeping up-to-date with the newest recommendations online (with particular attention to reddit.com/r/medicalschool and Student Doctor Network (SDN)), as well as recommendations from successful upperclassmen at your school.

In addition, "success" in medical school is ultimately what *you* make of it. To some, it may mean matching into plastic surgery at a highly renowned academic institution. To others, it may mean matching at a close-knit rural family medicine program at a program to which you have no ties. Therefore, we encourage you to get connected with upperclassmen and alumni who have achieved *your* specific goals. You should do this early in medical training: as early as the moment you choose to matriculate at your particular school.

*That said, you should take our recommendations for specific resources (e.g., Board Review Series (BRS) Gross Anatomy) with a grain of salt.* They are simply what worked for us when we went to medical school from ~2015 to 2020. In general, you should stay flexible and open-minded to whatever newer, more up-to-date resources are recommended by successful upperclassmen at your school.

With that disclaimer, we will now focus on the most broadly applicable strategies for success in medical school.

## 43.1 You Still Need a Schedule—Now More than Ever

Re-read the "Personal Schedule" section of Chapter 9, Timing, Class Structure, and Personal Schedules. Ideally, you'll have gotten into the habit of developing and sticking to a personal schedule before medical school. As discussed in Chapter 42, Real Talk on the Medical School Experience, self-organization is vital in medical school because the demands on your time increase dramatically. In addition, if you procrastinate for too long (e.g., miss 2 days' of lectures), then the "stack of pancakes" will become overwhelmingly large. Don't rely on motivation—just *do* the work, even if you don't feel like you're going to get much out of studying. Again, the material is not conceptually difficult; you just need to avoid procrastination, get started with that *first* flash card or practice problem of the day, and put the time in. One silver lining, at least, is that you don't have to spread your time across so many extracurriculars anymore.

- As discussed in Chapter 42, Real Talk on the Medical School Experience, you should expect to spend 5 to 10 hours studying each day for 5 to 7 days per week in your preclinical years (typically more in your second year compared to first year).
  - Don't focus so much on the number of hours. Instead, give yourself daily and weekly goals based on active learning objectives. We will discuss more about these specific active learning resources shortly.
- Again, avoid multitasking and prioritize deep work (and deep leisure—don't try to mix work and play. Instead, you should be fully committed to work when you're working and fully committed to leisure when you're unwinding).
- Break down large, intimidating tasks into small, concrete steps and give yourself a scheduled block of time for each small step (e.g., "Do all 200 question bank problems by the end of the week" becomes "Do 40 practice questions each day").
- Enter the non-negotiable "fixed time" items into your schedule first because you will have to work around them for the more flexible items (7–9 h of sleep, mandatory school stuff like Team Based Learning (TBL)/Problem Based Learning (PBL) and clinical encounters, self-care such as fixed leisure time at the end of the day).
  - Don't get out of shape. Aside from the damage to your health, it may also impact your residency application chances.[1]
  - *The bulk of your time during third year will be spent at rotation sites.* You will physically have to be there, and you can't always predict when you will be allowed to leave. You should be conservative in blocking off these times in your calendar. For example, schedule off "4:30 AM to 6:30 PM" for a day in surgery as the most realistic, worst-case scenario for that day, *including travel time to and from your clinical site.*
- Enter the non-negotiable "flexible" items (e.g., work-out times, meditation, research time, personal relationships, etc.).
  - If you're even remotely considering a competitive speciality (dermatology, orthopaedic surgery, plastic surgery, ophthalmology, urology, integrated interventional radiology, otolaryngology), then you should start doing research in that field early in medical school. Devote enough time each week to make demonstrable progress on the project each week. What this means will depend on the project, your aptitude for research, and the expectations and support of your mentor and research group.
    - The summer after the first year of medical school is typically your best opportunity (aside from a dedicated research year) to be maximally productive in research (i.e., churning out multiple abstracts, presentations, and publications). During this time, medical students frequently spend at least 40 hours per week on research. Some would also study for USMLE Step 1, but it's unclear whether this will be done now that it's pass/fail.
  - We strongly recommend continuing at least one **interesting hobby** throughout medical school. Ideally, it will be something that both allows you to destress and impress the ADCOM again come residency application season. Bonus points (but absolutely not expected) if you're able to obtain a demonstrable achievement with that hobby (e.g., winning "Battle of the Bands" or a baking competition).
- Your schedule will change throughout medical school, especially in the first few months as you are adjusting to your new life. It will also change *dramatically* throughout third and fourth year, as your schedule will be completely different each month per your rotation expectations.
- The Pomodoro technique is tremendously helpful for getting through hours of studying every day. We also recommend getting up and walking around (or even changing your study spot) every few hours or so to avoid getting fatigued.

## 43.2 You Still Need to Maintain Wellness—Now More than Ever

As thoroughly emphasized throughout this book, maintaining wellness is something that you need to be proactive and creative about. The demands of medical school—particularly the clinical years—makes it

---

[1] Maxfield CM, Thorpe MP, Desser TS. Bias in Radiology Resident Selection: Do We Discriminate Against the Obese and Unattractive? Acad Med 2019;94(11):1774-1780. Available at: https://pubmed.ncbi.nlm.nih.gov/31149924/. Accessed July 8, 2022.

much harder, but it's still something you need to make the time for. Unfortunately, this means that you have less mindless time for procrastination and goofing around. You will probably need to stick to a watertight schedule that includes studying, clinical duties, and self-care. Again, we refer to the general recommendations in Chapter 18, Self-Care and Wellness. We also offer the specific additional considerations to medical school:

- Try to form a quality friend group of medical students for social support. Medical school is a very odd environment, and people outside of it will not fully understand your struggles. It's good to have peers you can vent to. At the same time, recognize that the social dynamic in medical school is generally different from college and that it may be harder to make friends. Many people treat it more like a professional working environment than a college social atmosphere. People may be more focused on their personal spheres (e.g., children, spouses) and may not do as much spontaneous hanging out as was done in college.
- That said, it's also very helpful to have close friends outside of medical school. It can be easy to get fully caught up in the medical school bubble, and having friends in other contexts can help ground you and put your struggles and concerns into perspective.
- Do one thing—ideally every day—that you genuinely enjoy.

## 43.3 Exhaust All Active Learning Resources before Even Trying Passive Learning (If at All)

- As described in Chapter 42, Real Talk on the Medical School Experience, the material in medical school is not particularly conceptually difficult. There's just a ton of it. Your classmates are all going to be of roughly similar intelligence, and they'll all have access to the same educational materials (i.e., school syllabi and third-party resources). In addition, much of your performance is graded relative to others (e.g., board exam scores, class percentile if that's communicated on the Dean's Letter). As such, we maintain that academic success in medicine school = "high quality/active work" × "time". That is, a significant predictor of your success in medical school will be how much pure, brute force you're willing to put in *as long as that time is all or almost entirely active learning.*
  - In addition, our experience has been that the NBME exams (e.g., USMLE, shelf exams) reward memorization much more so than the MCAT. The MCAT felt much more like a heavy critical reasoning test, challenging students to abstract from first principles in the basic sciences. In contrast, the USMLE and shelf exams tended to emphasize recalling and applying (using fairly straightforward logic) obscure, specific facts from the student's enormous mental inventory of medical knowledge. Indeed, the literature demonstrates that while MCAT scores predict USMLE scores, the overall effect size is weak[2]—suggesting that the exams may emphasize different cognitive abilities.
- The strategies we are describing were applicable in 2020, but the landscape of medical education is rapidly changing. Before trying any of these principles, discuss and compare them to strategies used by successful upperclassmen (if preclinical) and recent alumni (if you're an upperclassman) from your school. In addition, if they recommend your medical school's academic advising, then you should also consider those suggestions.

### 43.3.1 Preclinical Years

You should aim to spend 5 to 10 hours each day on deep, active learning. This does not need to be done all at once; you can spread it throughout the day, especially if you choose not to attend lectures in person.

- **In-house material:** If your school is true pass/fail (i.e., no internal ranking of grades during preclinical years that affects things like AOA selection, Dean's letter comments), then you will have to decide how much effort to devote to in-house material. Some students will choose to completely ignore in-house material and focus solely on board prep. Because the board prep material is the "highest-yield" material (i.e., things that are most likely to be tested on standardized exams because

---

[2] Gauer JL, Wolff JM, Jackson JB. Do MCAT scores predict USMLE scores? An analysis on 5 years of medical student data. Med Educ Online 2016;21:31795. Available at: https://pubmed.ncbi.nlm.nih.gov/27702431/. Accessed July 8, 2022.

they are—in theory—the most relevant to clinical practice), students who only use board prep material tend to pass the in-house exams. On the other hand, board prep material does *not* cover all the material that could be tested on boards. In fact, it's common to have multiple questions on Step 1 and Step 2 CK on material covered in your school's syllabi but not on board prep material. That does not necessarily mean a strategy of dividing time between in-house and board-prep material is the best strategy, but it is a popular one. In addition, now that Step 1 is pass/fail, your priorities will likely shift. As such, we ultimately conclude that you'll hear different recommendations for dividing your attention between in-house and board-prep material, depending on your priorities (e.g., acing a pass/fail Step 1, integrating information across multiple sources, etc.). It's unclear which recommendation—if any—is "best." Experiment with different approaches early in med school and reassess and reimplement based on your results with respect to your specific goals.

- **Lectures:** If your school allows you to watch lectures remotely, then you should not feel pressured to physically go to lecture. In fact, we only recommend physically going to lecture if it uniquely aids you in sticking to a routine and improves your overall well-being (e.g., social aspect of seeing classmates in person). A common strategy is watching lectures from home at increased speed. However, don't feel pressured to watch at the highest speed possible. The most up-to-date research on comprehension suggests that there's *necessarily* a trade-off between speed of receiving information and comprehension; "speed reading" without compromising comprehension is impossible.[3] Watch the lecture at the fastest speed *for you* at which you can still deeply understand the material at a conceptual level.
  - There may be utility to paying attention to the lecturer's inflection, body language, and points of emphasis during a lecture to determine *which* material is highest-yield (i.e., most important to understand, retain, and most likely to be tested). Much of the medical school preclinical material was extremely information-dense, and it was hard to get a sense of the big picture on my first pass of the material. High-quality lecturers were great at providing the big picture overview and emphasizing *which* granular details were the most important to know and why.
- If your school models in-house questions after NBME questions (or uses NBME exams), then board-prep material will be much more applicable to your in-house exams. Therefore, you can consider spending less time solely on in-house material.

• Use the same active learning and studying techniques we described in Chapter 10, Obtaining a Solid GPA.
  - The specifics of implementing this will vary depending on which active learning tools you use for your preclinical education. Broadly speaking, the most popular ones make use of spaced repetition (e.g., Anki[4]), Method of Loci (SketchyMedical), high-yield lectures (Pathoma, Boards and Beyond), and integrative practice problems (question banks such as Kaplan, USMLE-Rx). In general, they all cover the same material, and there does not appear to be any good evidence that one method is overwhelmingly better than the others. **Our recommendation is to use a mix of these resources and to be persistent with them. Avoid resource overload—there is likely diminishing utility to adding more resources.**
  - For example, I used Anki, Pathoma, USMLE-Rx with a sprinkling of Boards and Beyond for difficult conceptual material consistently for 2 years—in addition to my school's in-house material.
  - **"USMLE World,[5] First Aid, Pathoma[6]"** was referred to as "UFAP"—the highest-yield materials for acing USMLE Step 1. Additional material from other resources (e.g., SketchyMedical, Boards and Beyond, BRS Physiology) has made its way into the holy grail of highest yield material.
    - Various premade Anki decks consolidate the information across these various sources. We will not name any here because the "best" ones change year-to-year. We recommend speaking to upperclassmen and academic advising at your medical school. The discussion at reddit.com/r/medicalschoolanki and reddit.com/r/medicalschool can also be illuminating.

---

[3] Rayner K, Schotter ER, Masson MEJ, Potter MC, Treiman R. So Much to Read, So Little Time: How Do We Read, and Can Speed Reading Help? Psychological Science in the Public Interest 2016;17(1):4-34. Available at: https://journals.sage-pub.com/doi/10.1177/1529100615623267. Accessed July 8, 2022.

[4] Anki. Available at: https://apps.ankiweb.net/. Accessed July 8, 2022.

[5] Quality Is Our Obsession—Start Your USMLE® Step 1 Prep With UWorld. Available at: https://medical.uworld.com/usmle/usmle-step-1/. Accessed July 8, 2022.

[6] Pathoma. Available at: https://www.pathoma.com/. Accessed July 8, 2022.

13. A 63-year-old man is brought to the emergency department because of a 4-day history of increasingly severe left leg pain and swelling of his left calf. He also has a 1-month history of increasingly severe upper midthoracic back pain. During this time, he has had a 9-kg (20-lb) weight loss despite no change in appetite. He has no history of major medical illness. His only medication is ibuprofen. He is 180 cm (5 ft 11 in) tall and weighs 82 kg (180 lb); BMI is 25 kg/m². His vital signs are within normal limits. On examination, lower extremity pulses are palpable bilaterally. The remainder of the physical examination shows no abnormalities. An x-ray of the thoracic spine shows no abnormalities. A CT scan of the abdomen shows a 3-cm mass in the body of the pancreas; there are liver metastases and encasement of the superior mesenteric artery. Ultrasonography of the left lower extremity shows a femoropopliteal venous clot. Which of the following is the most likely cause of this patient's symptoms?

    (A) Carcinoid syndrome
    (B) Hypercoagulability from advanced malignancy
    (C) Multiple endocrine neoplasia
    (D) Splenic artery aneurysm and embolic disease of the left lower extremity
    (E) Superior mesenteric artery syndrome

**Fig. 43.1** Sample medical boards question.

- In general, you should try to memorize everything in the First Aid and Pathoma chapter corresponding to your in-house block for USMLE Step 1 (and do the corresponding practice problems in USMLE-Rx,[7] Kaplan,[8] Pastest,[9] or other question banks).
- We generally recommend sticking to a single question bank (e.g., USMLE-Rx, Kaplan, or Pastest) that is **not USMLE World (UWorld)** throughout your preclinical courses. We recommend saving UWorld for your dedicated period because the questions are highly integrative and you will not learn from them optimally until you have gone through all of the prerequisite material. That said, some people do recommend using UWorld throughout the school year.[10]

- **How to approach questions in medical school**: Medical school may be your first exposure to clinical vignette questions. Unlike the short, discrete questions you were probably used to in undergrad, clinical vignettes are typically at least a paragraph long and give you both relevant and irrelevant information. They expect you to pick the "best" answer from incomplete information, challenging you to make good judgment in the face of uncertainty. Here, we will go through a sample[11] NBME USMLE Step 1 question with our recommendations for approaching these questions (▶ Fig. 43.1):
  - **Read the question (last sentence of the vignette) first, and THEN go back and read the rest of the vignette.** Reading the question ("Which of the following is the most likely cause of the patient's symptoms") first allows you to focus your attention on the most salient, relevant pieces of information in the vignette (weight loss, leg swelling, back pain, pancreatic mass with liver metastases).
  - Go through each answer choice and come up with a specific reason why each wrong answer choice is wrong.
  - Leave some time at the end of each test to go back and read your answers and go over your *thought process* for picking the right answer. Oftentimes, you may rush and be a bit more careless your first time reading through the exam to make sure you get to every question. Once you've actually answered all the questions, go back and be more deliberate in your reasoning.
- **Specific courses**—for acing your in-house exams, your in-house materials (syllabi, lectures, review sessions by instructors) will be all you need. That said, here are additional resources that helped us understand the big picture and the highest-yield information (your school and/or classmates will likely have free copies of these materials).

---

[7] High-Yield Tools to Help You Master Medical School. Available at: https://www.usmle-rx.com/. Accessed July 8, 2022.

[8] USMLE® Step 1 QBank: Get More Out Of Your QBank. Available at: https://www.kaptest.com/usmle/practice/usmle-step-1-qbank. Accessed July 8, 2022.

[9] USMLE Step 1. Available at: https://www.pastest.com/usmle-step-1/. Accessed July 8, 2022.

[10] How I Used My UWorld Subscription for MS1 and MS2. Available at: https://medical.uworld.com/blog/usmle/how-i-used-my-uworld-subscription-for-ms1-and-ms2/. Accessed July 8, 2022.

[12] From preclinical to wards, we're with you every step of the way! Available at: https://www.boardsbeyond.com/home-page. Accessed July 8, 2022.

[11] Sample Test Questions. Available at: https://usmle.org/pdfs/step-1/samples_step1_2020.pdf. Accessed July 8, 2022.

- As above, know the First Aid and Pathoma material for each course well. If you're having trouble understanding *concepts* in each course, Boards and Beyond[12] and BRS Physiology[13] (particularly for cardiology, renal, pulmonology, endocrine, and gastroenterology) are great supplementary resources.
- **Gross anatomy**—Netter's[14] and Rohen's[15] atlases are the go-to reference materials. Netter's provides high-quality drawings of gross anatomy, whereas Rohen's provides high-quality gross dissections. In fact, after a week or so, many students will skip anatomy dissection altogether to spend more time reviewing these atlases than meticulously dissecting through fat and fascia to find the anatomic structures of interest. e-Anatomy[16] is a fantastic resource for learning radiologic anatomy. BRS Gross Anatomy[17] is also fantastic for getting used to board-style questions early in medical school. It also points out the highest-yield material in anatomy for boards, which was invaluable because much of gross anatomy simply did not appear on boards (for us, at least).
- **Biochemistry and genetics**—Boards and Beyond is fantastic at breaking down complex biochemical pathways into the most important and basic conceptual principles. The biochemistry section of First Aid for USMLE Step 1 is also invaluable, and *you should know this section completely for Step 1.*[18]
- **Medical microbiology**—This is a ton of rote memorization, and Anki and question banks will be your friend here. Many students (myself not included) swear by the method of loci memorization technique used by SketchyMicro.[19] We recommend trying it to see if it works for you. The microbiology section of First Aid for USMLE Step 1 is also invaluable, and *you should know this section well for Step 1.*
- **Immunology**—In addition to Boards and Beyond, First Aid, question banks, and Anki, we recommend *How the Immune System Works*[20] as a quick read to understand the top-down, big picture perspective of immunology.
- **Pharmacology**—In addition to Boards and Beyond, First Aid, question banks, and Anki, many students recommend SketchyPharm.[21]
- **Pathology and histology**—In addition to First Aid, question banks, and Anki, Pathoma will be your best friend. Pathoma is the life-saver for medical students learning pathology and histology.

## 43.3.2 Clinical Years

We again emphasize following the "3 A's" described in Chapter 42, Real Talk on the Medical School Experience. Although there is great variation in terms of grading and expectations by superiors on rotations, physician-educators generally want to work with learners who:

- **... are proactive about self-improvement**. Early in your rotation, tell your resident and attending that you actively want to work on a specific learning goal (e.g., mastering the musculoskeletal exam in outpatient clinic, coordinating follow-up care at discharge on inpatient rotations) and then actively demonstrate that you are working on these objectives.

---

[12] From preclinical to wards, we're with you every step of the way! Available at: https://www.boardsbeyond.com/home-page. Accessed July 8, 2022.

[13] Costanzo LS. BRS Physiology (Board Review Series) 7th Edition. Available at: https://www.amazon.com/Physiology-Board-Review-Linda-Costanzo/dp/1496367618. Accessed July 8, 2022.

[14] Netter FH. Atlas of Human Anatomy (Netter Basic Science) 7th Edition. Available at: https://www.amazon.com/Atlas-Human-Anatomy-Netter-Science/dp/0323393225. Accessed July 8, 2022.

[15] Rohen JW, Yokochi C, Lütjen-Drecoll E. Anatomy: A Photographic Atlas (Color Atlas of Anatomy a Photographic Study of the Human Body) Eighth, North American Edition. Available at: https://www.amazon.com/Anatomy-Photographic-Atlas-Color-Study/dp/1451193181. Accessed July 8, 2022.

[16] Interactive anatomical atlas of the brain based on anatomical diagrams and CT and MRI medical imaging exams. Available at: https://www.imaios.com/en/e-Anatomy. Accessed July 8, 2022.

[17] Chung KW, Chung HM. Gross Anatomy (Board Review Series) 7th Edition. Available at: https://www.amazon.com/BRS-Gross-Anatomy-Board-Review/dp/1605477451. Accessed July 8, 2022.

[18] Le T, Bhushan V. First Aid For the USMLE Step 1 2020, 30th Edition. Available at: https://www.amazon.com/First-USMLE-Step-2020-Thirtieth/dp/1260462048. Accessed July 8, 2022.

[19] All-in-one Medical Program. Available at: https://sketchy.com/products/micro. Accessed July 8, 2022.

[20] Sompayrac LM. How the Immune System Works (The How it Works Series) 6th Edition. Available at: https://www.amazon.com/How-Immune-System-Works-dp-111954212X/dp/111954212X/ref=dp_ob_title_bk. Accessed July 8, 2022.

[21] All-in-one Medical Program. Available at: https://sketchy.com/products/pharm. Accessed July 8, 2022.

- Actively elicit feedback from superiors every week or so, e.g., "Early in the rotation, I mentioned that I wanted to work on X. How do you think I'm doing in terms of improving that? Anything you would recommend I do differently?"
- **... have great medical knowledge and are active learners**. Obviously, it helps to get as many pimp questions correct as you can. That said, it's really not the end of the world if you get them wrong. If you're unsure about the answer to a pimp question, demonstrate that you're making an educated guess, e.g., "I'm not sure, but based on the pathophysiology of the disease, I would expect X." It's arguably more important to demonstrate that you care about lifelong learning than actually getting the question right on the spot. Point out to your supervisor that they asked a good question and you'll have to do some more reading about the topic. Bonus points if you later bring up something interesting that you discover when doing more reading on the topic.
  - Don't reveal gross knowledge deficits on topics you "should" know about. For example, if you don't know high-yield material that is likely to be tested on the shelf exam (e.g., differential for shortness of breath, chronic cough, diabetes medications), do *not* demonstrate this to the team by asking for additional instruction. Do reading on your own time. Save your questions for things that require higher-level reasoning and synthesis of information, i.e., things that cannot be easily researched on your own time.
  - **OnlineMedEd**[22] is a popular resource for learning about the bread-and-butter cases in each medical specialty. Of note, some of the information is outdated; we generally recommend using **UpToDate**[23] (particularly the "Summary and Recommendations" section) for *anything* you will encounter on the floors as a "final" authoritative resource as a medical student. For example, if you are about to scrub in on a laparoscopic cholecystectomy, the UpToDate article is fantastic for reviewing basically every relevant topic that a medical student would be expected to know.
- **... deeply care about patients' well-being.** You'll shine if you go the extra mile for patients' well-being, e.g., actively following up with case management daily on a patient who's simply awaiting placement at an outside facility, speaking directly with the surgical team if they don't seem to be as concerned about a patient's prognosis as your team, or speaking directly with physical therapy about changing the patient's recommendation for placement if the patient is simply awaiting placement at a facility but you feel that the patient could be discharged to his/her house (vs. a facility).
- **... demonstrate superior clinical reasoning.** Your presentations and notes should have a well-formulated *assessment* and *plan*. Many medical students excel at organizing the history, physical exam, and lab + imaging findings into a cohesive narrative but struggle with offering their personal assessment of the overall clinical picture.
  - Your assessment should begin with a one-liner summary statement + /− a provisional diagnosis (e.g., "Mr. Smith is a 45 year old man with histories of obesity and nonalcoholic fatty liver disease who presents with 1 week of intermittent right upper quadrant pain most consistent with symptomatic gallstone disease"). You need to include a differential diagnosis of at least 3 diseases, as well as any relevant "must rule out" diagnoses and why you think they're less likely vs. additional work-up of those diagnoses in your plan.
  - "The differential includes peptic ulcer disease because of X and Y, hepatitis because of X and Y, and right lower lobe pneumonia because of X and Y. Perforated viscus is felt to be less likely given the absence of peritoneal signs and normal vital signs. I would like further work-up with..."
  - Demonstrating confidence and excellent public speaking skills[24] helps tremendously with presentations. If you struggle with public speaking, then watch famous speeches and consider public speaking lessons (e.g., Toastmasters[25]).
- **... are fantastic team players.** Ideally, you will get along with everyone on the team. Even if the interns don't directly grade you, the residents and attendings will likely ask for their input when evaluating you. Try to make personal connections with your teammates; ask them about their hobbies, where

---

[22] OnlineMedEd. Available at: https://home.onlinemeded.org/. Accessed July 8, 2022.

[23] UpToDate: Industry-leading clinical decision support. Available at: https://www.uptodate.com/. Accessed July 8, 2022.

[24] Schraeder TL. Public speaking and presentation skills. Available at: https://oxfordmedicine.com/view/10.1093/med/9780190882440.001.0001/med-9780190882440-chapter-3. Accessed July 8, 2022.

[25] What is Toastmasters? Available at: https://www.toastmasters.org/. Accessed July 8, 2022.

they're from, and why they chose their specialty during moments of down-time. It's not enough to be a fantastic doctor; the ideal medical student is also a great colleague and coworker.

- If you notice a potential learning point that multiple members of the team struggle with, offer to do a **presentation** for the team addressing that learning point. For example, you can do a presentation on common rashes seen in inpatient medicine because multiple team members were having trouble with rashes during your rotation.
- Systems-based care: coordination of care, handoffs (e.g., signout), discussing with consultants (and can even push-back on questionable recommendations).

• **... have fantastic clinical skills (e.g., history taking, physical exam, bedside manner).** Experience with a skilled teacher is going to be the best teacher for improving your clinical skills. Pay close attention in whatever clinical skills experiences you get, and take full advantage of physicians who are willing to teach you. The *JAMA Rational Clinical Examination*[26] series is fantastic for appreciating the statistical utility (i.e., sensitivity, specificity, and likelihood ratios) of various physical exam maneuvers. *Bates' Guide to Physical Examination and History Taking*[27] is the go-to reference material for proper history taking and physical examination skills. Stanford Medicine[28] also has excellent free videos on physical exam skills.

- That said, be careful when asking for evaluation and feedback. If you believe that your superior thinks you're incompetent, do *not* ask for feedback on a physical exam or history-taking skill that you're poor at. You're better off getting instruction on these deficits elsewhere (e.g., protected clinical skills session).

• **... are committed to professionalism.** Again, always show up slightly early (on time at latest) and stay as long as it's appropriate to do so. Never lie. Use professional language in professional settings. Most of this is about *not* doing inappropriate things.

• **... can read the room**. We can't guarantee that every attending will be receptive to each of these strategies. For example, some attendings are very laid-back and not pedantic at all. They may not be very receptive to your laying out specific learning objectives and periodically checking your progress on those expectations. Instead, they may simply grade you more holistically. You would do well to avoid coming off as overly nit-picky and type A to such an attending. *Be adaptable.*

- This means that you should highlight your best qualities depending on your social setting. Don't be fake, but recognize that different people will appreciate different aspects of your personality more than others. Emphasize those traits and contribute to the group's social cohesion.

You should ultimately *aim* to perform at the level of an intern, but you should recognize that this is virtually impossible. Much of medical training is based on direct experience, and it's simply unreasonable to expect that a new clinical medical student would perform at the level of a resident.

## 43.3.3 Shelf Exams

You should use whatever free time you have to study for the shelf exam at the end of the rotation, as you will generally need to do well on the shelf exam to get "honors" in the rotation. We emphasize using active learning techniques (e.g., practice problems, spaced repetition) because your time to study is limited, and you cannot afford to waste time on low-yield passive learning strategies. You should start studying for the shelf early in the rotation, and even the weekend before so you have some knowledge to impress with on arrival. Whenever possible, study for the shelf exam during your rotations *as long as you are confident that your seniors are ok with this—this comes after patient care and notes.*

---

[26] The Rational Clinical Examination. Available at: https://jamanetwork.com/collections/6257/the-rational-clinical-examination. Accessed July 8, 2022.

[27] Bickley LS. Bates' Guide to Physical Examination and History Taking Twelfth, North American Edition. Available at: https://www.amazon.com/Bates-Physical-Examination-History-Taking/dp/146989341X. Accessed July 8, 2022.

[28] Stanford Medicine 25. Available at: https://stanfordmedicine25.stanford.edu/. Accessed July 8, 2022.

- **UWorld for Step 2 CK**[29] is arguably the best question bank to do throughout your clerkships. Other question banks[30] are also available if you want more questions.
- Dedicated Anki decks are available for clerkships. Refer to upperclassmen and reddit.com/r/medicalschoolanki.
- We benefited from the following reference books for each rotation:
  - **Internal medicine**—*Step-up to Medicine*[31] is long but extremely high-yield. That said, it's doubtful that a single resource will contain everything needed to prepare for the medicine shelf. Your best preparation will be having prepared well for Step 1 and actively learning throughout the clerkship.
  - **Surgery**—*Dr. Pestana's Surgery Notes*[32] is the short, super high-yield pocket book that can help you with floor work and common pimp questions. De Virgilio's *Surgery: A Case Based Clinical Review*[33] is much longer and more comprehensive, but may be the **one of the most helpful**. It goes through high-yield surgical cases across every organ system and is a wonderful Socratic method with the relevant medical work-up and discussion of complications. The practice problems in the book were also very similar to the shelf questions..
  - **Pediatrics**—*BRS Pediatrics*[34] is also helpful for shelf and "pimp" questions.
  - **Psychiatry**—*First Aid for the Psychiatry Clerkship*[35] should be everything you need for the shelf. *Lange Q&A Psychiatry*[36] has additional questions if anyone wants more.
  - **OB/Gyn**—*Case Files Obstetrics and Gynecology*[37] and the APGO uWise OB/Gyn practice problems[38] (as a supplement to UWorld) were sufficient for the shelf.
  - **Family medicine**—AAFP board review questions[39] and *Case Files Family Medicine*[40] were sufficient for the shelf.
- It's relatively low yield, but skimming through the relevant chapters in First Aid for USMLE Step 1 can be helpful for the rare basic science questions on each shelf exam.

## 43.3.4 Dedicated Study Periods

In the weeks leading up to USMLE Step 1 and USMLE Step 2 CK, you will go into maximum overdrive in terms of studying. We each spent ~5 to 8 weeks of studying ~6 days a week, 10 to 12 hours each day to consolidate our knowledge before taking these extremely stressful exams. The specifics of these "dedicated" study periods are beyond the scope of this book. Refer to the recommendations on SDN, reddit.com/r/medicalschool, successful upperclassmen from your school, +/− your school's academic advising. That said, we have some general guidelines for approaching dedicated periods:

---

[29] Quality Is Our Obsession—Start Your USMLE® Step 2 CK Prep With UWorld. Available at: https://medical.uworld.com/usmle/usmle-step-2-ck/. Accessed July 8, 2022.

[30] USMLE® STEP 2 CK PREP. Available at: https://www.kaptest.com/usmle-step-2ck. Accessed July 8, 2022, USMLE Step 2 CK. Available at: https://www.pastest.com/usmle-step-2-ck/. Accessed July 8, 2022. Accessed July 8, 2022, USMLE. Available at: https://www.usmle-rx.com/products/step-2-test-prep-ck-qmax/. Accessed July 8, 2022.

[31] Agabegi SS, Agabegi ED. Step-Up to Medicine (Step-Up Series) 4th Edition. Available at: https://www.amazon.com/Step-Up-Medicine-Steven-S-Agabegi/dp/1496306147. Accessed July 8, 2022.

[32] Pestana C. Dr. Pestana's Surgery Notes, Fifth Edition. Available at: https://www.amazon.com/Dr-Pestanas-Surgery-Notes-Vignettes-dp-1506254349/dp/1506254349/ref=dp_ob_title_bk. Accessed July 8, 2022.

[33] de Virgilio C, Grigorian A. Surgery: A Case Based Clinical Review, 2nd ed. 2020 Edition. Available at: https://www.amazon.com/Surgery-Case-Based-Clinical-Review/dp/3030053865. Accessed July 8, 2022.

[34] Brown LJ, Miller LT. Pediatrics (Board Review Series) 1st Edition. Available at: https://www.amazon.com/Pediatrics-Board-Review-Lloyd-Brown/dp/0781721296. Accessed July 8, 2022.

[35] Ganti L, Kaufman M, Blitzstein S. First Aid for the Psychiatry Clerkship, 5th Edition. Available at: https://www.amazon.com/First-Aid-Psychiatry-Clerkship-Fifth/dp/1260143392. Accessed July 8, 2022.

[36] Blitzstein S. Lange Q&A Psychiatry, 11th Edition. Available at: https://www.amazon.com/Lange-Psychiatry-11th-Sean-Blitzstein/dp/1259643948. Accessed July 8, 2022.

[37] Toy E, Ross P, Baker B, Jennings J. Case Files Obstetrics and Gynecology, 5th Edition. Available at: https://www.amazon.com/Case-Files-Obstetrics-Gynecology-Fifth/dp/007184872X. Accessed July 8, 2022.

[38] uWISE v.3.5.2021. Available at: https://apgo.org/page/uwisev3-2. Accessed July 8, 2022.

[39] AAFP. Available at: https://www.aafp.org/cme/all/board-review-questions.html. Accessed July 8, 2022.

[40] Toy E, Briscoe D, Britton B, Heidelbaugh JJ. Case Files Family Medicine 5th Edition. Available at: https://www.amazon.com/Case-Files-Family-Medicine-5th-dp-1260468593/dp/1260468593/ref=dp_ob_title_bk. Accessed July 8, 2022.

- Maintaining wellness is absolutely essential. Dedicated periods are *extremely* stressful, and it's fairly common to experience some sort of breakdown. We'll reiterate our recommendations from Chapter 17, Crushing the MCAT: "Exercise often, sleep 6 to 8 hours a night, take appropriate time off (e.g., at least 1–2 days a week and *whenever you feel burnt out or as if you are not retaining material*), eat healthily (avoid simple sugars, alcohol). Again, it's a marathon, not a sprint, and you'll want to 'sharpen the saw' to the best of your ability.
  - Consider practicing stress reduction techniques (e.g., deep breathing exercises, meditation) early in your study period so that you can best use them to mitigate exam stress during your practice and real exams."
- Don't just think of the board exams as dumb, painful hurdles. Having a foundational, deep understanding of basic sciences and clinical reasoning is extremely helpful for actual patient care and distinguishes you from mid-level providers. If you are even remotely interested in research, it's also critical to have a broad and deep foundational vocabulary and understanding of medicine so that you can come up with intelligent, plausible testable hypotheses. In addition, having a deep, broad understanding of medicine helps tremendously with clerkships and distinguishes you in terms of medical knowledge when asked pimp questions. The knowledge base also carries over to shelf exams. So yes—dedicated study periods are extremely painful, but they actually help greatly in terms of crystallizing your medical knowledge.

## 43.4 Proactively Search for Your Passion

Medical school gives you a few years to determine what type of medicine you will practice for the rest of your life. While it's true that you can tailor your practice within a field down the line (or even retrain altogether), the decision to apply to a particular specialty in residency is arguably the most important career decision you will make as a physician. Many students go through broad divisions: adults vs. children? Surgery vs. nonsurgery? Pure intellectual vs. procedural (e.g., infectious disease vs. gastroenterology)? Do I need direct patient contact? How much do I care about lifestyle during residency training?

It is critical to explore all possibilities and minimize potential feelings of "what if..." before you commit to the medical specialty you will be practicing for the rest of your life. You will be much more motivated and likely to succeed if you have found an area of medicine that deeply interests you. As such, we recommend shadowing in as many specialties as possible in your preclinical years—even if you feel like you won't enjoy the specialty. Medical students are commonly surprised by what they end up liking, and your preferences will likely evolve throughout your career. For this reason, we recommend *continuing* to test your interest with repeated exposures at various stages in your training. For example, let's say that you fell in love with pediatrics as a first-year medical student. We encourage you to shadow again in second year and then to really test your limit by seeking out challenging clinical encounters during your pediatrics clerkship and acting internship (assuming you make it that far with your pediatrics interest). On the other hand, let's say you shadow a surgical specialty early in medical school and you hate it. We recommend re-exploring surgery with an open mind during your clerkship in third year because your appreciation might change at that later stage in training.

When doing this, really commit to exploring as many options as possible in your medical school. Seriously consider things like dual degrees and unconventional rotations (e.g., abroad, in rural areas, etc.). An underappreciated aspect of finding *your* specialty is that much of it relies on intangibles (e.g., culture of the specialty, how you *feel* working with the bread-and-butter pathology and patient population), and this requires direct experience to assess. In addition, you often don't know what you don't know about various specialties—diving in with an open mind and scrupulously assessing your state of mind as you engage with these specialties and experiences is vital. We also recommend *The Undifferentiated Medical Student*[41] podcast for a wealth of high-quality interviews with attending physicians across various specialties.

In this vein, we recommend paying close attention to the bread-and-butter cases in each field. It's easy to get attached to the captivating, most awe-inspiring aspects of each field, but the reality is that you will be spending most of your waking hours on the mundane. For example, the open aortic aneurysm repairs in vascular surgery might be exciting, but you need to be honest with yourself about how well you would tolerate the long hours and many endovascular procedures that come with the field.

---

[41] A Top-ranked Medicine Podcast in iTunes. Available at: https://www.undifferentiatedmedicalstudent.com/the-podcast/. Accessed July 8, 2022.

You should also figure out what your personal dealbreakers are (i.e., what you absolutely cannot tolerate in a job). For example, you might enjoy the variety in emergency medicine, but if you genuinely cannot tolerate constant circadian rhythm shifts, then it's probably not the best field for you. Also consider what values and features of the specialty would be consistent with your personal life. Many students will choose to forgo surgical training if they have multiple children to take care of and want to spend as much time as possible with them; this is a totally reasonable personal decision. That said, keep an open mind and recognize that you're probably more resilient than you think and that your specialty of interest probably has more flexibility than you think (depending on the particular residency program).

A very reassuring sign is genuine interest in the science behind the field. Whatever specialty you are going into, you will spend countless hours in residency studying the nuances of the basic science and clinical practice of that field. You will also be engaged in lifelong learning (i.e., critically evaluating new research) as an attending physician. Pay attention to the fields that you genuinely enjoy studying. Flip through the high-impact journals of each specialty and be mindful of which research articles/Wikipedia pages you could see yourself even browsing for fun.

Money shouldn't be a major consideration when choosing a medical specialty. Even if you have extremely high amounts of debt, you will be able to pay back your loans in some fashion (as per Chapter 37, Financial Aid). It's much more important that you genuinely enjoy and derive some sense of *meaning* from the specialty. Find the field that makes you feel fulfilled—on some level—to come into work early in the morning for terrible hours as a resident (or doing overnight shifts, working call, etc.).

If you still haven't found something that genuinely interests you as you near residency application, consider taking a year off (e.g., paid research year) to continue soul-searching. Speak to academic advisors throughout the process to bounce ideas and get recommendations for unconventional areas of medical practice (e.g., aerospace medicine, occupational medicine, transgender health, etc.) The beautiful thing about a medical career is that there is tremendous flexibility in how you can make best use of your medical degree. You can even pursue nonclinical careers (more in Chapter 46, Nonclinical Careers) if you genuinely believe that clinical medicine would not be the best use of your talents. Ultimately, what matters is that you find something that gives you meaning, that you can tolerate for the rest of your career, and aligns best with your natural abilities.

## 43.5 Summary

The medical school material is not conceptually difficult; you just need to avoid procrastination, get started with that *first* flash card or practice problem of the day, and put the time in.
Expect to:
- Spend 5 to 10 hours studying each day for 5 to 7 days per week, but the hours are not hard cutoffs.
- Give yourself daily and weekly goals based on active learning objectives.
- Be fully committed to work when you're working and fully committed to leisure when you're unwinding—prioritize deep studying.
- Actively focus on keeping an accurate schedule to assist in prioritizing.
- Avoid overcommitting to responsibilities for the first several months.
- Take some time for friends and other things you enjoy almost every day, even if it's just a few minutes.

A significant predictor of your success in medical school will be how much pure, brute force you're willing to put in, *as long as that time is all or almost entirely active learning.* Avoid passive learning as much as possible. Experiment with different approaches to learning, and which resources you are using, early in med school and reassess and reimplement based on your results with respect to your specific goals. No single resource works best for every subject or rotation; consider switching based on the best available opinion when approaching a new section.

When you get to clinical rotations, focus on being active and learning about your patients and their conditions in your spare time. UpToDate is a great resource during clinical rotations. Focus on going the extra mile and building a relationship with patients so that you can add value to their care. Showing your clinical reasoning is important as well, as is incorporating feedback rapidly. All of these things will make up the bulk of your subjective evaluations. Dedicated study periods are useful for reviewing and permanently crystallizing pertinent information.

# 44 A Peek at the Residency Application Process

*Joel Thomas and Neal K. Ramchandani*

Your career in medicine will have a lot of applications and interviews. This means a lot of wearing a suit, walking around in a hospital, and enthusiastically answering "Tell me about yourself." Applying to residency is very similar to applying to medical school, but there are also a few key differences. Additionally, similar to the medical school interview trail, the logistics of the residency interview trail were also upended in the wake of the COVID-19 pandemic. As of 2022, most (if not all) programs are only offering online interviews. While much of the advice in this chapter still stands, we recommend reviewing Chapter 34, Interviews for specific advice regarding the logistics of online interviews. That said, we hope this chapter proves useful if/when programs resume in-person interviews.

## 44.1 Residency Application Cycle: The Big Picture

- Decide you're actually ready to apply to residency (~third year of medical school).
  - Depending on specialty, participate in subinternships (July–September of fourth year of medical school).
- Gather application materials (ERAS, letters of recommendation) in August to mid-October of fourth year of medical school.
- Apply to residency programs +/– separate intern years (September/October of fourth year of medical school).
- Receive and schedule interview invites (October–January of fourth year of medical school).
- Travel to and interview at various programs (October–January of fourth year of medical school).
- *Rank* programs (February of fourth year of medical school).
- Receive Match results (March of fourth year of medical school).
- Begin residency as part of binding agreement (July after graduating medical school).

First, you need to ask yourself, "Am I actually ready to apply to residency?" This may sound like an odd question because residency appears to be the logical next step after 4 years of medical school. Many applicants, however, will choose to delay applying to residency to either make themselves more competitive or to enter a different career trajectory altogether. The most competitive medical specialties (i.e., dermatology, plastic surgery, orthopaedic surgery, otolaryngology) seek applicants from prestigious medical schools with extremely high board scores and extensive research (typically 10+ published papers/abstracts/presentations). Applicants who aren't as competitive often choose to delay graduation and their application to residency to pursue additional research (a research year). This is because applying to residency programs as a fourth-year medical student gives you a tremendous advantage for residency applications compared to—say—graduating and applying afterward (e.g., as a postgraduate research assistant). In addition, some graduates choose to avoid/defer clinical medicine altogether[1] and enter other careers such as management consulting.

So let's assume you're moving forward with applying to residency. If you're applying to a highly competitive specialty, your planning will have started early in medical school, and you'll have ideally developed meaningful relationships with faculty, been productive in research in that field, and completed acting internships at multiple institutions (i.e., "away rotations") to make yourself a competitive applicant. Acting internships are intense rotations in which you attempt to function at the level of a first-year resident (i.e., intern) in that specialty. They are extremely stressful because the expectations for interns are dramatically higher than those of medical students. In addition, you are under constant pressure because you are constantly under evaluation to obtain the best possible letter of recommendation for your specialty.

Some specialties (dermatology, radiology, radiation oncology, physical medicine and rehabilitation, and some anesthesiology and neurology programs) also require a separate intern year. While not necessary, you would benefit from getting "honors" in an acting internship in internal medicine or surgery[2] before

---

[1] Innovative careers for doctors, scientists, and healthcare professionals. Available at: https://www.docjobs.com/. Accessed July 8, 2022. Doctors at McKinsey. Available at: https://www.mckinsey.com/about-us/new-at-mckinsey-blog/doctors-at-mckinsey. Accessed July 8, 2022.

[2] An acting internship is typically required by all medical schools before graduation, anyway

you submit your residency application so that competitive intern year programs (i.e., the "cush" ones with less scutwork,[3] more elective time, and supportive ancillary staff who are paid to *do* aforementioned scutwork) review your application favorably.

You will next compile your application materials, beginning with the letters of recommendation. Ideally, you will have identified several attending physicians who will write strong, positive letters of recommendation for you. You should contact them at least 4 weeks[4] in advance of the deadline for letter submission, and you will likely have to gently remind them and/or their administrative assistants as you get closer to the application deadline. Academic attending physicians tend to be extremely busy, but they are usually also punctual. You will likely experience some gut wrenching dread several days before the application deadline, only to experience blissful relief as your letter is uploaded at the last possible moment.

The next step is the ERAS application, which is the primary application for the residency match. This is essentially a watered-down, bare-bone version of the medical school primary application. Most of it is simply biographic information, but key areas to polish include:

- **Photo**—You need a professional-quality headshot in a suit or other professional attire, *not* your white coat.
- **Personal statement**—Limited to 28,000 characters (including spaces). Explain how you decided on the specialty to which you're applying, as well as your professional aspirations. While your personal statement has to be good, there is much less pressure on it compared to medical school applications. The vast majority of personal statements for residency are "fine," and many advisors will tell you that it's better to write something that's overall unremarkable and "fine" compared to taking a risk and inadvertently writing something off-putting. Avoid overly flowery, meaningless drivel. Attending physicians are extremely busy, and they're used to the brevity of medical documentation. Economy of language will win you major points.
- **Volunteer, work, and research experiences**—Describe your extracurricular activities. Overall, these are less important for residency admissions, but you will want to demonstrate that you're a well-rounded, interesting person. You have 1,020 characters to explain each activity.
  - **Publications**—Arguably the most important part of the "extracurriculars" section. Your number of publications (partially weighted by the impact factor of the journal) will likely be heavily scrutinized for competitive specialties.
- **Hobbies and interests**—This is a small, tucked-away portion of the application, but it is *extremely* important in distinguishing yourself among the sea of applicants with high board scores and clinical research. If you have interesting hobbies, *sell yourself strongly*. Even if you don't have interesting hobbies, *highlight the most interesting/"wow" factor aspects of those hobbies*.
  - For example, "I play guitar" becomes "I play progressive rock and jazz guitar, and I enjoy composing jazz fusion/progressive rock music."

Other "most important" components of your residency application[5] include Step 1 score, letters of recommendation in the specialty, the MSPE (medical student performance evaluation—basically the narrative transcript of your medical school performance), and selection to Alpha Omega Alpha (AOA), the medical honors society. The criteria for AOA selection vary greatly by school, ranging from pure academia criteria (i.e., clerkship grades, Step 1 score) to purely peer selection, to a combination of peer selection, academics, and extracurricular achievement. In addition, MD vs. DO vs. international (e.g., Caribbean) school status is tremendously important, especially for competitive specialties. It is virtually impossible to match integrated plastic surgery, for example, as a DO student compared to an MD student (although it theoretically can happen. There were only 12 total DO applicants for plastic surgery between 2016 and 2020, so we don't have a great sample size).[6]

---

[3] E.g., transporting patients, drawing your own labs, wasting time on tedious orders through an inefficient electronic medical record, calling to make follow-up appointments, taking routine vital signs, sending faxes.

[4] Earlier is even better. Attending academic physicians tend to be extremely busy.

[5] Results of the 2018 NRMP Program Director Survey. Available at: https://www.nrmp.org/wp-content/uploads/2018/07/NRMP-2018-Program-Director-Survey-for-WWW.pdf. Accessed July 8, 2022.

[6] Residency Match Report. Available at: https://com.tu.edu/TUCOM%202016-2020%20Residency%20Match%20Report.pdf. Accessed July 8, 2022.

One *extremely* important variable in residency match outcomes, however, is *connections*. This is hinted at by "letters of recommendation" being one of the most important variables. More explicitly: the author of the letter is just as, if not more important, than the quality. This is especially the case for smaller specialties in which prominent faculty know each other and meet regularly at conferences. This greatly differs from medical school applications. Most medical school applicants simply will not have had the opportunity to forge meaningful relationships with "persons of interest" for medical school admissions (e.g., prominent academic medical faculty). In contrast, medical students actively pursue opportunities to work closely with academic physicians (e.g., acting internships, medical school research) to obtain influential letters of recommendation. In this vein, the prestige of your medical school—as a proxy for the number of influential faculty members—*tremendously* affects your odds of getting into competitive specialties. The most successful applicants will have glowing letters of recommendation from esteemed faculty members in their fields. While academics alone may get you into *a* program, breaking into the uppermost echelon will likely require playing the game of medical school politics well to be on "hot-shot" faculty's radars.[7]

In addition, *regional ties* are very important, especially for programs on the West Coast. Essentially, if your application screams "I was born and raised in the Midwest," you will stand a poor shot at getting interviews at West Coast programs—especially when the West Coast is a highly competitive region to match in, period. To maximize your odds of getting an interview at a different region, you will need a tie such as family in the area or *away rotation* done in the region. Some applicants will do away rotations in other regions simply to "unlock" the region.

After you finalize your ERAS application, you will need to decide *which* programs to apply to. Depending on your specialty, this can differ dramatically from medical school applications. For medical school, you likely applied to 25 to 35 schools. For relatively noncompetitive[8] specialties (e.g., pediatrics, internal medicine, family medicine), applicants typically apply to just over 20 programs.[9] For competitive specialties, however, applicants frequently apply to *every* residency program in the field (e.g., 70–90 programs) to maximize their odds of getting enough interviews to gain *any* residency spot. As with medical school interviews, we recommend paying more for more opportunities. In the grand scheme of things, a few extra thousand dollars spent on applications will be a drop in the bucket, and you may forever ask "What if?" if you choose not to apply to that reach program you really wanted to attend.

This brings us to the next and arguably most important difference between medical school and residency applications: the Match. Residency applicants are "matched" to programs through a sorting algorithm that uses applicants' and programs' "rank list" preferences.[10] Applicants can go on as many interviews as they want, but they will ultimately rank the programs they interviewed at with hopes for matching at a *single* program—ideally one that they ranked highly. Likewise, programs hope to not go too far down their list of ranked applicants to fill their residency class. The sorting algorithm favors applicants. That is, applicants are encouraged to rank programs according to their *true* preferences, and multiple mathematical analyses have verified that it's in their best interest to do so (regardless of whatever postinterview communication they may receive from programs). The National Resident Matching Program (NRMP) beautifully explains how the process works,[11] but the key differences compared to medical school applications are seen in ▶ Table 44.1.

## 44.2 Couples Match

Medical training can be hard on your personal life. You might meet your soulmate in medical school, only to be thrust across the country by the vagaries of the residency match. Fortunately, we've got the Couples Match, which is an option for "couples" to group their residency applications, and becomes a package deal for programs.

---

[7] This is much more important for small, procedural fields (neurosurgery, plastics).

[8] Every specialty is competitive at the top, however. Matching pediatrics or internal medicine at Penn, for example, is likely to be as competitive as matching dermatology or orthopaedic surgery at a "mid-tier" program.

[9] Determining the Optimal Number of Program Applications. Available at: https://www.acponline.org/about-acp/about-internal-medicine/career-paths/medical-student-career-path/determining-the-optimal-number-of-program-applications#:~:text=In%20recent%20years%20the%20number,over%20the%20past%205%20years. Accessed July 8, 2022.

[10] TMDSAS uses essentially the same algorithm, which is based on the "stable marriage problem" in economics.

[11] The Matching Algorithm. Available at: https://www.nrmp.org/matching-algorithm/. Accessed July 8, 2022.

**Table 44.1** Medical school versus residency admissions

| Residency | Medical school |
|---|---|
| You do not find out whether you've matched at any program until the end of the application cycle. This incentivizes you to go on as many interviews as possible—potentially to too many "match" and "safety" programs—to maximize your odds of matching, even if it means fewer interviews for other applicants | You can find out early in the application cycle that you've gotten in "somewhere", allowing you to give up interviews at other "safety" and "match" schools, freeing them up for other applicants who may be better fits for those programs and allowing you to focus more on "reach" programs |
| You can only order your rank preferences. Once you match, you are committed to a binding agreement to that program. Therefore, you should only rank programs that you would see yourself (at least) tolerating. Do not rank a program no.15 on your list if you strongly believe you would be miserable there—it's probably better to go unmatched and scramble somewhere else (although this is obviously a personal decision—at the end of the day, you may have to decide whether you would prefer to train at a place where you **might** be unhappy (and even then, perception is often different from what ends up happening in reality) but pursue your dream specialty vs. training at a place that would make you dramatically happier but in a different specialty) | You can choose among multiple schools that have accepted you |

After applying, you anxiously await interview invites. Thankfully, you do not need to worry about secondary applications. Similar to medical school applications, interview slots are allocated on a first-come, first-serve basis, so you should be hypervigilant about ERAS and program communications. You then interview at programs throughout the country in your intended specialty/ies[12] and ultimately submit your rank list. The algorithm ultimately decides your fate, and then you start at your new home in July!

Regarding logistics: we recommend many—if not all—of the same travel strategies described in Chapter 35, Interview Trail Travel and Attire. A key difference is that residency programs do not typically host applicants like medical school interviews do.

The actual interview process, however, is dramatically different compared to medical school applications. First, essentially all residency interviews are 2-day affairs. Almost all programs will have an "optional but highly encouraged" (aka mandatory) preinterview dinner (pre-COVID times). *Treat this like its own interview.* This is an opportunity for the residents to see how you interact in a "normal" (read: highly artificial, structured, and pressured) social setting. Your travel plans should accommodate arriving early enough to make the preinterview dinner, so you should aim to arrive by 4 to 5 PM at latest to allow for travel time to the dinner. Fortunately, most programs will allow you to bring your luggage to the dinner and interview. You will be seated with other applicants and current residents, and you will be treated to a fantastic dinner, courtesy of the program. Faculty (i.e., attendings) *should not* be present; it should only be you and the residents. Alcoholic beverages will likely be consumed. You will be asked "What questions do you have for me?" *multiple times.*

Most programs genuinely have good intentions with the preinterview dinner. Applicants are worn out from travel, and many would appreciate a free, high-quality meal, as well as time to relax. They would probably also enjoy having insider, intimate information about the program from current residents about the culture and day-to-day life. Unfortunately, the actual execution of the preinterview dinner suffers from many problems—largely related to asynchrony of information. That is, applicants have much more at stake to lose, some programs are not totally forthcoming about the function of the interview dinner

---

[12] I.e., separate intern year for the select specialties mentioned earlier. In addition, some applicants will choose to apply to *multiple* specialties in the same application cycle. This requires multiple personal statements, as well as more letters of recommendation (at least, additional letters from the other specialty). This is most often done by applicants applying to a hypercompetitive specialty plus a "back-up" less-competitive specialty (e.g., plastic surgery and general surgery). Applicants who are genuinely on-the-fence about multiple specialties, however, have also been known to use this strategy to come to a more informed decision throughout the application cycle. Oftentimes, getting first-hand knowledge from residents at various programs will push these applicants toward one specialty.

(and applicants have no way of knowing which programs are dishonest in this regard). We have several thoughts about the preinterview dinner:

- **It can be weirdly Machiavellian.** Most residents sign up for the dinners because they genuinely enjoy talking to applicants and getting a free, nice dinner. In addition, at most programs, residents' input from the dinner won't make or break your application unless you did something egregiously inappropriate. Most residents are simply trying to have a good time and meet interesting applicants who may become future colleagues. Most residents will not be analyzing your every action and utterance. A small minority of programs, however, encourage residents to meticulously (over)analyze social cues to identify unenthusiastic, bored (read: introverted) applicants who may not be "good fits" (read: people whom you may be biased against) for the program based on very arbitrary subjective judgments.
  - Again, going back to the asynchrony of information—it's virtually impossible for an applicant to determine *which* programs do this. So many applicants end up on the defensive—feeling much more guarded and rigid than they otherwise would be to avoid potentially offending residents at the aforementioned programs.
  - Many applicants who are tired from constant travel would like to relax on their own terms to decompress before the interview day. Sitting at dinner with the pressure of having your social interactions meticulously scrutinized is *not* relaxing. Emerging evidence on analyzing body language suggests that the Dunning-Kruger effect is *strong*—most people who believe themselves experts at it are not much better than chance.[13] It's very easy to write off an applicant who's more introverted at baseline as "not interested in the program," especially if he/she doesn't ask generic questions for the sake of asking questions when prompted with "What questions do you have for me?"
  - At the same time, we recognize that abiding by social niceties is simply playing the game. Residency programs rightfully want applicants who can adhere to social expectations because much of being a physician is acting/playing the role that patients expect from you. Essentially, putting on an act is part of the job description.
- **Be careful with how much you drink.** In general, if you *do* drink, drink no more than what the residents drink. Do not order drinks unless at least one resident does so. If you do order a drink, don't order something outlandish or outrageously expensive. Do *not* get visibly intoxicated, and—*please*—do not do or say anything inappropriate while intoxicated. If you have a history of doing so and cannot 100% trust yourself to not risk this, then don't drink. Also, remember that you may need to drive to your lodgings after dinner.
- **You need to put effort in (don't "just be yourself"), but don't try *too* hard.** That is, don't try to dominate the conversation or be extra loud to be extra memorable. Don't try to impress people by alluding to your CV. Just maintain light-hearted conversations. Make sure you're talking at least 20 to 30% of the time throughout dinner. Demonstrate active listening when other people are talking (e.g., maintaining eye contact, smiling, nodding appropriately). *Minimize looking at your phone* during the dinner—give the residents and your coapplicants your undivided attention.
  - If you rotated at the program—or if it's your home program—don't alienate coapplicants by consistently bringing up insider info about the program with current residents.
  - Wear business casual unless the program tells you otherwise.
- **It's ok to be late.** Travel plans are notoriously unpredictable. Just let the residents/program coordinator know!
- **Questions we encourage asking during the dinner:** Ask where residents live, impressions of call and night schedules, fun things to do in the area, how receptive the program is to change, protected research and education opportunities, alumni outcomes, free food, helpfulness of the program coordinator (a great program coordinator is an underappreciated asset; he/she will make your life immeasurably easier!), resident lounge/call areas, board prep and outcomes, integration/relationships with the rest of the departments in the hospital, opportunities to engage with medical students, major changes being planned or recently initiated in the program, favorite and least favorite things about the program, "What surprised you the most about this program?" "Why did you choose this program?" "How do you plan on specializing/shaping your career?" favorite faculty member and why.

---

[13] At Airports, a Misplaced Faith in Body Language. Available at: https://www.nytimes.com/2014/03/25/science/in-airport-screening-body-language-is-faulted-as-behavior-sleuth.html. Accessed July 8, 2022.

The next day, you will participate in the formal interview day. In reality, the interview dinner was the first day of the interview. Interview day schedule varies from program-to-program. Generally, the day begins in the morning or afternoon with light refreshments, followed by orientations from faculty + /– residents + /– administration. Some applicants will interview, whereas others will be given a tour of the department + hospital. The two groups will then switch. Next is typically lunch, followed by a farewell presentation.

## 44.3  How Do Residency Interviews Work?

Residency interviews vary greatly from program to program, and the general attitude of the interviews varies across specialties. For example, diagnostic radiology interviews may be overwhelmingly casual and relaxed while medicine intern year interviews can be much more formal, with the trend being difficult "behavioral" interview questions. Likewise, there are anecdotal reports of those applying to surgical specialties reporting more stressful interviews—and even some tests of manual dexterity!

The most striking difference is the *number* of interviews. At some locations, you will interview with 203 people, but in others, you may interview with 6 to 15 different faculty members for a shorter duration, round-robin style. You will likely be asked, "What questions do you have for me?" by most, if not all of these interviewers. As such, you will need to learn how to give succinct answers to questions in a rapid-fire fashion, as well as how to immediately present yourself well and identify a conversational topic that captivates your interviewer and allows you to deeply connect. At the end of the day, recognize that getting an interview suggests that you're academically qualified for the program. At this point, the program is essentially trying to gauge fit. That said, the vast majority of applicants—as with medical school admissions—do not significantly help or hurt their application on interview day. Again, holistic review seals the deal; the admissions committee will ultimately evaluate your application as a whole, and the reality is that most applicants' fates are dictated by factors that led them to get the interview in the first place, i.e., board scores, letters of recommendation, research, and medical school prestige.

And yes, thank you emails. As with medical school interviews (more in Chapter 34, Interviews), you should email everyone who interviewed you with a short, personalized email thanking them for their time (unless explicitly told not to).

## 44.4  What Do I Do When I'm Done with Interviews?

You need to finalize your rank list. Again, no matter what you may read on the internet or what programs communicate to you after the interview, *you need to rank based on your true preferences*. The match algorithm is rigorously designed to favor your preferences when ranking; you do *not* stand any lower chance of matching at a program lower on your rank list, even if you've stacked the top of your list with "reach" programs. Creating your rank list is an incredibly personal decision, but we recommend the following considerations:

- **Academic vs. community vs. hybrid**. This is a personal decision that you have hopefully explored in-depth throughout medical school. If in doubt, consider academics, as it's much easier to switch from an academic program to a community setting than vice versa.
  - Academic programs—which tend to be tertiary and quaternary referral centers—generally have more exposure to extremely rare diseases. They tend to have highly subspecialized physicians actively involved in research. At the same time, many—but not all—place greater emphasis on training of fellows than residents. For example, Academic Program X may have more exposure to a rare surgical disease, but the value of this may be diminished if the resident is not getting opportunities to scrub in on that disease because the fellows cover them.
- **Do NOT rank purely on prestige**. It's more useful to think about tiers of programs, e.g., "top 5," "top 20," "top 50." Programs within each tier are largely interchangeable and do not have significant differences in terms of clinical training, research opportunities, etc. So you should *not* rank the #19 program on Doximity higher than the #21 program purely on rankings. Instead, consider the specific differences between the programs (e.g., would you enjoy living in the Midwest vs. the East Coast) and how much they matter to *you*.
  - This is incredibly hard for many people in medicine because we're so used to caring so much about prestige and reputation throughout our careers—especially so if we've attended elite institutions

throughout our lives. At the end of the day, recognize that you're *still* going to become a physician. The difference in prestige between being a "Mayo Clinic"-trained physician vs. a UCSD-trained physician worth it if you can't stand the cold (or the Midwest) and your entire family is in California?
- Do you have a family? If so, will your significant other be able to find employment in the city in which you choose to train? Is it in a safe area? Would you find cultural communities in which you thrive? Are the school districts adequate for your children?

• **Really evaluate the specific quality of life differences between programs** (e.g., call and night schedule, supportive ancillary staff, vacation time, protected academic or research time, educational budget, employer-matched retirement plan (*this is huge*), health insurance benefits, salary relative to cost of living, etc.).

Once that's done, what do you do?

You relax. Hard. You've reached the promised land of medical school: the second half of fourth year. *Please* use this time to relax as much as possible. Take vacations. See friends and family. Play video games until your brain oozes out of your ears. Whatever you do, do *not* try to prepare as much as possible by cramming medicine before intern year. It will hardly make a difference, and whatever small advantage you gain would be dwarfed by the opportunity cost of missing one of the last few protected times for relaxation before the onslaught of residency. Do your future self a favor and prioritize your wellness. Treat yourself! You've worked extremely hard up till this point, and you deserve a break.

## 44.5 Final Thoughts

As hectic and disorienting as the residency trail can be at times, you should try to enjoy it above all else. We again emphasize that most applicants will not dramatically improve or worsen their applications in interviews. Use this as an opportunity to travel throughout the country, meet your future colleagues, and get excited about the field you've chosen! You're going to be a doctor! You're visiting amazing life-saving healthcare centers throughout the country, and you're going to be at the heart of their operations as a *licensed physician*. You're going to eat delicious food and drink cocktails with some of the most accomplished, interesting people you'll ever meet! Keep a photo album! Give yourself some time—whenever feasible—to just explore the various cities. Kick back and put your feet up in airport lounges! I still remember many amazing plane conversations with random strangers, as well as spectacular sites that have filled my photo albums. Relish the journey, and be proud of the outcome—your hard work and determination will pay off in the end.

# 45  A Day in the Life in Medicine

*Joel Thomas, Phillip Wagner, Ray Funahashi, Nitin Agarwal, and Vamsi Reddy*

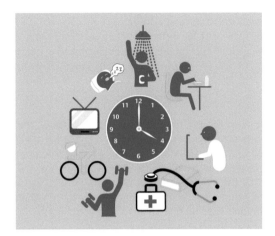

As discussed throughout the book, a "typical day" in medicine will vary tremendously depending on stage in training, specialty, and even the specific niche within that specialty (e.g., even within neuro-ophthalmology, you can focus on an operative vs. nonoperative career). In this chapter, we will walk through a day in the life of several authors at specific points in their training.

## 45.1  Vamsi Reddy—Fourth-Year Medical Student (MS4) at Medical College of Georgia

### 45.1.1  Preclinical

- 5:30 AM: Wake up, go to the gym.
- 5:45–6:30 AM: Work out.
- 6:30–7:30 AM: Go home, shower, get ready.
- 8 AM–12 PM: Class.
- 12 PM–1 PM: Go home, eat lunch.
- 1 PM–3 PM: Research/Extracurricular responsibilities.
- 3 PM–7:30 PM: Study for class.
- 7:30 PM–8 PM: Dinner.
- 8 PM–10 PM: Finish up any other responsibilities/Study more.
- 10 PM–10:30 PM: Chill.
- ~10:30 PM–11 PM: Fall asleep.

### 45.1.2  Clinical (Depends on Rotation)

- 5:30 AM: Wake up, get dressed.
- 6 AM–7 AM: Get to hospital, preround on patients.
- 7 AM–8 AM: Round with the team (the length of rounding depends on the rotation you are on).
- 8 AM–12 PM: OR, Clinic.
- 12 PM–12:30 PM: Lunch.
- 12:30 PM–5 PM: Scut work, check on admitted patients, study if possible.
- 5 PM: Sign off patients to the night team.
- 5:30 PM–6 PM: Go to gym.
- 6 PM–7 PM: Go home, shower, eat dinner.

- 7 PM–11 PM: Study as much as possible.
- ~11 PM–11:30 PM: Fall asleep.

## 45.2 Phillip Wagner, MD—Third-Year Resident (PGY3) in Internal Medicine at University of Pittsburgh Medical Center (UPMC)

- 5:30 AM: Wake up.
- 5:45 AM: Start drive to hospital.
- 6:00 AM: Arrive at parking garage.
- 6:15 AM: Arrive in lounge to get sign-out on overnight patients.
- 6:30 AM: Arrive in your Team room.
- 6:30 AM–8:00 AM: Electronic chart review (prerounding).
- 8:00 AM–9:00 AM: Visit and examine all patients (intern); attend daily case conference (resident).
- 9:00 AM–9:15 AM: Preround with case management and social work.
- 9:15 AM–11:30 AM: Walk rounds (seeing patients and explaining daily plans as a team).
- 11:30 AM–12:00 PM: Start notes, call consultant teams, place orders.
- 12:00 PM–1:00 PM: Noon educational conference (or continuation of work, depending on workflow).
- 1:00 PM–3:00 PM: Finish writing notes, elective procedures (line placement, discharge planning, family conversations and updates).
- 3:00 PM–4:00 PM: Teaching rounds and afternoon table rounding with the attending MD.
- 4:00 PM–5:30 PM: Finish writing notes, elective procedures (e.g., line placement), discharge planning, family conversations and updates, following up with consultants.
- 5:30 PM–6:00 PM (IF no admissions, sign out to night team) OR 5:30 PM–7:00 PM: Admit new patients.
- 6:30 PM–7:30 PM: Arrive home (depending on workflow).
- 7:15 PM–8:00 PM: Exercise.
- 8:00 PM–8:15 PM: Shower.
- 8:15 PM–8:30 PM: Dinner.
- 8:30 PM–10:00 PM: Watch TV while reviewing charts from the day, ensuring plans were carried out, and reading up on new guidelines, research, and more deeply about patients' diagnoses.
- 10:00 PM: Sleep.
- 2:00 AM: Wake up when you think you hear your pager going off, but you were just dreaming.
- 4:00 AM: Wake up in a sweat thinking you forgot to order something, and check the electronic medical record.
- 5:30 AM: Repeat.

Roughly 1 day off per week for chores, errands, cleaning, social activities (pre-COVID).

## 45.3 Nitin Agarwal, MD—Seventh-Year Chief Resident (PGY7) in Neurosurgery at University of Pittsburgh Medical Center (UPMC)

On a typical non-cal day:
- 5:00 AM: Alarm.
- 5:15 AM: Out the door on the way to UPMC Presbyterian Hospital.
- 5:30 AM: Chart review via the electronic medical record.
- 6:00 AM: Morning film rounds to review all the new consults as well as update imaging.
- 6:15 AM: ICU rounds with the Critical Care Medicine Team.
- 6:45 AM: Staff patients with attendings.
- 7:00 AM: Examine the patient in the preoperative holding area for first case.
- 7:10 AM: Re-review imaging for case and operative plan with attending.
- 7:30 AM: Position patient on OR table after intubation, lines, neurophysiological monitoring baselines are obtained.
- Surgical cases throughout the day of various lengths and complexity.
- 6:00 PM: Typically start evening rounds and family meetings.
- 7:00 PM: Discuss pertinent updates with attendings.

- 8:00 PM: Run the list with the team and on-call resident.
- 8:30 PM: Return home.
- 8:45 PM: Quick shower.
- 9:00 PM: Prepare for surgical case for following day.
- 9:30 PM: Lights out.

## 45.4 Joel Thomas, MD—Transitional Year Resident (PGY1) at Indiana University Methodist

As discussed in Chapter 44, A Peek at the Residency Application Process, certain medical specialties (radiology, dermatology, physical medicine and rehabilitation, radiation oncology, and some neurology and anesthesia programs) require you to do a separate intern year. Most trainees do a year of medicine or surgery (essentially equivalent to intern year in internal medicine or general surgery). A minority pursue a year of pediatrics (essentially equivalent to an intern year in pediatrics).

The most competitive option is a transitional year, in which the intern "transitions" through various rotations to gain a very broad exposure to medical specialties. The responsibilities, hours worked, and call burden tend to be much lower, as you rotate on more electives vs. heavy inpatient rotations. Here are two examples of rotations I had during my transitional year before starting diagnostic radiology training (PGY2–PGY5) at Washington University in St. Louis.

**Autopsy pathology:** I spent a month on autopsy pathology, assisting the team with dissections and postmortem examination of patients who died unexpectedly in the hospital for unknown reasons.
- **Monday**
  - 7:30 AM: Alarm.
  - 8:00 AM: Get a text from the pathology team that there are no cases for the day. Spend the rest of the day doing whatever I want (e.g., watching TV, working on this book, working out, playing guitar, reading for fun, playing video games, baking, Zooming with friends and family, mindless online shopping).
- **Tuesday**
  - 7:30 AM: Alarm.
  - 8:00 AM: Get a text that there's an autopsy for the day.
  - 8:15–11:30/12: Assist with the autopsy:
    - Write any and all findings on the chalkboard and autopsy note sheet.
    - Slice organs into cross-sections and grossly examine them for signs of pathology (e.g., ischemia/infarction, fat necrosis, tumors, blood clots in the lungs and coronary arteries).
    - Cut fine little sections of each organ into slides for microscopic examination.
    - Review anatomy and pathology with the pathology residents and attendings.
  - **Variations:**
    - Pediatric autopsies typically only took about 2 hours.
    - Brain-cutting days (fine dissection of whole brains) also took about 1 to 2 hours, total. These were great opportunities for neuroanatomy and neuropathology review (e.g., blood vessels, cranial nerves, postmortem normal changes in the brain).
- Repeat for the rest of the week through Friday. Typically, I would have 1 to 3 days off depending on whether there was a case for the day. *One week, I only worked 3.5 hours total.*[1]

Overall, this was a very relaxed rotation with great opportunities for hands-on work and significant teaching and anatomy review from the residents and attendings.

**Inpatient pediatrics:** I spent a month on inpatient pediatrics, basically being a hospital doctor for children with a variety of medical conditions (meningitis, pyelonephritis, pneumonia, failure to thrive, "BRUE" or brief resolved unexplained events, questionable seizure, dehydration from gastroenteritis). This was the most work-heavy rotation I had the entire year, as it was the **only** month I had all year with call or nights.[2]

---

[1] This is why transitional year programs are so competitive.

[2] Again, why transitional year programs are supercompetitive. I would highly recommend Indiana University Methodist to anyone looking for a great transitional year with fantastic learning opportunities and minimal busywork. When I was at work, residents and faculty were extremely eager to teach and incorporate me into the team.

- **Days: 3 weeks, 6 days a week.**
  - 6:00 AM: Alarm.
  - 7:00 AM: Receive sign-out from the night team and review overnight events, vitals, labs, imaging, and consult notes from the previous day on established patients. Do extensive chart review on new patients. See established patients and their family to perform a focused history and physical exam. Spend more time with new patients to hear their story in their and parents' own words (it's poor practice to purely base your decision making on the medical record).
  - 8:00 AM–10:30/11 AM: Round on all of the patients with the team (other interns, resident, +/− attending physician).
    - Pediatrics uses "family centered rounds," in which you explain what has happened with the patient, what the medical team thinks is going on, the plan is for the day, and the big-picture plans (i.e., discharge, follow-up, red flags to look out for that would warrant returning to the ED) *to the patient's family* in layperson terms (vs. medical jargon, as is typically done in rounds). Many people do not enjoy family-centered rounds because they feel that it is harder to communicate and discuss more nuanced information. That said, I was fine with it, as we clarified any possible points of confusion outside the room with the attending, using normal medical jargon.
    - If the attending is not physically present during rounds, the resident will typically communicate the agreed-upon plan from rounds to the attending.
  - 11:00 AM–1:00 PM: Now that the plan has been discussed and approved by the resident and attending, the interns will execute the plan. This includes calling consultant physicians to evaluate and treat the patient, ordering labs and imaging, and communicating the plan to nursing. During this time, the interns will also write notes.
    - Patients that are getting discharged will have their discharge orders and instructions completed (e.g., instructions postdischarge, including education about red flags that would warrant returning to the ED, discharge prescriptions, follow-up instructions).
  - 12:00–1:00 PM: Lunch would be provided, and there would be an educational conference running in the background. If you completed your work by 12:00, you're encouraged to pay attention to the conference. Otherwise, you're free to continue working on notes and clinical duties.
  - 1:00 PM–1:30 PM: "Run the list" with the attending. That is, discussing the plan again with the attending who may have new recommendations/changes since the morning. Attendings will spend additional time on their own reviewing records, evaluating the patient, and discussing with their colleagues, and they may modify the plan from the morning accordingly.
  - 1:30 PM–5:00 PM: During this time, the day is much less regimented. If there's nothing to do, you could basically just hang out and check up on your patients as needed. Typically, you would also respond to messages (our institution switched from 100% pagers to an in-house instant messaging system that made things **so** much easier) from nurses, dieticians, physical therapists, case management, and other physicians throughout the day. I spent much of this time studying for USMLE Step 3.
    - 2:00–3:30 PM: Neurology and psychiatry rounds. The pediatric neurology and pediatric psychiatry teams would come to the team room and discuss their assessment and plans for patients that were on our service. During this time, they would also provide education.
    - If there are new admissions, then an intern will do an admission history and physical exam, come up with an assessment and plan for the patient, discuss with the resident and attending, and place admission orders (e.g., vital signs every 4 h, IV medications, "code status" or whether the patient's family wants full CPR and intubation, etc.). Of note, admissions can show up any time throughout the day (including during rounds), and interns should always be ready to take an admission.
    - Complete sign-out before 5:00 PM. Basically, you fill out an online standardized system (using "IPASS": Illness severity, Patient summary, Action list, Situation awareness and contingency plans —"if the patient has respiratory distress, get a STAT chest X-ray and EKG and low threshold to intubate, and Synthesis by receiver) for each of your patients to be given to the night team.
  - 5:00 PM–5:15/5:30 PM: Give sign-out to the night-team. The online sign-out that you completed will be printed out, and you will verbally explain your sign-out to the night team.
  - 5:30 PM–9:00 PM: Go home, hang out, relax, +/− study for Step 3 and work out.
  - 10:00 PM: Sleep.
- **Short call:** Every 4 days, you will stay beyond 5:00 until 9:00 PM (at earliest) on "short call." During this time, you will take new admissions. There tend to be *many* admissions from 5:00 PM to 9:00 PM.

Typically, I would leave at ~10 PM because I had to tidy up things for the admissions (calling consults, placing orders, communicating to nursing, staffing with the attending) before I could go.

- Fortunately, the residents and attendings were *very* understanding of the fact that I was a transitional resident (and therefore *not* with several months of pediatrics experience) on short call. Specifically, they were very patient with my knowledge gaps and tactfully provided education to fill in those gaps.
- On short call days, you also took the "CART" pager throughout the day (7 AM–5 PM). This is the pager that gets called anytime there was a "code," or critical event (potential cardiopulmonary arrest) requiring a rapid response. I got CART pages typically 0 to 2 times per short call shift. I never had to actually perform CPR, as other providers got to the scene before me every time (even though I tried to get to the scene as quickly as possible). The intern on call was also expected to write a note for the CART event, but I only ended up having to do this once, as the other providers that arrived before me typically told me that they would write the note for me.

- **Weekends:** If you weren't on call, you could leave at around 10:30 to 11 AM after rounds. You simply signed out your patients to the intern on call.
  - If you were on short call during weekends, then good luck. You hold onto the CART pager from 7:00 AM to 5:00 PM. You also take *another pager* corresponding to the teams signing out to you after morning rounds. So from late morning to 5:00 PM, you're fielding pages for both rapid responses *and* whatever issues that the primary teams signed out to you. *This was* **maddening**—*I remember running around like a chicken with his head cut off, responding to non-stop pages left and right. Most of these pages were for fairly minor issues (pain control, "can this patient eat?" "is this patient going home today?"), but I still had to discuss with my senior to make sure I wasn't inadvertently missing something dangerous. I would frequently get pages en route to another page, and each time I would have to stop what I was doing and immediately respond to the new page to make sure I wasn't missing anything emergent.* It was essentially the opposite of flow[3] because of the constant interruptions and inability to focus deeply on any given task.
    - At 5:00 PM, you were relieved of both pagers and left to simply take admissions until 9:00 PM at latest.

- **Nights: 1 week (6 days):** Night float on pediatrics was—by far—my worst experience in residency so far.
  - 7:30 AM to 2–3:30 PM: Try my absolute hardest to get quality sleep in my apartment with blackout curtains, facemask, and earplugs. I suffer from sleep-onset insomnia at baseline, and it was extremely hard to get used to sleeping during the day as other people in my apartment building loved to make noise throughout the day.
  - 5:00 PM–5:15/5:30 PM: Arrive at the hospital and take sign-out from the day team. Take the pager corresponding to the teams you're covering.
  - 5:15/5:30 PM–9:00 PM: You're only responding to pages and messages on issues relating to the day team. You're protected until 9:00 PM from new admissions because the short-call interns are taking admissions. That said, if a short-call intern admits a patient, he/she will sign-out that patient to you, and you will field whatever acute issues arise with the patient.
  - 9:00 PM–12:00 AM: There were usually a *ton* of admissions during this time. Admit patients.
  - 12:00 AM: Eat my "lunch" and drink my energy drink.
  - 12:00 AM–2:00 AM: Typically, acute issues (pages, messages) would arise for the patients during this time, +/– scattered admissions.
  - 2:00 AM–7:00 AM: Usually it would be fairly relaxed during this time.
    - Some interns would try to get some sleep, but it was essentially impossible for me to fall asleep during this time in the hospital. I would try to get scattered 20-minute periods of shut-eye whenever I felt utterly exhausted, but I never truly fell asleep. I wonder if some part of me was too anxious about falling into a deep sleep and missing a page or message. As a result, I spent most of this time mindlessly watching TV (*lots* of *90 Day Fiance*) and YouTube on my phone to pass the time. One day, I brought in my Xbox controller and played Skyrim on my laptop when it was particularly slow.
    - By around 3:00–4:00 AM, the delirium of being awake started to set in, and all of the interns would tend to tell really dumb jokes to each other and crack each other up. Overall, it was a very odd experience, and being the intern on call overnight at a pediatrics hospital felt very bizarre (given that I was going into radiology). Nonetheless, it was a good learning experience on the types of acute issues that arose overnight, as well as the general hospital experience after hours.

---

[3] Oppland M. 8 Characteristics of Flow According to Mihaly Csikszentmihalyi. Available at: https://positivepsychology.com/mihaly-csikszentmihalyi-father-of-flow/. Accessed July 8, 2022.

- It was also a great learning experience in teamwork. Everyone tried his/her hardest to lighten the load for others because it was universally understood that the night float was miserable. This meant that residents and attendings weren't nearly as formal and pedantic during the days. Nursing and other staff tended to be very much to-the-point and efficient in messaging, and late-night messages were kept to a minimum, "as needed" basis. There also tended to be a lot of wonderful snacks.
- 7:00 AM: Sign out to the day team. Carefully drive home and try to fall asleep.
  - I had meal-prepped all of my food for the week before starting nights. Most of the other interns ate from the cafeteria, as we had free meals on our employee badge for nights.

## 45.5 Summary

Depending on what you want to go into, your training (and therefore your life) can be vastly different. Factor these things in when you are picking your field.

# 46 Nonclinical Careers

*Ray Funahashi*

## 46.1 Yes, Some People Don't Pursue a Clinical Career after Medical School

As you know by now, after graduating from medical school you are a "doctor." But this doesn't mean you are a licensed physician—a professional who can independently diagnose and treat patients.

Becoming a physician requires further formal clinical education and training at a residency program. Only then can you be considered a clinician, surgeon, or physician.

A **nonclinical career** means that you are doing work that is not direct patient care. You will see that this encompasses a wide range of jobs, but their realistic availability will narrow the choices for a typical medical graduate.

## 46.2 Why Do People Choose Nonclinical Careers?

Many medical students graduate with debt, and paying off those loans depends on having a decent income. *Practicing as a physician is the safest bet to attain the level of income to pay off loans.*

So you might be wondering then, why do some graduates go on to nonclinical careers?

The reasons vary from person to person, but we will look at the major reasons below:
- Original plan.
- Skillset/Interest mismatch.
- Burnout/Lifestyle.
- Failed residency/Admission.

### 46.2.1 Original Plan

For some people, not going into a clinical career is part of their grand plan from the beginning. The plan is to obtain medical knowledge or intimate first-hand understanding of the healthcare system to leverage in nonclinical careers. That said, this is a tremendously costly investment in time, money, and effort. So, in general, we don't recommend people go to medical school for the exclusive purpose of pursuing a nonclinical career.

For medical school graduates who do pursue nonclinical careers, a significant portion will go into business (Healthcare, Biotech, Pharma, or Management Consulting) or academic research. We will describe these careers in more detail later.

Importantly, many graduates that follow these pathways get a dual-degree (i.e., MD/PhD, MD/MBA—as discussed in Chapter 25, Dual-Degree Programs: MD/PhD, MPH, MBA, JD, and Others) and find ways to minimize their school loans (so requiring a high salary to pay off debt isn't the primary concern).

Those pursuing the business pathway will pursue an MBA degree concurrent with their MD. Many schools offer MD/MBA dual-degree programs. While the MBA degree usually requires additional tuition, the benefit in career options (and networking) is seen as worthwhile. Students may pursue scholarships to lower the amount of debt they accumulate in medical school.

Those pursuing the research pathway will pursue a PhD degree concurrent with their MD. Many schools offer MD/PhD dual-degree programs.

### 46.2.2 Skillset/Interest Mismatch or Pull in a Different Direction

Some people realize their true passion actually doesn't lie with medicine. Having the desire to go to medical school, doing medical school, and practicing medicine are all VERY different things. As described in Chapter 41, Real Talk on a Medical Career, much of how medicine is actually practiced can't be appreciated until experienced firsthand. You might do a 180 about wanting to pursue a medical career because you were kidding yourself about your passion for medicine, forced to go into medicine from external pressure, or didn't realize medicine wasn't for you until too late. This reason can be exacerbated when combined with the reasons below (e.g., burnout/demanding lifestyle).

### 46.2.3 Burnout/Lifestyle

For some people, the hours, emotional toll, constant paperwork, and personal and relationship sacrifices become too much—especially during residency when you are being paid very little per hour. There is a reason "lifestyle" specialties such as dermatology are among the most competitive to get into.

### 46.2.4 Failed Residency/Admission

Some people are forced to go into a nonclinical career because they fail to match into residency (usually multiple times) or they fail out of a residency program.

## 46.3 Pivot Points: When Do People Switch to Nonclinical Careers?

The timing varies from person to person, but they can be categorized into the following:
• Before residency.
• During residency.
• After residency.

### 46.3.1 Before Residency aka During or After Medical School

Some people drop out of medical school or pivot to pursue a nonclinical career after medical school. In this situation, most clinical jobs are not an option because of the lack of residency training. Common reasons for people who pivot during this period are **original plan**, **interest mismatch**, **burnout**, and less commonly **failed residency admission**.

### 46.3.2 During Residency

Residency is a very trying time in terms of lifestyle and emotional toll. The advantage of pivoting during this period is that other clinical jobs (e.g., as a side gig) and jobs that require clinical knowledge (e.g., EMR review/working for health insurance companies) will now be open to you. Common reasons for people who pivot during this period are **interest mismatch**, **burnout**, and less commonly **failed residency**.

### 46.3.3 After Residency

As an attending, lifestyle is generally better compared to residency. However, people do pivot during this period too. Some people pivot immediately after residency utilizing the fact that they are now board-certified as a backup for their career. As with pivoting during residency, the advantage of pivoting during this period is that you qualify for clinical knowledge-dependent jobs, unlike a medical school-only graduate. **Job options greatly open up when pivoting jobs from being or having been a board-certified clinician**. This cannot be understated. The downside is that most options open to you to pivot to will likely be less pay than your clinical job, at least in the beginning. Also, if you know clinical medicine isn't your passion from an early stage, the trade to reach this stage is years of misery and losing years that could have been spent toward building a career in your true interest. Common reasons for people who pivot during this period are **interest mismatch**, **burnout**, and less commonly **original plan**.

## 46.4 What Are the Typical Nonclinical Jobs?

Most nonclinical jobs medical graduates and career-switchers pursue fall into the following categories:
• Consulting (business strategy and management).
• Biotech.
• Pharma.
• Research (academia).
• Data science (biomedical informatics).
• Health insurance/Chart reviewing.
• Hospital management.

- Healthcare policy.
- Graduate and medical school admissions consulting.
- Medical writing/Medical education content producer.
- Investing/Venture capital (VC).
- Entrepreneur.
- Limited practice.

### Big Brands

For some jobs, for better or for worse, having Big Brands on your CV gives you a big advantage. Big Brands are schools, organizations, businesses, honors that are prestigious and widely known.
Some examples:
- Schools: Harvard, Oxford, Stanford, MIT, Penn, Columbia, etc.
- Businesses: Google, Amazon, Apple, Microsoft, etc.
- Organizations: United Nations, NASA, NIH, World Bank, Bill and Melinda Gates Foundation
- Honors: Rode Scholarship, Marshall Scholarship

### Quantitative (aka Quant / Math) skills

For some jobs, you will need to demonstrate proficiency in mathematics and statistics. These are colloquially referred to as "quant" skills. The way companies and institutions identify if you have requisite quant skills is often through your school transcripts, and occasionally, administered tests and on-the-spot problems during technical interviews. The exact quant skills you need to apply for a particular job will vary, but they can include Calculus, Probability and Statistics, and Linear Algebra. This means that you need to plan accordingly to meet these requirements before applying to jobs that require them. This is not an issue for applicants who already have engineering, computer science, physics, or mathematics background.

## 46.4.1 Consulting (Business Strategy and Management)

Management consulting is the most popular option for people who pivot after medical school or during residency.

Consulting is essentially "brain rental" for businesses. You will be hired to analyze or advise a business on what to do to fix a problem. You can work independently (which is difficult without previous experience) or you will work as an employee and part of a team for a consulting firm.

As a consultant, you may work in areas such as healthcare, investment, legal matters, electronic medical record (EMR). Your MD/DO background is mainly leveraged for credibility, and surprisingly, depending on your project assignment, you may or may not use your medical knowledge at all!

## Pros

- Consulting jobs are one of the highest paying among nonclinical options. If you are working for McKinsey, Bain, or Boston Consulting Group, then it is very reasonable to make at least $200,000 per year out of medical school, with annual increases of 10-20%. This is the case even if you didn't attend a prestigious medical school or undergraduate program.[1] If you have medical school debt, this would be something to consider.
- Typically you will have a variety of projects you are assigned to, so you may have exposure to fields you otherwise wouldn't have any interaction with. Depending on your preference, this can keep things interesting or overwhelming.
- Consulting jobs (at firms) have decent upward mobility and often it opens many doors to other career pathways and options.

---

[1] https://managementconsulted.com/management-consulting-what-is-it/

## Cons

- You may or may not utilize your medical knowledge depending on the firm and projects you are assigned.
  - At a general business management consulting firm, for example, you could be assigned to helping an automaker make a business decision, but assigned to helping a medical insurance company in another assignment.
  - Large consulting companies can assign you work on projects in which you have no background knowledge of because they have their own large network of true experts that they expect you to consult and learn what you need to know quickly. Or a senior member of the team may already have a relevant background and they will be supervising you.
- The lifestyle for entry-level consultants is notoriously bad due to constant assigned travel and long hours. How much you travel will depend on the firm. Generally speaking, as a low-ranking associate, you are often sent to meet in person with the client and be "on-site" to conduct studies and observations. The traveling can be novel in the beginning but can become exhausting pretty quickly. As you advance in the ranks, the lifestyle may improve. However, this is partly why many people choose to do consulting as a stepping stone onto other careers with similar to slightly-lower income with substantially better lifestyle.
- For general business management consulting firms, an MD, regardless of your experience, will likely be hired as an Associate, which is an entry-level position for postgraduate candidates. Candidates who don't have a graduate degree often start in the position below this, as Business Analysts.
  - This means that, whether you are a fresh MD out of medical school, or a seasoned attending with 15 years of experience, you will likely be starting in the Associate position.
  - For this reason, pivoting to management consulting is less popular for attending physicians because the starting pay is lower than an attending salary. Keep in mind, however, that you will be making much more money than a resident if coming straight out of medical school, with opportunities to make as much as - or more than - attending physicians if you stay the track.
- As an Associate, you will be doing a fair share of creating PowerPoints and excel spreadsheets.

## Recommendation

- The competition for entry into this field is fierce. You will be competing with post-MBA applicants. You may be asked to take a math exam and an interview where you demonstrate solving business case problems, called Case Interviews. You cannot simply decide to apply on a whim. You will need to prepare weeks to months to perform well with case interviews.
  - For case interviews, consult an MBA student for the latest popular resources (e.g., https://www.craftingcases.com/, https://www.rocketblocks.me/), and seek practice partners (e.g., via https://www.preplounge.com/en) to build your skills.
- In addition to clearing interview hurdles, you will need to show previous business experience to be competitive for these jobs.
  - Having an MBA could substitute for this, which is why doing an MD-MBA would be a great advantage.
- For top-tier management consulting firms (such as McKinsey, BCG, Bain), big brands on your CV matter.
- Your standardized test scores will somewhat matter for these top-tier firms.
- Having quant skills is highly recommended.
- Network as much as you can (especially by reaching out to recruiters seeking to hire physicians), keep a record of your contacts, and try to get as many warm introductions as possible.

## 46.4.2  Biotechnology (Bio-Tech/Med-Tech)

Biotech and med-tech companies will hire MDs to work in sales, consulting, business analysis, research, and liaison roles. For people who have completed residency, working in biotech/med-tech or pharmaceutical companies are popular for career pivoting. Unlike in management consulting, having clinical training and experience actually does influence your pay and ability to bypass entry-level positions.

## Pros

- Pay can be moderate to high, depending on the job. If you have medical school debt, this would be something to consider.
- There is usually decent upward mobility and the experience can open doors to other opportunities.
- You may utilize some of your medical knowledge.

## Cons

- You may need to travel extensively, depending on the job.
- You may be involved in work and projects that don't rely on your medical background.

## Recommendation

- You will often need to have previous business experience to be competitive for these jobs.
  - If you decide to pivot to this route during medical school, intern at a biotech company sometime before graduating. This will help you stand out from MD's with no experience in biotech.
  - A lesser option would be to intern at your university's research commercialization institute to gain market analysis and commercialization experience.
- Having previous research experience relevant to the company's focus makes you a better candidate.
- Getting a dual-degree during medical school, such as PhD, MBA, or MS (i.e., bioengineering) helps greatly.
- Network as much as you can and try to get as many warm introductions as possible.

### 46.4.3 Pharmaceutics (Pharma)

Pharmaceutical companies will hire MDs to work in sales, consulting, business analysis, research, and liaison roles. For people who have completed residency, working in biotech/med-tech or pharmaceutical companies are popular for career pivoting. Unlike in management consulting, having clinical training and experience actually does influence your pay and ability to bypass entry-level positions.

## Pros

- Pay can be moderate to high, depending on the job. If you have medical school debt, this would be something to consider.
- There is usually decent upward mobility and the experience can open doors to other opportunities.
- You may utilize some of your medical knowledge.

## Cons

- You may need to travel extensively, depending on the job.
- You may be involved in work and projects that don't rely on your medical background.

## Recommendation

- You will often need to have previous business experience to be competitive for these jobs.
  - If you decide to pivot to this route during medical school, intern at a pharmaceutical company sometime before graduating. This will help you stand out from MDs with no experience in pharma.
  - A lesser option would be to intern at your university's research commercialization institute to gain market analysis and commercialization experience.
- Having previous research experience relevant to the company's focus makes you a better candidate.
- Getting a dual-degree during medical school, such as PhD, MBA, or MS (i.e., bioengineering) helps greatly.
- Network as much as you can, keep a record of your contacts, and try to get as many warm introductions as possible.

## 46.4.4 Research (Academia, Pharmaceutical Industry, or Government)

For people interested in making research the focus of their career, becoming an academic or federal (i.e., NIH) researcher is the goal. Typically, medical graduates will pursue a postdoctoral research fellowship and/or research grants in order to become a Principal Investigator (PI) at a university or federal institution. Having a history of producing research publications is key for entering this job field. Deans at medical schools typically have a research background.

### Pros

- You will gain deep and cutting-edge expertise in a specific knowledge field.
- You get the opportunity to make an impact and advance knowledge.
- It is intellectually challenging.
- With sufficient experience, there is an option to transition to industry, if desired.

### Cons

- The pay is typically relatively low (unless you are in pharma) and that makes it difficult to pay off debt unless you go the MD/PhD route (no debt).
- Faculty positions are limited and highly competitive; becoming a PI is difficult.
- There is constant pressure to produce as many publications as possible.

### Recommendation

- Research and publish as much as possible during medical school and residency.
- If you want to do clinical research for a career, you will need to build experience first.
- Having big brands on your CV matters.
- Getting a dual-degree during medical school, such as PhD, MPH, or MS (i.e., field of research interest) helps greatly.
- Try to amass presentations, talks, and grants to put on your CV.
- Find and work with experienced and supportive research mentors as early as possible.
- Network as much as you can, keep a record of your contacts, and try to get as many warm introductions as possible.

## 46.4.5 Data Science (Biomedical/Clinical Informatics)

People who are interested in making biomedical data useful or gathering actionable clinical insights from data can pursue a career in biomedical informatics. With the explosion in the technologies of Machine Learning (ML) and Artificial Intelligence (AI), bioinformatics is a hot field that will continue to grow. The field is wide, with analysis being conducted in fields such as genomics and proteomics in addition to clinical informatics such as EMR and clinical trials, personalized medicine. Having clinical knowledge and direct experience using the EMR gives a tremendous advantage when working in the field of clinical informatics.

### Pros

- You will gain deep and cutting-edge expertise in a specific knowledge field.
- You have the opportunity to generate impact and advance knowledge.
- It is intellectually challenging.
- Opportunity to apply medical knowledge and computational methods.
- Pay can be moderate to high, depending on the job. If you have medical school debt, this would be something to consider.
- You will gain transferable skills and the job could open other doors, both in academia and industry.

## Cons

- These jobs typically require additional training and study (often a master's degree or PhD).

## Recommendation

- Dual degree (MD/MS or MD/PhD in computer Science, biomedical informatics or data science are tremendously advantageous).
- Quant skills are mandatory.
- Computer science (CS) skills are mandatory (i.e., often at minimum a BS in computer science, biomedical informatics, data science, or engineering unless you already have an alternative requisite background).
- Research and publish as much as possible during medical school and residency.
- Try to amass presentations, talks, and grants to put on your CV.
- Find and work with experienced and supportive research mentors as early as possible.
- Network as much as you can, keep a record of your contacts, and try to get as many warm introductions as possible.

## 46.4.6 Health Insurance/Chart Reviewing

Working for a Health Insurance company is a popular option for experienced physicians with burnout or looking to transition away from clinical care. Because of the necessity for clinical experience, this job category is often not an option for pre-residency pivoters (aka medical students or fresh medical school graduates).

## Pros

- Both part-time and full-time jobs are possible.
- You will be using your medical knowledge and expertise.
- Pay can be moderately high depending on job and experience.
- Lifestyle: work schedule can be tailored more or less to your preference.

## Cons

- Some people may feel conflicted about doing work that includes denying medical insurance claims.
- The work may feel repetitive.
- No seeing patients.

## Recommendation

- Network as much as you can, keep a record of your contacts, and try to get as many warm introductions as possible.

## 46.4.7 Hospital Management

Working in hospital management is a popular option for experienced physicians with interests in business management, looking to transition away from clinical care, or experiencing burnout. Because of the necessity for clinical experience and knowledge about the workings of a hospital or clinic, this job category is often not an option for pre-residency pivoters (aka medical students or fresh medical school graduates). Previous business experience is a key advantage for those who want to enter this job field.

## Pros

- Both part-time and full-time jobs are possible.
- You will be using your medical knowledge and expertise.
- Pay can be moderately high depending on job and experience.

## Cons

- Some people may feel conflicted about having to work with costs and profit motive in healthcare.

## Recommendation

- You will need to have previous business experience to be competitive for these jobs.
  - Having an MBA is valued, so doing an MD-MBA dual degree would be an advantage.
  - With the right networking at your hospital, you can take on business management-type projects and assignments as an attending and slowly build experience and responsibility over time before applying to full-time hospital management jobs.
- Having big brands on your CV matters.
- Network as much as you can, keep a record of your contacts, and try to get as many warm introductions as possible.

### 46.4.8 Healthcare Policy

This is a popular option for people who had an original plan to pursue a career in healthcare policy or have a strong desire to affect social change and the health of populations through governmental policies. Entering jobs in healthcare policy often requires previous experience, relevant research, or a supporting degree.

## Pros

- Both part-time and full-time jobs are possible.
- You may use your medical knowledge and expertise.
- You get the opportunity to make an impact through changes in governmental and healthcare policy.
- The work can be intellectually intensive.
- The work may have variety.

## Cons

- Pay can be on the lower end.
- Additional study (e.g., MPH) may be necessary.

## Recommendation

- A dual-degree or second degree (JD, MPH, or MPP) may be advantageous in policy work.
- Having big brands on your CV matters for establishing immediate credibility.
- Research and publish as much as possible in your field of choice (the more related to policy, the better).
- Seek an internship at a think-tank or policy-research institution if possible.
- Network as much as you can, keep a record of your contacts, and try to get as many warm introductions as possible.

### 46.4.9 Graduate and Medical School Admissions Consulting

If you want to help pre-medical students and graduate students pursue their dreams of a career in medicine, you might become a graduate/medical school admissions consultant. You can work as an independent consultant or you could also work for an admissions consulting company. If working independently you will earn higher pay but you will need to work on marketing and attracting students yourself. If working with a company, your pay will be lower but the company will supply you with students to work with.

## Pros

- Both part-time and full-time jobs are possible.
- You get the opportunity to make an impact by helping aspiring graduate and medical students.
- Low barrier of entry.

## Cons

- It may be difficult to maintain this as a full-time job due to its seasonal/cyclic nature.
- You probably will not use your medical knowledge.
- Pay per hour may be high, but total pay may be low due to the inconsistent volume of applicant customers.

## Recommendation

- Look to serve on the admissions committee of your medical school because former admissions committee or interviewer experience gives you a tremendous advantage when applying to jobs in Admissions Counseling.
- Having big brands on your CV matters.
- Build testimonials over time by helping as many students as possible whenever you can and save their testimonials to promote your services in the future.

## 46.4.10 Medical Writing/Medical Education Content Producer

Those who are interested in using their medical knowledge for writing (often nonacademic) publications can pursue a career in medical writing. In a related sense, those who are interested in writing medical education test questions for standardized tests or commercial question banks, or producing medical education multimedia can pursue a career as a medical education content producer. This can be pursued independently or by working for a company. Depending on the subject knowledge necessary, this job can be open to medical graduates and clinicians of all levels.

## Pros

- Both part-time and full-time jobs are possible.
- You get the opportunity to make an impact by creating educational medical content or writing.
- You may use your medical knowledge and expertise.

## Cons

- It may be difficult to maintain this as a full-time job due to relatively low pay.
- The work can be time-intensive.
- The lower pay may make it difficult to pay off loan debt.

## Recommendation

- Network as much as you can, keep a record of your contacts, and try to get as many warm introductions as possible.
- Publish articles and papers as much as possible to build your portfolio.

## 46.4.11 Investing/Venture Capital

People who are interested in healthcare technology investing can pursue a career investment and venture capital by working at firms. Technically, although a career in this space can be pursued by anyone with a bachelor's degree, the catch-22 is that it is extremely difficult to obtain a job without prior relevant experience (preferably at reputable firms).

## Pros

- Technically, this career can be pursued at any time.
- The pay is moderate to high depending on the job. If you have medical school debt, this would be something to consider.
- You will utilize knowledge about healthcare fields and trends.

## Cons

- The field is very difficult to break into—venture capital is notoriously difficult.
- Lifestyle: Similar to management consulting, work-life balance may not be very good, especially at the entry-level.

## Recommendation

- The competition for entry into this field is fierce. You will be competing with post-MBA applicants.
- You will need to show previous business experience to be competitive for these jobs.
  - Having an MBA will NOT substitute for this, though doing an MD-MBA would still be a great advantage.
  - The best thing you can do to make yourself competitive for these jobs is to intern at investment and venture capital firms. Some medical students can pull this off during a summer of off-year during medical school. However, those students usually have undergraduate business backgrounds.
- Having big brands on your CV matters.
- Having quant skills is highly recommended.
- Network as much as you can, keep a record of your contacts, and try to get as many warm introductions as possible.

## 46.4.12 Entrepreneur/Start-up

People who are entrepreneurial at heart may start or join start-ups. Typically successful entrepreneurs are individuals who are extremely tenacious, passionate about a problem, obsessed with innovative problem-solving, and have a very high risk and reward tolerance. The entrepreneur is not limited to solving only problems in the medical space; however, this would be most applicable given an MD/DO background. Start-ups require great sacrifice in time, effort, finances, and they have a high fail-risk. Because of this, unless you have an intense passion and desire for solving a particular problem with a start-up, we don't recommend this career path.

## Pros

- You get the opportunity to make an impact by creating something that will address a societal or commercial need.
- You will have the ultimate agency over your career and life, if successful.
- You may utilize medical knowledge, depending on your innovation/venture.
- You can technically pursue this career at any point, whether you are a seasoned physician or a noob fresh out of medical school.

## Cons

- A majority of start-ups fail.
- Lifestyle: Long hours with low pay, especially in the beginning.
- Because of the low pay (unless you eventually succeed), it is difficult to pay off loan debt.

## Recommendation

- Getting a dual-degree during medical school, such as an MBA (for business foundational knowledge and networking), or another degree related to your innovation (e.g., MS or PhD) will help greatly.
  - Gaining prior business experience will help. The easiest way to do this would be internships as businesses during medical school (summer or off-year).
  - Consider relocating to an entrepreneur-friendly city (aka a city with abundant and willing investors) to network during your off-year while working on your innovation.
- Find as many funding sources as a medical student, if possible since many people will be willing to talk to you.

- Fail fast with product iterations and test rapidly. Learn from feedback and keep adjusting or pivoting your idea or product. Try to produce a working prototype as soon as possible.
- For excellent free general entrepreneurship classes and advice, check out the StartUp School on YouTube run by Y Combinator.
- Network as much as you can, keep a record of your contacts, and try to get as many warm introductions as possible.

## 46.4.13 Limited Practice

Okay, so limiting clinical practice is not really a career pivot, but it often is the financial bridge while transitioning to other careers. Some people will continue to keep a part-time clinical job indefinitely while working other jobs, lower the clinical work volume to avoid burnout, address lifestyle issues, and devote time to other interests.

### Pros

- You still get to apply and maintain your clinical knowledge and skills.
- Lifestyle: you choose the weekly total hours.
- High hourly pay:
  - Locum tenems (part-time traveling clinical work) earns very high hourly pay, and you can do it for a few days or even months out of the year, depending on the company.

### Cons

- The travel can get tiresome, and the locations you are assigned to may not be desirable.

### Recommendation

- Network as much as you can, keep a record of your contacts, and try to get as many warm introductions as possible.

## 46.5 Summary

There are a variety of reasons medical students elect to not go into residency. Sometimes they weren't competitive enough to match, but often it's that, for a multitude of reasons, they would rather do something else. Once you know exactly the type of field you would like to transition to, you can use your time in medical school (if you plan on finishing) to continue specializing. This can be done with a dual degree (MBA, MPH, etc.), or by using your off time to gain experience/specialization or gain networking contacts in your eventual field. Some fields are easier and more lucrative to transition to than others, but an MD might be a major selling point for prospective employers—more of a bonus than a professional detour.

# 47 Stories of Inspiration

## 47.1 Joel Thomas—"Fake Pneumonia"

I was about halfway through my inpatient adult medicine rotation. The expectations and responsibilities had ramped up dramatically compared to my medical school rotations. I had just started to feel somewhat comfortable managing six to eight medically complex patients. I was expected to know every little detail about each patient and come up with a reasonable assessment and plan. I was expected to follow-up on the status of every plan by keeping in active communication with every member of the healthcare team (e.g., consultant physicians, dieticians, physical and occupational therapy, case management). I was expected to be both thorough and quick. Mind you, this was only my second month as a doctor (and my first month as a doctor on an inpatient rotation).

It was an especially busy day when I was given this new admitted patient. By this point, my workflow for new patients consisted of trusting and reviewing other clinicians' assessments and independently verifying. For the most part, I trusted other clinicians' judgment. After all, what reason would I have to trust myself (after about a month of residency training) over the admitting emergency physician with decades of experience in patient care?

The ED note said that he had been experiencing cough and fatigue for several days. His chest X-ray was read as having some opacities (areas of abnormal density/whiteness) suggestive of pneumonia. There's really only one reasonable diagnosis in an elderly man with cough and chest X-ray findings consistent with pneumonia. Hint hint, it's pneumonia.

So he was started on IV antibiotics and admitted to our general medicine service. For the sake of completeness, I went down and personally interviewed him and performed a physical exam. I also attempted to review his imaging myself. Several things made me pause. First, I really couldn't appreciate any opacities on his chest X-ray that would suggest pneumonia. I wasn't sure what to make of this because I didn't have a whole lot of experience reading chest X-rays, and I felt that I should trust the judgment of the radiologist who has probably read thousands of chest X-rays. The patient also didn't really have a classic clinical presentation of pneumonia. He didn't have overt shortness of breath. He didn't have a fever. His lung examination was essentially normal. In fact, he really only complained of chronic cough, and on further questioning, he reported many allergy symptoms (runny nose, itchy and watery eyes, nasal congestion). He had also been using a steroid inhaler typically used for allergies many years ago but stopped prior to the onset of these symptoms. His symptoms had also been going on for weeks, versus a typically acute to subacute onset for pneumonia.

My attending physician had warned me about the preponderance of "fake pneumonias" in the hospital. He explained that it was very easy for ED physicians to "see" opacities on the chest X-ray that weren't really there and to admit and treat the patient for pneumonia. It's a fairly risk-averse strategy, and it provides an actionable explanation for the patient's symptoms. In addition, pneumonia is extremely common and can be fatal if not rapidly treated. So from the ED's perspective, it's totally reasonable to be trigger-happy and treat "fake pneumonia." Moreover, ED physicians are typically swamped with patients and have to make quick treatment decisions off of limited information.

The internist, however, has time to be more discerning. If you have to squint really hard to see the pneumonia, my attending explained, then it's probably *not there*. Instead, you need to dig deeper and find an alternative explanation for the patient's symptoms. In this case, I had immediate initial doubts about the pneumonia diagnosis and felt that the patient had allergic rhinitis causing postnasal drip (aka upper airway cough syndrome), one of the most common causes of chronic cough. My attending felt this was a reasonable explanation, and we stopped antibiotics. To everyone's relief, the patient's symptoms improved dramatically over time with inhaled steroids.

The story could end here, and I would still fondly remember it as a case for trusting my own clinical judgment and scientific skepticism. But—of course—there's more.

When I initially interviewed the patient, he had offhandedly mentioned that he was experiencing fatigue, unintentional weight loss, and occasional heart palpitations for several weeks. I also noticed that his heart rate was elevated and had been elevated for several weeks. From my studies, I knew that it was appropriate to check thyroid function levels and to get an EKG, given his palpitations and elevated heart rate. I was essentially certain that they would be normal, as *every* patient with palpitations that I had done this for had normal thyroid levels. Still, the recommendations were clear that it was worth checking, and I felt that it was good to practice evidence-based medicine to be thorough and complete.

Imagine my surprise when his thyroid function tests were *grossly* abnormal. This was an elderly African American man with no known personal or family history of thyroid or autoimmune disease presenting with potential severe hyperthyroidism. The textbook presentation for hyperthyroidism is a young to middle-aged White woman, often with bulging eyes and wet, sweaty skin. No one on my team—myself included—expected this result. We immediately followed up with an extensive endocrine evaluation. The patient was ultimately diagnosed with severe Graves disease and started on appropriate treatment. He now follows with endocrinology for his new diagnosis of Graves disease and responded extremely well to treatment.

This was one of my most memorable experiences as a doctor. I was just over a month into my intern year (and 2 weeks into my training as an inpatient medicine doctor) when I diagnosed severe Graves disease in a *very* unlikely patient. I had originally felt sheepish even suggesting the thyroid function tests, as I expected them to be stone-cold normal. Still, the patient *had* reported palpitations, fatigue, and unintentional weight loss, and the recommendations for work-up were clear—even if seemingly very academic and low yield. This was someone who could have been treated for and discharged with an illness he did not have. Instead, my careful history-taking revealed subtle symptoms that were initially missed, leading to a completely different diagnostic work-up that revealed a serious treatable condition. I truly felt like a doctor in that moment, as my training and attention to detail made a genuine difference that could have been—and *was*—missed by other providers.

I experienced a renewed appreciation for medicine. Up till that point, I often felt that my role as an intern was largely to "move the meat," i.e., writing notes, ensuring timely admissions and discharge, placing orders, calling consults, and other secretarial tasks. I figured that much of the deep diagnostic reasoning wouldn't be emphasized until later in my training. But even as an early intern, I saw that the individual physician's efforts could make a tremendous impact on patients' outcomes. I realized that although much of patient care can feel algorithmic and mindless, the ceiling is essentially limitless in terms of the individual physician's efforts and contributions. In the true spirit of academic medicine, I was inspired to continue carrying that level of scientific skepticism to all of my patients moving forward. It still stands as a core principle of my approach to doctoring: the physician ultimately has the responsibility to carefully collect and synthesize all the relevant information. Even as a future radiologist, I wholeheartedly agree with Sir William Osler's adage that you should "listen to the patient, as he is telling you the diagnosis."[1]

## 47.2 Phillip Wagner—"The Bigger Picture"

She did not look well. She was sitting in her bed with her husband by her side. The sign-out from the ED was that she had fallen off her porch. Her story was reasonable, and involved drinking and friends and a clumsy tendency. Imaging showed a fractured pelvis, but it was nondisplaced, so no surgery was needed. I gave her the diagnosis, detailed how we would treat her pain, and told her she would be evaluated by our physical therapy team in the morning. She was grateful, agreeable, but also seemed at times uninterested or preoccupied. I noticed her urine drug screen was positive for heroin and cocaine, and attributed her lack of attention to a combination of intoxication, pain, and as it was 2 AM-fatigue. Her husband was polite, but curt, and spent most of the time hovering awkwardly in the corner.

As I was documenting her exam, I read about her previous hospitalizations. She was absolutely a frequent flyer. Four admissions in as many months, all for some sort of trauma. Falls, car accidents, robberies. The last admission was 6 weeks ago where she was reportedly the pedestrian half of a hit and run, no police report, no witnesses. Urine drug screens were positive for multiple illicit substances. She had been referred for rehabilitation services countless times, and labs from her last visit indicated a high probability of her having hepatitis C.

---

[1] William Osler: A Life in Medicine. BMJ 2000;321:1087. Available at: https://www.bmj.com/content/321/7268/1087.2/rr/760724. Accessed July 8, 2022.

While Hepatitis C can certainly be transmitted by contaminated needles, there is a nonzero chance of it being an STD as well. Sharing a positive diagnosis therefore can be complicated. You aren't just telling someone they have a serious disease, but also possibly telling them something about their relationship or their partner that may be more impactful. So, while this patient was "OK" with us sharing medical information in front of her husband, this is the type of information that tends to be shared privately. Only, privacy never seemed to be on the table.

She needed to stay in the hospital for days so we could manage her pain. Yet, at 6 AM when I walked in the hospital, during rounds, on my way to coffee at mid-afternoon, and on the way out the door at night, her husband was at her bedside. There is supportive, and then there is ever-present. And while it isn't unreasonable for a family member to never leave the hospital—it happens from time to time—this felt different. He was close when I was in the room, but was somehow not involved. He was polite, but only spoke when spoken to.

Eventually, the nursing staff and medical team alike grew suspicious. Stepwise, the evidence of domestic abuse accumulated, first circumstantial, and then substantial. Nurses ran interference while we ordered fake tests that required she be transported to another floor. While there, she hinted at what concerned us most, but came up short of admitting it frankly. We shared her Hepatitis C diagnosis, and she made us promise not to tell her husband. She was discharged with a phony appointment for a mammogram, which was actually a number for a women's shelter should she need it. She thanked us, and they left together.

Roughly one week later, our patient called. She was calling from the ground in her apartment. Her husband had broken her wheelchair, stolen her pain medication, and abandoned her. She had called the police. Once she was back in the hospital, we verified her husband was in police custody. She admitted to everything—the broken pelvis, the falls, the car accident—was actually her husband.

The second hospitalization felt how medicine is supposed to feel. A person needs help, and item by item, you assess, fix, find others that can be fixed, and guide. People leave better than when you first meet them. And, by the time she had left several days later, she looked like a new person, and we felt like we had helped with that. She looked so much better that I didn't even worry when she missed our scheduled follow-up appointment. And then she missed her second appointment.

The next time I saw her, it was almost a year later. She was thin, weary, and I don't think she remembered who I was, even though she said she did. She came in with an infection, likely from a return to drug use. And, in her room, sitting in the corner, legs crossed, hovering but not doting—was her husband. I asked him to leave the room, and she stopped me. "No, I want him here."

I've had a lot of good moments in medicine—they aren't infrequent. But I can already tell there are not enough of them alone to want to do this job, at least for me. There has to be some pleasure, or at least a measure of satisfaction, in the process—even when the outcome you want doesn't happen. I don't know how this patient is doing right now—if she has gotten away from her abusive relationship, if she has been able to win her battle with addiction, or if her family still talks to her. I've heard she has come in several times since, so I have to trust that the fight continues, hopefully with providers that will have more luck than I. I don't know that we, for all our effort, were able to overcome the constraints, incentives, and reality of her life. But I'm certainly happy we tried, and that has to be enough sometimes.

## 47.3 Nitin Agarwal—"The Axon to Neurological Surgery"

While family members in medicine provided an early exposure to health sciences, another foremost formative influence was attending boarding school, where I was surrounded by extremely high-caliber and talented peers. There is an infectious energy to high achievement. The Lawrenceville School further cemented my interest in medicine, a field full of driven individuals.

To this end, upon graduation from boarding school, I enrolled at the accelerated 7-year BA/MD program with medical school at Rutgers New Jersey Medical School, where I had an incredibly rewarding mentorship with the faculty neurosurgeons. Going into medical school, I already had a strong inclination toward surgery. As with other things in my life, I simply found something I was passionate about, kept at it, and maintained the momentum. Several experiences reinforced this interest. At the beginning of medical school, I found myself in the emergency room of the Level 1 Trauma Center in Newark, where I assisted the neurosurgery resident to place an external ventricular drain in a patient who suffered a severe traumatic brain injury. In addition, I had the opportunity to participate in basic science and translational research to improve outcomes following spinal cord injury. In my experience, most people in neurosurgery note some substantial clinical or research exposure to the field and simply cannot imagine doing anything else. Fortunately, I was lucky enough to be given the opportunity to train at the University of Pittsburgh Medical Center where I, at the time of this writing, serve as a Chief Resident in Neurological Surgery.

In retrospect, I find myself pleasantly surprised by how quickly 7 years of training has passed. I can still vividly picture first being the intern learning the ropes and then the junior resident on call as the first contact for the inpatient neurosurgical service. Neurosurgery training may be cited as long and arduous. Residents are typically the first service to enter and the last to leave the hospital each day. Every patient encounter becomes another humbling moment. To this end, I credit my martial arts training from a young age with providing me the mental and physical stamina to enact relentless, top-notch patient care.

One case remains fresh in my mind as a testament to this fact. Early in my training as a junior resident, I was scrubbed into a common procedure in the operating room—a straightforward decompression to remove an abscess from a patient's back. Everything was moving smoothly as if on autopilot. However, all of a sudden I was engulfed by an overwhelming sense of terror. I thought I had violated the spinal cord and instantly caused permanent neurologic damage. I was terrified at the thought that I alone had hurt someone so gravely with my own hands.

With years of experience, my attending just chuckled knowing all was still well. What I mistook as a terrible complication was thankfully only minor bleeding. Nevertheless, my recollection of the case constantly reminds me that patient care especially in the operating theater is always high stakes. At the same time, it highlighted the importance of the mentorship that makes this field so special to me. The privileged opportunity to operate on the brain and spine necessitates the length and complexity of our training.

Despite this constant sense of gravity, I remain excited to come into work every day amid the challenges of hospital-based medicine. In the trenches, my coresidents bring an abundance of joy and camaraderie. Most importantly, I cannot express enough unwavering gratitude to my mentors and patients for all the training I continue to receive.

# Section V

## Appendix

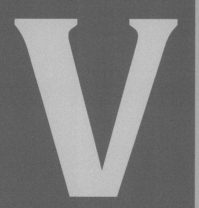

# Appendix A: Resources

There are a lot of useful pre-med resources. This book compiles the best recommendations from multiple sources and also offers original commentary on conflicting strategies across the different resources. Still, we recommend exploring these other resources if you're still hungry for more perspectives. We maintain an up-to-date list of these resources at http://www.premedicine.co/. As always, we urge you to weigh the *evidence* behind what you read and whether it's *applicable* to your particular circumstances.

## A.1 Student Doctor Network (SDN) Forum

For US pre-meds, the SDN forums dominate online discussion. It is the largest collection of user-driven content on US medical schools. If you have questions about anything related to being pre-med, you can post them and get feedback almost immediately. More importantly, you will frequently have ADCOM members posting and replying in real time.

That said, you should generally read their recommendations with a grain of salt. SDN has a reputation for being overly harsh and pessimistic in their expectations for the successful applicant. A (somewhat accurate) caricature of the typical SDN post is a pre-med with a 3.9 GPA and 90th percentile MCAT worrying about getting into medical school because they "had a slight downtrend GPA trend." In addition, you will find many differing recommendations from different users on various topics, and it's difficult to gauge the "best" advice—especially when it's given by non-ADCOM members. The SDN community is also non-representative of medicine as a whole. While many people in medicine have heard of it, very few actually post on it (or at least admit to doing so, anyway).

The school-specific threads deserve their own mention. Current medical students at medical schools frequently post on them and answer whatever questions are asked. They are also updated in real time during the application cycle. Because of the SDN forums, one of the authors actually found out that he was accepted to Pitt before the "official" decision release date; the Pitt thread had announced that admissions decisions were prematurely released.

Ultimately, SDN can be an extremely valuable source of "insider" information about medical schools because anonymous medical students and physicians—including ADCOM members—post on the website. At the same time, there is *no* guarantee that whoever is posting is entirely honest. Be skeptical when you read posts. If there's an overwhelming amount of negativity, step back and ask whether the poster may have some ulterior motive or whether there's more to the story that isn't being shared. If a product is heavily advertised (or slandered), consider whether the poster has commercial ties. *Verify* whatever information is posted with more legitimate sources; if you're unable to, do more research before trusting the post blindly.

## A.2 Reddit

Specifically, reddit.com/r/premed, reddit.com/r/medicalschool, reddit.com/r/medicine, reddit.com/r/residency, reddit.com/r/medicalschoolanki.

Reddit is a discussion website divided into various individual "subreddits," e.g., reddit.com/r/premed, reddit.com/r/food. Each subreddit functions as its own autonomous discussion board and is maintained by moderators. Users can post and comment on various threads, and their threads and comments are "upvoted"; highly upvoted posts and comments earn more visibility. You do not need to make an account to view Reddit content.

Reddit.com/r/premed is *extremely* helpful, and much of the content we discuss in this book is echoed there. Like SDN, you can post about virtually anything and get immediate feedback from users. Reddit.com/r/premed allows you to engage in conversation with (self-proclaimed) medical students, residents, and attendings. Admittedly, you will simply have to trust users at their word that they are actually medical students and doctors, but it's fairly obvious that they are given the breadth and depth to which they cover topics related to medical training. As with SDN (and any other site with nonverified users), you should be open minded to advice but independently verify. While the anonymity of discussion boards allows for a level of open discussion that may not be otherwise obtained, you should always be cautious about possible sources of bias (e.g., uncovered advertisers) when assessing actionable advice.

Reddit is updated in real time, and the medicine subreddits are extremely active. The medicine subreddits are also extremely entertaining, and users frequently post memes about relatable struggles on the medical journey. You will also find many "Ask Me Anything" (AMA) threads, which can be incredibly enlightening if you have an especially candid medical student or resident (bonus points if they have ADCOM experience).

Reddit.com/r/medicalschoolanki deserves its own mention, as several highly popular Anki decks were born on this website. The author personally used the "Zanki" deck to prepare for medical school exams and Step 1, as well as other decks for Step 2 CK and Step 3. We strongly recommend this subreddit for anyone seeking free, high-quality USMLE prep.

Reddit.com/r/medicalschool, reddit.com/r/residency, and reddit.com/r/medicine are also interesting because they provide rich discussion about contemporary topics related to medical school, residency, and medicine as a whole. Again, you will find high-quality memes about shared struggles. You will also gain a better understanding of the specific grievances faced by medical trainees, as the website allows for anonymous venting. Keep in mind that these—again—are nonrepresentative samples of medical trainees. Like Yelp ratings, people are more likely to post on Reddit when they're extremely happy or extremely upset. As such, don't let yourself believe that medicine is all gloom and doom vs. all rainbows and sunshine based on the popular posts you find.

You will probably also find a subreddit for your undergrad, e.g., "reddit.com/r/cornell." This can be helpful for making new friends (e.g., I found other musicians to jam with through the Pitt subreddit), getting advice from upperclassmen, and having a laugh about high-quality memes about your school.

As with SDN, there is no guarantee that you're getting honest, credible information. Verify recommendations whenever you can, and keep an air of healthy skepticism.

## A.3  MD Applicants

MD Applicants is a database of user-submitted application cycle profiles and outcomes. A user will submit his GPA, MCAT, and extracurricular activities, as well as which schools he applied to, as well as the resultant outcomes (e.g., application complete—rejected, invited for interview—withdrew, attended interview—waitlisted, accepted, accepted off waitlist). You can search the database by GPA, MCAT, and particular schools (e.g., received interview at Harvard Medical School, accepted at NYU). You don't need an account to view the database.

This can be incredibly useful for getting a sense of what a successful applicant to a specific school looks like. It can also be helpful for understanding—in a general sense—how successful an applicant with the same GPA and MCAT score will be in the application cycle (assuming all other factors are similar).

A major caveat is that the data is user submitted. As a result, while most profiles are probably accurate (if you choose to trust the goodwill of the pre-med community), there are definitely profiles that are fake (e.g., 1.00 GPA accepted to all top 20 medical schools). In addition, there is definitely selection bias in terms of *who* decides to share their profile on this website. We hypothesize that applicants at either extreme of competitiveness are more likely to post compared to "average" applicants. As a result, don't extrapolate *too* much from the data on this site.

## A.4  AMCAS, AAMC, AACOM, TMDSAS

These are the official websites. They contain a wealth of information and data related to virtually every aspect of the journey to becoming a physician. These are the most authoritative sources, and if you encounter any inconsistencies with other sources, you should *generally* defer to the official websites.

## A.5  MSAR

This is a document released every year by the AAMC compiling official application data (e.g., GPA, MCAT) for every US MD school. Think of it as a verified version of MD Applicants but with depersonalized, aggregate data instead.

## A.6  Med School Insiders

Med School Insiders is a company started by former plastic surgeon resident turned physician-entrepreneur Kevin Jubbal that releases extremely high-quality content (e.g., blog posts, YouTube videos, educational resources such as Memm) about everything and anything related to medicine. We frequently cite their content, as it's very similar to our approach of using the most up-to-date evidence across multiple fields to make general recommendations while also remaining mindful of the need for individual trial and error. They also have a heavy emphasis on evidence-based self-improvement, which is useful to any reader.

## A.7  Khan Academy

This is a free online educational platform with high-quality lectures across virtually every field. Many students use it to supplement studying for pre-reqs and the MCAT.

## A.8  Organic Chemistry as a Second Language

Organic chemistry is hard and very nonintuitive for many students. Many students swear by this celebrated study guide for organic chemistry.

## A.9  Resources during Medical School

We go into more detail in the individual chapters, but high-yield third-party resources are essential during medical school. While we encourage everyone to try out a bunch of resources and see what works for their learning style, the resources we insist everyone try are:

- **First Aid and Boards and Beyond**: The backbone of every successful step 1 prep.
- **Online MedEd**: A brilliant collection of high-yield chalk talks that get you through MS2-MS4 in medical school and into intern year.
- **Sketchy Micro and Pharm**: Essential for those high-yield memorization topics—no one does microbiology better.
- **Pathoma**: A video series on medical pathology based on the text of Dr. Hussain Sattar; great for supplementing institutional resources when they fall short.

# Appendix B: Medical Specialties and Subspecialties

Here is a comprehensive list of fellowship opportunities available in each specialty.[1] Note that this is *not* exhaustive; there are many custom/nonaccredited fellowships and opportunities available for every medical specialty.

- Anesthesiology:
  - Adult cardiothoracic anesthesiology.
  - Critical care medicine.
  - Neuroanesthesia.
  - Obstetric anesthesiology.
  - Pain medicine *(can also be pursued through physical medicine and rehabilitation, psychiatry, neurology, and diagnostic radiology)*.
  - Pediatric anesthesiology.
  - Regional anesthesiology.
  - Undersea and hyperbaric medicine.
- Anatomic pathology:
  - Bone and soft tissue pathology.
  - Dermatopathology *(can also be pursued through dermatology)*.
  - Gastrointestinal pathology.
  - Gynecologic pathology.
  - Forensic pathology.
  - Head and neck pathology.
  - Hematopathology.
  - Neuropathology.
  - Pediatric pathology.
  - Renal pathology.
  - Surgical pathology.
  - Thoracic pathology.
- Clinical pathology:
  - Blood banking-transfusion medicine.
  - Chemical pathology.
  - Cytopathology.
  - Medical microbiology.
  - Molecular genetic pathology.
  - Pathology informatics.
- Dermatology:
  - Cosmetic dermatology.
  - Dermatopathology *(can also be pursued through pathology but without the clinical dermatology aspect)*.
  - Itch.
  - Micrographic surgery and dermatologic oncology.
  - Pediatric dermatology.
- Diagnostic radiology:
  - Abdominal radiology.
  - Breast radiology.
  - Cardiothoracic radiology.
  - Endocrinology, diabetes, and metabolism.
  - Musculoskeletal radiology.
  - Neuroradiology:
    - Endovascular surgical neuroradiology *(can also be pursued through neurosurgery)*.
  - Nuclear radiology (can also be pursued as its own residency).

---

[1]  Specialty Profiles. Available at: https://www.aamc.org/cim/explore-options/specialty-profiles. Accessed July 8, 2022.

- Pediatric radiology.
- Radiology informatics.
- Vascular and interventional radiology (now its own residency).
- Emergency medicine:
  - Administration.
  - Medical toxicology.
  - Pediatric emergency medicine.
- Family medicine: *Family medicine has MANY opportunities for subspecialization. This list is not exhaustive.*
  - Academic fellowship.
  - Adolescent medicine.
  - Addiction medicine.
  - Aerospace medicine (*can also be pursued through a wide variety of specialties including internal medicine, surgery, psychiatry, neurology, emergency medicine*).
  - Community medicine.
  - Geriatrics.
  - Hospice and palliative care.
  - Integrative medicine.
  - Obstetrics.
  - Reproductive health.
  - Sleep medicine.
  - Sports medicine (*can also be pursued through emergency medicine, physical medicine and rehabilitation, and orthopaedics*).
  - Women's health.
  - Wilderness medicine (*can also be pursued through emergency medicine*).
- General surgery:
  - Breast surgery.
  - Colon and rectal surgery.
  - (Cardio)thoracic surgery (*note that in many places, these surgeons will do either cardiac or thoracic surgery and not necessarily both*).
    - Congenital cardiac surgery.
  - Hand surgery.
  - Minimally invasive/bariatrics.
  - Pediatric nerve.
  - Surgical critical care (trauma surgery).
  - Surgical oncology.
  - Transplant surgery.
  - Vascular surgery.
- Internal medicine:
  - Allergy and immunology.
  - Addiction medicine.
  - Cardiology:
    - Adult congenital heart disease.
    - Advanced heart failure and transplant cardiology.
    - Cardiac electrophysiology.
    - Interventional cardiology.
  - Critical care medicine.
  - Gastroenterology:
    - Transplant hepatology.
  - Geriatrics (can also be pursued through family medicine).
  - Hematology and oncology (note that you can do hematology or oncology alone, but most people specialize in both).
  - Hospice and palliative medicine (can also be pursued through family medicine).
  - Infectious disease.
  - Nephrology.

- Pulmonology (many specialize in pulmonology + critical care medicine).
- Rheumatology.
- Sleep medicine (can also be pursued through neurology and psychiatry).
- Internal medicine/pediatrics (can do any internal medicine or pediatric fellowship).
- Medical genetics:
  - Biochemical genetics.
- Neurology:
  - Autonomic disorders.
  - Balance disorders.
  - Child neurology (*can also be pursued as its own residency*).
  - Clinical neurophysiology.
  - Epilepsy.
  - Geriatric neurology.
  - Headache.
  - Movement disorders.
  - Neurocritical care.
  - Neuroendocrinology.
  - Neurogenetics.
  - Neuroimaging
  - Neuroimmunology (multiple sclerosis).
  - Neuromuscular medicine.
  - Neuro-oncology.
  - Neuro-ophthalmology.
  - Neuro-otology.
  - Neuropharmacology.
  - Neuropsychiatry (*can also be pursued through psychiatry*).
  - Pain medicine.
  - Sleep medicine.
  - Surgical endovascular neuroradiology.
- Neurosurgery:
  - Endovascular surgical neuroradiology (*can also be pursued through neurology and neuroradiology*).
  - Functional neurosurgery.
  - Neurotrauma and neurocritical care.
  - Neuro-oncology/image-guided neurosurgery.
  - Pediatric neurosurgery.
  - Peripheral nerve (*can also be pursued through orthopedic surgery or plastic surgery*).
  - Skull base.
  - Spinal neurosurgery.
- Nuclear medicine.
- Obstetrics and gynecology:
  - Family planning.
  - Female pelvic medicine and reconstruction.
  - Gynecologic oncology.
  - Maternal/fetal medicine.
  - Minimally invasive gynecologic surgery.
  - Reproductive endocrinology and infertility.
  - Urogynecology.
- Ophthalmology:
  - Cornea.
  - Glaucoma.
  - Neuro-ophthalmology (*can also be pursued through neurology*).
  - Ophthalmic plastic and reconstructive surgery.
  - Pediatric ophthalmology.
  - Retina, medical.
  - Retina, surgical.

- Uveitis, inflammatory disease.
- Orthopedic surgery:
  - Adult reconstruction.
  - Foot and ankle.
  - Hand surgery (*can also be pursued through general and plastic surgery*).
  - Musculoskeletal oncology.
  - Orthopedic spine.
  - Orthopedic sports medicine.
  - Orthopedic trauma.
  - Pediatric orthopadics.[2]
- Otolaryngology:
  - Facial plastics and reconstructive surgery.
  - Head and neck oncology.
  - Laryngology.
  - Otology-neurotology.
  - Pediatric otolaryngology.
  - Rhinology.
  - Sleep medicine surgery fellowship.
  - Voice, swallowing, and upper airway.
- Pediatrics:
  - Adolescent medicine.
  - Cardiology, pediatric.
  - Child abuse pediatrics.
  - Critical care, pediatric.
  - Developmental and behavioral pediatrics.
  - Emergency medicine, pediatric.
  - Endocrinology, pediatric.
  - Gastroenterology, pediatric:
    - Transplant hepatology, pediatrics.
  - Hematology and oncology, pediatric.
  - Hospitalist, pediatric (*now—controversially—becoming required to become board certified in pediatric hospital medicine*[3]).
  - Infectious disease, pediatric.
  - Neonatal-perinatal medicine.
  - Nephrology, pediatric.
  - Pulmonology, pediatric.
  - Rheumatology, pediatric.
  - Sports medicine, pediatric.
- Physical medicine and rehabilitation:
  - Brain injury medicine.
  - Cancer rehabilitation.
  - Electrodiagnostic.
  - Multiple sclerosis.
  - Neuromuscular medicine (*can also be pursued through neurology*).
  - Neurorehabilitation.
  - Pain medicine (*can also be pursued through anesthesiology, psychiatry, neurology, and diagnostic radiology*).
  - Pediatric rehabilitation.
  - Spinal cord injury medicine.

---

[2] Etymologically redundant: "orthopaedics" means straight child, or "ortho" (straight) "paed" (child), after its historic development in the correction of developmental orthopaedic anomalies.

[3] Beresford L. Pediatric hospital medicine marches toward subspecialty recognition. Available at: https://www.the-hospitalist.org/hospitalist/article/142861/pediatrics/pediatric-hospital-medicine-marches-toward-subspecialty. Accessed July 8, 2022.

- Sports medicine.
- Spine.
- Stroke.
- Plastic surgery (*can also be pursued as a fellowship from general surgery, but this takes longer*):
  - Burn surgery (can also be pursued through general surgery).
  - Complex gender surgery.
  - Cosmetic plastic surgery.
  - Craniofacial surgery.
  - Facial plastic surgery.
  - Hand surgery.
  - Neuroplastic and reconstructive surgery.
  - Pediatric plastic surgery.
  - Reconstructive microsurgery.
- Preventive medicine.
- Psychiatry:
  - Addiction psychiatry.
  - Child and adolescent psychiatry (*can also be pursued as its own residency*).
  - Community psychiatry.
  - Consultation-liaison psychiatry.
  - Forensic psychiatry.
  - Geriatric psychiatry.
  - Neuropsychiatry (*can also be pursued through neurology*).
  - Women's mental health.
- Radiation oncology:
  - Brachytherapy.
  - Hematologic radiation oncology.
  - Proton therapy.
  - Pediatric proton therapy.
- Urology:
  - Advanced robotic and laparoscopic.
  - Endourology/advanced stone disease.
  - Genitourinary reconstruction and prosthetics.
  - Kidney and pancreas transplant.
  - Male infertility, microsurgery, and andrology.
  - Pediatric urology.
  - Urologic oncology.
  - Voiding dysfunction.
- Vascular surgery (*can also be pursued as a fellowship from general surgery, although this takes longer*).

Most specialties also have training options available in global and/or community health.

# Index

*Note:* Page numbers set **bold** or *italic* indicate headings or figures, respectively.

# Index